Textbook of contraceptive practice

To John Peel, without whose inspiration
the first edition
would never have appeared

Textbook of

CONTRACEPTIVE PRACTICE

Second edition

MALCOLM POTTS
President, Family Health International

PETER DIGGORY
Consultant Gynaecologist, Kingston Hospital, Surrey

Illustrations by Jayne Diggory

CAMBRIDGE UNIVERSITY PRESS

Cambridge

London New York New Rochelle

Melbourne Sydney

CAMBRIDGE UNIVERSITY PRESS
Cambridge, New York, Melbourne, Madrid, Cape Town,
Singapore, São Paulo, Delhi, Tokyo, Mexico City

Cambridge University Press
The Edinburgh Building, Cambridge CB2 8RU, UK

Published in the United States of America by Cambridge University Press, New York

www.cambridge.org
Information on this title: www.cambridge.org/9780521270854

First published 1969
Reprinted with corrections 1970
First paperback edition 1970
Reprinted 1971
Second edition 1983
Re-issued 2011

A catalogue record for this publication is available from the British Library

Library of Congress Catalogue Card Number: 83-5295

ISBN 978-0-521-24934-8 Hardback
ISBN 978-0-521-27085-4 Paperback

Contents

	Foreword	ix
	Preface	xi
1	The history of contraception	1
2	Patterns of family planning	17
3	The population explosion	37
4	The safety and effectiveness of contraceptive methods	53
5	Traditional methods	74
6	Contraception and lactation	84
7	Periodic abstinence	97
8	The condom	106
9	Vaginal contraceptives: chemical and barrier	119
10	Steroidal contraceptives	136
11	The intrauterine device	216
12	Voluntary sterilization	245
13	Abortion	274
14	Medical aspects	322
15	Legal and administrative aspects of family planning	347
16	Conspectus	368
	References	402
	Index	457

Foreword

by Professor Sir Dugald Baird, M.D, F R.C.O.G.

There is little doubt that the second edition of *Contraceptive Practice* will prove to be as popular as the first. There is a vast amount of new information, great care has been taken to assess the validity of conclusions and the clarity of the writing should enable it to be read with profit and enjoyment by those with little knowledge of medicine and statistics as well as by doctors and nurses. The world situation is described in detail by one of the authors who has spent many years studying the problem of contraception on location in many parts of the Third World. The fact that the situation in Europe and more particularly in Britain is discussed by a leading obstetrician and gynaecologist actively engaged in practice has resulted in a colourful, realistic and first-hand account of contemporary problems related to contraception and sex.

It took the FPA and three generations of wives, husbands, doctors and politicians over 50 years to persuade the Government to take financial responsibility for providing the women of Britain with help so that they could have children by desire rather than by accident. Progress has been rapid since 1967 and in Britain today, even in social class V (unskilled manual workers), very few families contain more than three children, while the net reproductive rate in many countries in Europe is less than one. This is a particularly fortunate trend in view of the increasing automation in industry. The methods by which this is achieved, including sterilization and abortion, are discussed in detail and the knowledge and social insight of a first-class clinician combined with an understanding of the uses of epidemiology make this a particularly valuable account.

As far as the long-term future is concerned, one cannot do better than quote from the Conspectus. It is possible that in 100, or even 500 years' time, women may still be using a systemically active method of contra-ception, at least for some part of their reproductive lives, both to prevent pregnancy and to mimic those changes in the life-long pattern of reproduction associated with protection against breast cancer and from forms of reproductive pathology which occur when pregnancy is delayed or never takes place at all.

It is a fact of life that men still use their reproductive systems as did their stone-age ancestors and in much the same way as evolution programmed it. Men are not faced with the complex, interlocking and difficult-to-predict pathologies which face women in the modern world.

Preface

In 1969, when the first edition of this book was published, contraception was still regarded as therapy for 'disease' – namely excess fertility. Therefore, the book was written primarily for doctors (always referred to in the masculine gender) who would advise and prescribe contraceptive techniques for their patients. In particular, therapeutic abortion was justified by reference to an extensive list of medical indications. This second edition presents family planning in all its aspects as a series of choices offered to clients or consumers.

We believe that the pregnant woman herself is, when she has had an opportunity to consider her options and to discuss them with her consort and friends, the person best placed to decide whether to continue an unintended pregnancy or to seek an early abortion.

In the last fourteen years a great deal more effort and work has gone into surveillance of the Pill, IUDs, abortion techniques and sterilization than was devoted to the initial development of these forms of contraception. As a result we have expanded the text and greatly increased the literature references in this second edition and adopted a new layout in the chapters on steroidal contraceptives in order to accommodate the additional information. We now know more of the dangers and, more recently, the positive benefits of the oral contraceptive, which has been greatly improved and made safer by lowered dosage levels. The second generation of IUDs performs somewhat better than the first, but no really fundamental breakthrough has occurred. Sterilization has proved more popular than was envisaged in the 1960s and there have been important technical simplifications in its application to women. Surgical abortion techniques have proved far safer and more acceptable than could possibly be anticipated when the abortion laws were liberalized in Britain and the US. On the other hand, the 'breakthroughs' which might confidently have been expected in the 1970s have largely failed to materialize; there is no male Pill on the market and no medical method for routinely inducing delayed menstruation. In real terms, investment in contraceptive research and development has suffered an unforeseen decline in recent years.

The ideal of making wide contraceptive choice universally available has encountered many barriers. Political leaders of nations, or of racial or other minority groups, often see contraception as desirable only for others; overtly or covertly, they oppose its availability within their own sphere of influence. Modern effective contraceptives inevitably carry some risk to their users. Within the developed world these risks are closely monitored and are widely publicized in the media. A great deal of medical time and effort is devoted to locating and protecting women most at risk from any particular technique. Liberals and feminists have combined to proclaim that women in the Third World must be similarly protected, forgetting that medical manpower is totally inadequate for such a task, that the risks of an unintended pregnancy are many times greater and that it may be ethically and clinically important to put such medical skills as are available into other areas of medical care such as paediatrics. Within the West, particularly within the US, medico-legal fears have come to influence the clinical decisions of doctors concerning contraception and sterilization to the ultimate detriment of the couple at risk of an unintended pregnancy.

We have tried to take a global view of contraceptive practice whilst still placing emphasis on the everyday problems primarily encountered in the West. We have attempted to establish a reasonable framework for contraceptive usage based on the increased biological and clinical data available. We explicitly avoid getting bogged down in some of the necessary, but rapidly changing, clinical guidelines for contraceptive use which, from time to time, are recommended by national and international institutions concerned with health and family planning. We try to provide a framework within which such guidelines can be judged and the interests of the couple balanced against the increasing pressure on the medical team to practise defensive medicine. We also hope this broader approach will be useful in third world countries faced with a need for local decisions to meet local situations.

Probably the most important development in family planning since the first edition has been the systematic accumulation of evidence, particularly through the World Fertility Survey, that the majority of couples all over the world genuinely desire to control their fertility. A large part of this demand was always there but development and modernization have increased it. The need for family planning has increased but some administrative and political leaders, and even some community groups, have taken big steps backwards. The provision of contraceptive advice to teenagers has been restricted within the US and the Abortion Act in Britain regularly comes under attack. The Pill has acquired a worse reputation than it deserves and injectable contraceptives have been banned in many countries on the grounds of increased immorality and insecurity about human sexuality, which was documented in the opening chapter of the first edition (and which is retained in this second edition) appears to be increasing, inflamed in part by the rapid change and insecurity of the contemporary world. The first and most important need of the 1980s is to spread information on the dangers of uncontrolled fertility and to put into perspective the small unavoidable risks associated with effective contraception.

We would like to thank Messrs MacDonald and Evans for permission to reproduce diagrams and tables from *Society and Fertility* by Potts & Selman. We would also like to thank: Rebecca Cook for legal advice, Heather Estall, Beryl Hales and Jean Pain, who have not only typed and retyped the manuscript but have commented upon and improved it; Drs Pouru Bhiwandiwala, Peter Donaldson, Peter Miller and Steve Mumford, who read and commented on various parts of the text; Mr William Barrows and Ms Nell Mincey for helping to find and confirm references and Marcia Jaffe for assistance in preparing the manuscript. We have a special debt to Louise Sanders of Cambridge University Press, whose editing detected and thereby removed innumerable errors and greatly improved our text.

We are particularly grateful to Sir Dugald Baird who agreed to write the foreword for this edition as he did for the first.

April 1983   Malcolm Potts
                                                  Peter Diggory

In early 1983 the International Fertility Research Program (IFRP) changed its name to Family Health International (FHI). It was not possible to indicate this change at all points in the text.

1

The history of contraception

Classical and mediaeval beginnings

Reproduction and its control have proved to be the last aspect of biology and clinical medicine to come under objective scientific scrutiny.

In antiquity a continuous tradition of contraceptive knowledge existed from the works of Aristotle in the fourth century BC., through a variety of Greek and Roman authors, to Pliny the Elder and Dioscorides in the first century AD. In the second century, Soranus, a Greek doctor practising in Rome, advanced in his *Gynaecia* both contraceptive technique and theory to a level surpassed only in the last 70 years. But such knowledge was never widely disseminated and rational techniques were discussed alongside magical recipes. Nevertheless, it was from this beginning that the contraceptive methods which were to be popularized in Europe during the nineteenth and twentieth centuries first came, though the derivation was secondary and via Islamic sources.[29]

Medical theory and practice in mediaeval Europe were developed within a Christian ethos which associated sex with sin. Even after the Reformation, Protestants and Catholics alike condemned contraception. One eighteenth-century writer, for example, declared that 'to publish methods of prevention smells so rank of the libertine and free-thinker that it ought not to be allowed in a Christian country'. When Soranus's *Gynaecia* was eventually resurrected and transcribed the contraceptive passages were entirely omitted.[35]

Only a fragmentary insight can be gained into the methods of fertility control used in mediaeval and early modern times, but occasionally the words and actions of individuals from a pre-industrial, peasant society come down across the ages. When the Inquisition examined the Cathar heretics of the Pyrenean village of Montaillou (1318–25) the mistress of the local priest recalls asking her lover 'What shall I do if I become pregnant by you? I shall be ashamed and lost.' 'I have a certain herb,' replied the priest. 'If a man wears it when he mingles his body with that of woman he cannot engender, nor she conceive.'[19]

Quaife has analysed depositions relating to paternity that were presented to the civil and ecclesiastical courts in Somerset, England between 1601 and 1660, covering high Puritan times. Only one in 200 unplanned pregnancies occurred to girls under the age of 17 and illegitimate births fell to exceedingly low levels, although 20 – 30% of first baptisms occurred less than nine months after marriage.[27] However, contraception and abortion were used, and one local herbalist publically names an unmarried woman who had used an abortifacient successfully because 'the whore should have paid for it'.

While known and available, the means of fertility regulation were almost universally condemned in the western world. Only in the twentieth century, and even then with stumbling reluctance, have the loving as well as procreative aspects of human sexual behaviour been acknowledged as good and acceptable in western society. The final seal of Catholic theological approval was given at the Second Vatican Council (1962–65) with the Council's statement on the Church in the modern world (*Gaudium et Spes*) describing marriage as a 'community of love'.

The nineteenth-century birth control movement

The first altruistic attempts of those with the privilege of knowledge and experience to share it with others were made in the early nineteenth century, but it was only freethinkers such as Francis Place (1771–1854) and John Stuart Mill (1806–1873) who had the vision and courage to embark on such a task.[12] Place's 'Diabolical Handbills'[8] were perhaps the earliest vehicle of domiciliary family planning advice and in distributing them the young Mill became entangled with the police. Place records that, in framing his Handbills, he sought the advice of 'accouchers of the first respectability and surgeons of great eminence'; unfortunately he provides no clue to their identity. Contraceptive practice was to remain outside the sphere of medical literature for many more decades.

The Reverend Thomas Malthus's (1766–1834) *Essay on Population* (1798) was the intellectual hinge in the understanding of population change and its economic implications, but it proposed nothing more realistic than 'moral restraint' for individuals struggling to control their own fertility. Charles Darwin, however, in a characteristically perspicacious way understood the main biological factors controlling human fertility more clearly than any of his nineteenth-century colleagues. He wrote: 'Malthus has discussed these several (population) checks, but he does not lay stress enough on what is probably the most important of all, namely infanticide, especially of female infants, and the habit of procuring abortion.'[10]

As the nineteenth century progressed, rapid urbanization and industrialization increased the pressure to control fertility. In the US achieved family size fell from 7.04 in 1800 to 3.56 in 1900. There was a massive and visible increase in criminally induced abortion. In France (1868) one commentator called it 'a veritable industry', and in Michigan (1873) a physician pointed out that abortion has become so frequent it is rare to find a married woman who passes through the childbearing period who has not had one or more'. In 1868, Lord Amberley (1842–1876), father of Bertrand Russell, presided over a meeting of the London Dialectical Society at which James Laurie (1832–1904), Charles Bradlaugh (1833–1891) and George Drysdale (1829–1907) all spoke. In summing up Amberley called for a medical contribution to the problem under discussion.[28] The *British Medical Journal* and the *Medical Times and Gazette* were instantly critical of this 'most scandalous insult' to the medical profession. At the annual meeting of the British Medical Association (BMA) in the following year, Dr. Beatty (d. 1872) condemned 'the beastly contrivances for limiting the numbers of offspring', and the *Lancet* commented: 'We do not think that the practices to which we have been compelled to refer would be tolerated even as subjects for discussion by more than a very small number of medical men.'

In several ways, the United States was ahead of Europe. An active birth control movement had been initiated in the 1830s by Robert Dale Owen (1801–1877), son of the English co-operative pioneer, and Dr Charles Knowlton (1800–1850). Owen's *Moral Physiology* (1831)[24] was the first book on birth control to be published in America and Knowlton's *Fruits of Philosophy*[18] (1832) was perhaps the most influential contraceptive pamphlet ever to appear. Technically, it was an advance on anything which had been published before and superior to most which appeared in the next 50 years. In the United States as in England, the birth control movement attracted a number of eccentric protagonists but, unlike its English counterpart, it had the firm support of a number of eminent physicians, including A. M. Mauriceau, R. T. Trall (1812–1877), Edward Bliss Foote (1829–1906), Edward Bond Foote (1854–1912) and Alice B. Stockham (1833–1912).

However, as in Europe, the second half of the nineteenth century saw a polarization of views. Anthony Comstock (1844–1915) was both a driving force and a symbol of the late nineteenth-century opposition to reproductive freedom.[4,7] He was the head of the New York Society for the Suppression of Vice and claimed to have personally arrested 3873 persons of whom 2911 were convicted. In 1873 he successfully lobbied the US Congress to pass 'an Act of the Suppression of Trade in and the Circulation of, Obscene Literature and Articles of immoral use', which encompassed literature deemed to be pornographic, medicines and articles for causing abortion and contraceptives. The first draft of the Act contained the clause 'except from a physician in good standing' but this was omitted from the final legislation and for nearly a century the Comstock legislation devastated family planning in America. When asked why he classified contraceptives with pornography he replied 'If you open the door to anything, the filth will pour in and the degradation of youth will follow.' It seems probable that Mr Comstock would feel at home with the contemporary Moral Majority in America.

The prosecutions which the Comstock Act triggered induced a certain caution in the medical profession. However, it did not prevent journals such as the *Michigan Medical News* (1882) and the *Medical and Surgical Reporter* (1888) from publishing articles on contraception.[25]

The twentieth-century transition

The 50 years from 1870 to 1920 were key ones for western fertility decline; they were years when illegally-induced abortion was rampant and posed a major public health problem. It was during these years also that *all* the methods of contraception now in use came to be understood and were first open to scientific analysis. The opportunity for research and development was missed and the contemporary world still lives under the shadow of the confused and antagonistic attitudes towards family planning which characterized these years. Achievable technical advances based on sound biological knowledge were frustrated, needed services were not devised and emerging knowledge of contraceptive side-effects became items of political criticism rather than the basis of reasoned debate.

The grounds for opposition to contraception were basically moral. The use of adjectives such as 'lustful', 'selfish' and 'immoral' seem to have been obligatory in any mention of the subject. Even the barrier methods of contraception were claimed to induce 'galloping cancer, sterility and nymphomania' in women and 'mental decay and cardiac palpitations' in men; in both sexes contraceptive practice was said to produce mania leading to suicide. There was a noticeable tendency to confuse abortion and contraception. In 1887, for example, the General Medical Council struck the name of Arthur Allbutt off the British Medical Register for publishing an inoffensive little manual on domestic hygiene entitled *The Wife's Handbook*, which included chapters on antenatal care, pregnancy, the management of the baby and one called 'How to prevent conception'.[1]

Yet the decades between 1870 and 1920 were those when bacterial diseases began to be controlled, when great advances in public health took place, when asepsis and antisepsis entered surgery and the first chemotherapeutic drug, Salvarsan, was introduced. It is a major tragedy of recent history, whose reverberations now extend to every corner of the contemporary world, that in the progress of western medicine the technology of birth control was virtually halted by western Christendom's inability to handle human sexuality in an objective and humane way, at the very time when the technology of death control moved ahead in what must be judged one of the most successful outcomes of western civilisation.

Despite outward hostility to contraception from both the Church and the medical profession, the idea of family limitation gained increasing acceptance with individuals from within these two groups. Doctors were among the first to restrict their own fertility (see Chapter 2) and the British National Birth Rate Commission in 1914 stated that it had become 'almost a rule' for doctors to advocate the spacing of pregnancies. Few doctors seem to have educated parents in contraceptive techniques because such action would have been contrary to the medical ethos of the time. There was a wide variety of commercial products available and the main problem must have been to select wisely because there was no control of product advertising and manufacturers' claims greatly exceeded actual efficacy. In 1909 the BMA supported Lord Braye's Bill in Parliament which attempted to outlaw the sale of contraceptives. By contrast, the Council of the Malthusian League compiled a leaflet, entitled *Hygienic Methods of Family Limitation*,[20] 'for the benefit of those desirous of limiting their families but who are ignorant of the means of doing so and unable to get medical advice on the subject'. It achieved wide distribution and underwent numerous revisions.

The First World War was perhaps the most important solvent of public prejudice, transforming attitudes to sexual questions generally and to birth control in particular. The concessions to feminism, a growing concern with infant and maternal mortality, the first open discussion of venereal disease, the literary impact of Freud (1855–1939), Lawrence (1885–1930), Carpenter (1844–1929) and Joyce (1882–1941), and above all the publication of Havelock Ellis's (1859–1939) *Studies in the Psychology of Sex* all helped the emerging birth control movement. *Studies in the Psychology of Sex* banned as 'a bawdy, scandalous and obscene libel' in the 1890s, became the 'classic and dictionary of the twenties'. Slowly and reluctantly doctors responded to the changing outlook. The 1916 Report of the National Birth Rate Commission provided assurances on the safety of at least some methods of contraception and drew a careful distinction between contraception and abortion. However, extreme caution persisted and it was suggested that two medical practitioners should be required to give approval for the use of contraceptives. (An identical requirement was written into the British Abortion law 50 years later.) When this suggestion was first advanced by a gynaecologist at a meeting of the Medico-Legal Society, Earl Russell pointed out that 'it would be embarrassing and expensive to have to use contraceptives only in the presence of two members of the medical profession'. Both the *Lancet* and the *British Medical Journal* published favourable reviews of Marie Stopes's *Married Love* (1918)[33] but omitted references to the passages on birth control. However, her subsequent volume, *Wise Parenthood*[32] (also published in 1918), which developed the subject of contraception more fully, was advertised on the front page of the *Lancet*.

Nowhere are the conflicts surrounding family planning symbolized more clearly than in the life of Marie Stopes (1880–1958).[13] Born in Edinburgh, she showed a precocious scientific ability and established a sound reputation as a palaeontologist. She was one of the first women to obtain a doctorate of science and the first woman to receive a travel grant from the Royal Society. Yet when her first tragic marriage was unconsummated, she literally had to take herself to the British Museum Library in order to discover what should have taken place in the marital bed. 'I should go mad', she wrote, adding 'Why have I a scientific brain and all my scientific knowledge, if it is not to find out the things that seem to puzzle everybody.' This traumatic experience and her subsequent divorce inspired the writing of *Married Love*. It is a remarkable document for a woman who was 38 and still a virgin. The book is basically a hymn to the right of women to enjoy sexual satisfaction. The sections on birth control were added, almost as an afterthought, following a meeting in Highgate, London with Margaret Sanger, the US family planning pioneer, at a time when the latter was fleeing from legal persecution in New York.

Stopes subsequently married H. V. Roe of the aircraft manufacturing company, and with his financial support began her crusade for contraceptive services. She remained highly individualistic in her belief, convinced that women absorbed some essential element from the semen without which they could not be truly feminine or healthy. For this reason, she passionately promoted the cervical cap as opposed to the condom or vaginal diaphragm, both of which she believed prevented this magical process from taking place. She was hysterically opposed to abortion and in *Birth Control Today* (1934) described women who had abortions as 'a danger to the human race'.

Despite entrenched opposition, the early twentieth century saw considerable progress towards liberalization in the attitude of society towards contraception; such changes have been particularly marked in the periods immediately following the two world wars. With regard to abortion, the change in attitude came later, really only after the Second World War but legislation followed this change more rapidly and now 62% of the world's population live in countries with liberal abortion laws or freely available abortion (Fig. 1.1).

In a lecture entitled 'The Problem of Birth Control', given in 1918, Dr Killick Millard stressed the desirability of birth control on public health grounds and added that he had recently asked 80 colleagues for their views. Six had pleaded lack of knowledge and among the rest 'those who regarded birth control as being harmless were five times the more numerous'. Millard conducted a second enquiry, three years later, among gynaecologists and women doctors; of those who replied, 37 approved of married couples using contraceptive methods on medical and social grounds and only 13 disapproved.

In the slow progress of the twentieth-century birth control movement, an outstanding landmark in Britain was the outspoken address of Lord Dawson of Penn (1864–1945) to the 1921 Church Congress in Birmingham.[38] While still a medical student, Penn had signed a petition to the General Medical Council protesting at its treatment of Allbutt in 1887. His 1921 speech was a reasoned defence of 'artificial birth control' on medical, social and, especially, personal grounds; he challenged the more common objections to the practice, condemned abstinence as 'pernicious' and called on the Church to revise its opinions. Dawson was the King's physician and he virtually put the monarchy on the side of family limitation. 'Probably no utterance of recent times', declared the *Malthusian*, 'has so profoundly stirred the press and public as this outspoken declaration from such a high authority . . .' Poignantly, almost exactly a century earlier, in 1841, Queen Victoria had written to her uncle of the universal need to control human fertility:

> I think, dearest Uncle, you cannot *really* wish me to be the '*Mamma d'une nombreuse famille*', for I think you will see with me the great inconvenience a *large* family would be to us all, and particularly to the country, independent of the hardship and inconvenience to myself; men never think, at least seldom think, what a hard task it is for us women to go through this *very often*.[36]

Family planning services in developed countries only really came of age in the 1970s, and then with a good deal of turmoil. In Britain, the Family Planning Act (1967) followed the reform of abortion legislation. By 1973 contraception had been brought into the National Health Service, and for a

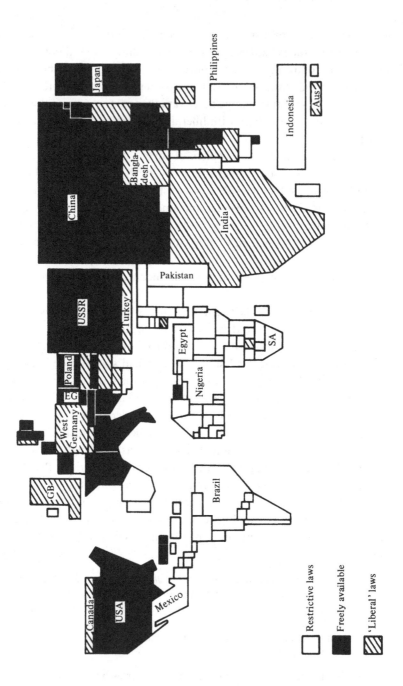

Fig. 1.1. The legal status of abortion in 1982. Countries drawn proportional to their population.

brief interval the country even enjoyed a Minister for Population. The medical profession, once opposed to contraception, has successfully lobbied for extra payments for contraceptive advice and sterilizing operations, a policy that has not won universal approval in a country where item-of-service payments for health care are unusual. The first US Federal legislation occurred in 1962 and was extended by a number of Acts, with Congress voting the so-called Title X in the 1970 Public Health Service Act. By 1968 more than 800000 couples were receiving family planning services from organized programmes in the United States and by 1972 $125 million was being spent a year and 3 million couples were being served.[17] Unhappily, the Reagan administration impeded the progress of these previously successful programmes.

Scientific review

A remarkable lack of scientific objectivity characterized most statements about contraception made in the 1920s and 1930s. Limited medical knowledge was backed up with simplistic moralizing, eugenic and demographic prognostications and totally unsupported generalizations regarding probable parental motivation. In the medical world, as elsewhere, the most vocal viewpoints tended to be those of the extremists, and many practising doctors probably behaved in a more reasonable manner than either the radical or conservative standpoints so widely expressed in public. In a celebrated medical novel of the period, A. J. Cronin provides what is presumably intended to represent the attitude of a family doctor.[9] Though Manson, the doctor hero, is portrayed as an enlightened and progressive young physician struggling against the bigotry and humbug of his profession, he is nevertheless revolted when asked by the local minister for contraceptive advice.

A Report of the Medical Committee of the National Birth Rate Commission (1927) drew attention to the lack of scientific knowledge of the efficacy of contraceptives[23] and a Birth Control Investigation Committee (BCIC) was formed 'to investigate the sociological and medical principles of contraception; the possible effects of the practice on physical and mental health; and the merits and demerits of all possible methods'. During the 12 years of its existence, with generous financial support from the Eugenics Society, this Committee carried out an ambitious and comprehensive research programme. The organization developed as a predominantly lay-inspired voluntary movement and operated 12 clinics in England and Scotland. Nine of these, which were affiliated to The Society for the Provision of Birth Control Clinics (SPBCC), collected data on 13000 new patients and 17000 return cases concerning the method of contraception used. The recommended method was the spring-rim vaginal diaphragm used in combination with spermicidal jelly and douching. Characteristically, those providing services recommended such elaborate methods that a large number of users appear to have been unable to persevere with the technique offered.[15] Nevertheless, this Society was the first to recognize the inevitable self-selecting nature of groups of contraceptive clinic clients and therefore made an early attempt to assess the knowledge about the usage of contraception by sending 500 postal questionnaires to 'members of the general public'. In his introduction to the foreword to the subsequent publication, Harold Laski commented: 'Books like this are a happy proof that the birth control movement is passing rapidly from the stage of enthusiasm to the stage of science.'[6]

In historical terms, science had come late to family planning. Professor Howard Florey was one of those whose research on uterine activity was supported by the BCIC.[5] Within his lifetime, he was to win the Nobel Prize for the discovery of penicillin, but no comparable advance was to arise in the field of birth control for many decades. Perhaps the most significant project that was supported by the BCIC was research at Oxford by Dr J. R. Baker into chemical contraception, which led to the elaboration of the spermicide Volpar[2] and to the development of scientific tests for spermicidal activity. However, work of this type was always pushed to the scientific periphery and when the nature of Baker's research in the Department of Zoology was discovered by his professor, he was denied laboratory space and the whole project would have ended if Professor Florey had not intervened. For Baker, contraceptive research in the 1920s was symbolized in his recollection of assembling his apparatus and reagents on a handcart and trundling them from the one department to the other through the streets of Oxford.[3] In 1930, the BCIC was reconstituted as The National Birth Control Association and by this time medical opinion had been sufficiently transformed to allow Sir Thomas Horder to become its first president.

The birth control clinic movement

The world's first birth control clinic was opened in Holland in 1882. By 1913 the Malthusian League was canvassing the need for family planning clinics in Britain although it was only in 1921 that Marie Stopes was able to open the 'first birth control clinic in the British Empire' and the League opened its first clinic in Walworth a few months later.

Margaret Sanger (1879–1965) was more pragmatic than Marie Stopes.[11] Born of a freethinker with Irish Catholic links, she trained as a public health nurse and her dramatic conversion to the promotion of family planning occurred as she cared for Mrs Sadie Sachs, who was suffering from a criminal abortion in the slums of New York.

Sanger always remembered with bitterness the flippant words of the attending physician: 'Any more such capers, young woman, and there will be no need to send for me'. His only response to the woman's query 'How do I stop getting pregnant?' was 'Tell Jake to sleep on the roof.' Margaret postponed going to see Mrs Sachs again as she had no advice to offer. However, she was called back three months later. Mrs Sachs died from this second abortion.

With courage and energy, the frail Margaret and her equally brave sister, Ethel, opened the first birth control clinic in Brooklyn in 1916. Although it was quickly closed down as a public nuisance by the New York police, it proved a milestone in contraceptive history. (It was at this time that Margaret fled to Europe and met with Marie Stopes.) Fortunately, Mrs Sanger had an extraordinary capacity for dramatic presentation of her theme. She persisted with the Brooklyn clinic and although she served a term of imprisonment, she eventually secured a decision in the Court of Appeals which enabled medically qualified personnel to give contraceptive advice legally 'for the cure and prevention of disease', a phrase which was liberally interpreted.

In 1930, contraception in Britain attained a legitimate and permanent place in preventive medicine through the publication of the Ministry of Health Memorandum 153MCW which empowered local authorities to provide birth control advice to limited numbers of women when necessary under medical circumstances. It was the only Governmental concession to the birth control movement in Britain until the 1967 Family Planning Act.

The clinic movement was always involved in controversy. For example, in 1932 the *British Medical Journal* was still refusing advertisements for doctors to work in Marie Stopes's clinic. It was particularly hazardous for women doctors, whose position within the profession was still a precarious one, to risk association with such dubious enterprises. In Britain and particularly in Marie Stopes's clinic, nurses played a major role in providing contraceptive advice. The nature of the United States legal decision allowing Margaret Sanger's work to continue forced a greater involvement of physicians in the provision of family planning, a trend which has continued until modern times.

A general rule of the medical profession, to which few exceptions are made, is that a doctor will not treat another doctor's patient except at the latter's request or in an emergency. The underlying philosophy is not that the doctor owns patients and resents competition but that when more expert help is needed the patient's own doctor is far more able than another to select the speciality and the individual best suited to the circumstances. Patients, however, have a right to select their medical advisors and a right to absolute privacy, but this can cause conflict and controversy. For example, when venereal disease clinics were first established they were set up on a basis of self-referral and total confidentiality to encourage their use; not even the client's regular doctor is informed except with permission. Those who started family planning clinics held that the need to encourage easy access and to respect privacy meant that such clinics must also breach the normal convention and allow self-referral; indeed in 1926 the Aberdeen Clinic was disaffiliated from the SPBCC because its medical staff refused to see clients except with their doctors' consent.[31] Ethical issues of a similar nature have arisen concerning contraceptive advice to minors and abortion counselling.

The provision of family planning services is frequently controversial although the nature of the debate remains very much the same at different times and in different places. The sophistication with which arguments are made may vary but the objective of society extending services to individuals to meet private fertility goals frequently involves perceived issues of morality and competitive breeding between different ethnic, social or economic groups.

In 1926 the British House of Lords debated whether the local authority welfare centres which had been set up after the First World War should offer family planning services.[30] Those who opposed the move held that a woman 'should do her duty to her husband and to the country'. It was suggested that birth control advice might somehow get to the 'undeserving' and even to 'the indolent and vicious' and family planning was held to be absolutely contrary to the moral and natural law. Those supporting the availability of family planning services cited the then high illegal abortion rate and the basic injustice of denying the poor information that the rich already had. Lord Buckmaster suggested: 'The Church must remember that it is no longer living in the days when it could compel Galileo to come upon his knees and say that the sun went around the earth.' And in that debate, more than 50 years ago, was one of the first and still clearest statements of the basic human rights that fertility control represents. Earl Russell, brother of Bertrand Russell the philosopher, concluded: 'It is for a woman who bears the child to settle not with her husband or with the state, but entirely with her own conscience whether she will bear a child or not. This is the liberty to which every woman is entitled. . .'

In the US Margaret Sanger had several able and distinguished medical associates, including Dr R. L. Dickinson (1861–1950), Drs Abraham and

Hannah Stone and Dr Alan Guttmacher. In 1920, as President of the American Gynecological Society, Dickinson pressed for more research on contraceptive techniques and three years later published the first authoritative article on contraception which he posted to physicians all over the country in order to challenge the Comstock Act. Dickinson founded, and was for a number of years Secretary to the National Committee on Maternal Health, and through the work of this organization the important relation between family planning and maternal health became clearly established in America. Abraham Stone edited the first medical journal devoted to contraception, *The Journal of Contraception*, from 1935 onwards, and with the sociologist Norman Himes co-authored what was for many years the standard birth control textbook. His wife made a singular contribution to the development of family planning by importing, in 1936, a package of contraceptive materials, and in the course of the protracted legal proceedings which followed succeeded in removing the 'federal handcuffs shackling the medical prescription of contraception'. Alan Guttmacher (1898–1974) was an able and prominent gynaecologist who, in later life, took an increasing interest in family planning and followed Margaret Sanger as President of the International Planned Parenthood Federation. As well as being an international leader in family planning, he was a prime mover in abortion reform in the US.

Those involved in family planning had had a long history of international concern and collaboration going back to the 1880s, but Margaret Sanger was the chief architect of the international family planning movement. In 1927 she organized, in Geneva, the first World Population Conference, which was attended by leading scientists, sociologists and physicians from Europe and America. It resulted in the formation of two important committees, the International Medical Group and the International Union for the Scientific Study of Population (IUSSP). The latter has survived as the official association of professional demographers. In 1952, Margaret Sanger brought together delegates from 23 countries as the first step in forming the International Planned Parenthood Federation (IPPF), of which she was the first President.[34, 16] The first government support for IPPF work came from Sweden in 1965 and General William Draper, Jr (1894–1974) brought the first significant US funds into both the IPPF and the United Nations Fund for Population Activities (UNFPA), founded in 1969. Dr Reimart T. Ravenholt, a civil servant of remarkable courage and vision, worked closely with Draper and turned an initially unpopular Aid for International Development (AID) project into one of the most successful international assistance programmes in history.

Medical education

In 1923 the editor of the *Practitioner* had declared: 'The subject of birth control is not taught in the medical schools and in the case of schools for male students it is safe to predict that it never will be; for women are more practical and less hypocritical than most men.'[26] In 1930 a senior medical student at Newcastle invited the doctor from the local birth control clinic to address the Student Medical Society on the clinic's work but the Society's committee was warned that any student attending the lecture would run the risk of failure in his final examination. The meeting was cancelled. It was not until 1936 that the first British medical school began to provide a single annual lecture on the subject; nor were the academic authorities anxious to allow students to obtain birth control knowledge from other sources.

In 1949 the Deans of 24 British medical schools replied to questions by the Federation of Medical Women on whether instruction on contraceptive technique was given to students,[21] and at only four schools was information given. Practical experience in the fitting of caps was provided in a few cases by attendance at the local voluntary or municipal clinics. Only two teaching hospitals ran special sessions for out-patients where contraceptive advice was given, but a number held fertility clinics.

From the 1960s onwards, a number of factors brought about significant changes in this situation. In the first place, the advent of the oral contraceptive provided the doctor with a therapeutic agent which clearly justified professional concern. Secondly, within the profession as a whole there was a greater emphasis on preventive medicine.

By 1976, an enquiry amongst British general practitioners found that 93% advised individuals on contraceptive matters although only 32% had received either undergraduate or postgraduate instruction in contraceptive technique. Amongst those qualified before 1950 this latter proportion was as low as 18% rising to 56% amongst those qualified after that date.[37]

Finally, the 1967 Family Planning Act in Britain and the Title X legislation in the US legitimized a situation that many doctors previously regarded as equivocal.

An inadequate starting place?

In 1863 James Young Simpson, the obstetrician who gave Queen Victoria chloroform during childbirth, described the use of a hand-held syringe and a metal cannula for uterine evacuation. It is the world's first description of vacuum aspiration abortion or menstrual regulation and he commented: 'It is in some cases attended with striking results.' In 1909

Richter described the use of intrauterine contraceptive devices and by 1923 one physician had inserted over 20 000 of them. In 1921 Ludwig Haberlandt described the physiological basis for oral contraception. The first voluntary female sterilization was performed at least as early as 1880. Sir Astley Cooper (1768–1848) experimented with vasectomy in dogs in 1823 and the first human vasectomies, performed for confused non-contraceptive reasons, were carried out in 1894.[14]

In short, biological, surgical and clinical knowledge of all the methods of fertility regulation now in use existed 50 or more years ago. The logistics of providing services and some of the problems of access of different socio-economic groups were all apparent within a few years, if not a few months, of opening the first birth control clinics in Europe and North America. Unfortunately, however, the potential for meaningful progress was very inadequately developed. The demographic transition in the West took place despite obstructive attitudes by governments and by the medical profession, so that when the population of developing countries exploded in the 1950s and 1960s the world as a whole was forced to respond by cobbling together a largely untested collection of methods and services.

The full tragedy of the western antagonism to sex is perhaps best appreciated by a final quotation from the freethinker Robert Dale Owen's *Moral Physiology* (1831) describing sexual intercourse:

> Controlled by reason, and chastened by good feeling, it gives to social intercourse much of its charm and zest, but directed by selfishness or governed by force it is prolific of misery and degradation. In itself, it appears to be the most social and least selfish of all instincts. It fits us to give even while receiving pleasure, and among cultivated beings the former power is even more highly valued than the latter. Not one of our instincts perhaps affords larger scope for the exercise of disinterestedness or fitter play for the best moral feelings of our race. Not one gives birth to relations more gentle, more humanising and endearing, not one lies more immediately at the root of the kindliest charities and most generous impulses that honour and bless human nature. It is a much more noble, because less purely selfish, instinct than hunger or thirst. It is an instinct that entwines itself around the warmest feelings and best affections of the heart.

If Owen's wisdom had been accepted, instead of the cant that was to follow, and still too often spills from the prejudiced and those lacking in social compassion, then the waste of pain and death from a century and a half of induced abortion could have been greatly reduced, the health of women improved, the happiness of marital relationships enormously expanded and the contemporary world would not have had to accommodate to such a terrifying growth in numbers. Specialist skills could have been devoted to achieving incremental improvements in contraceptive practice rather than having to ask, have we even arrived at a satisfactory starting place for our work?

When political acceptance finally arrived, it was often almost too late to help. At the UN Population Commission in 1981, Mgr James McHugh stated that it is 'morally acceptable for a nation to moderate its population growth to keep pace with its development strategies, food and economic resources and socio-economic policies'. As an official spokesman for the Vatican he also said that population policies should be 'respectful of human dignity and responsive to human needs',[22] a poetic and sincere summary of the goals of everyone working in family planning and words which would have brought worldwide applause had they been spoken in 1951 instead of 1981.

2

Patterns of family planning

Fecundity and fertility

Childbirth is the outward and public sign of a series of private and intimate decisions and actions to engage in intercourse, to use or not to use contraception and to accept or reject abortion. There is no evidence that human fecundity, the biological capacity for procreation, has varied significantly either from society to society or from one century to another. In the pre-industrialized world, until about two hundred years ago, the major restraints on fertility were the natural intervals of anovulation associated with breast-feeding supplemented by certain traditional methods of birth control; nevertheless they could be remarkably successful.[15] Since that time, the balance has been reversed and today the achieved family size is more fundamentally influenced by artificial means of fertility regulation than by physiological variations. As the biological extremes of sterility and hyper-fecundity are progressively mitigated, so the number of children born becomes almost entirely a volitional act. A similar revolution has begun in the Third World over the last 20 years and, to a significant extent, the future welfare of mankind depends upon the rate at which it is developed.

Even where the artificial control of fertility is predominant, natural regulatory mechanisms remain important and the interrelation between biological and social restraints on fertility, the use of contraception, abortion and voluntary sterilization, needs to be clearly understood. The age of the menarche has declined from a mean of over 17 years in northern Europe in the early nineteenth century to approximately 13 years in the contemporary US and Britain.[23] One of the factors influencing the onset of first menstruation appears to be a combination of critical body weight and reserves of subcutaneous fat.[11, 12] A likely explanation for these recent changes is probably improved childhood nutrition. Severe malnutrition in young women leads to anovulation as does anorexia nervosa. The average age at the menopause was thought to be about 45 years in the 1920s but it appears to have become slightly later in the last half century so that the normal menopause now occurs at about the age of 50 in the United Kingdom and the US.[9, 13] This added span of reproductive life under conditions of sustained good nutrition may have been a good evolutionary tactic for the species but it now presents an additional need for contraceptive responsibility in developed and developing countries.

For a woman to conceive, she must ovulate and have intercourse although the relation of these two events is such that several months of coitus must take place before the average woman becomes pregnant. When intercourse takes place daily, or more frequently, an average of three months elapses between the initiation of coitus and conception, while when sex occurs less frequently than 10 times per cycle, this interval is increased to approximately six months[37] (Fig. 2.1). The probability of getting

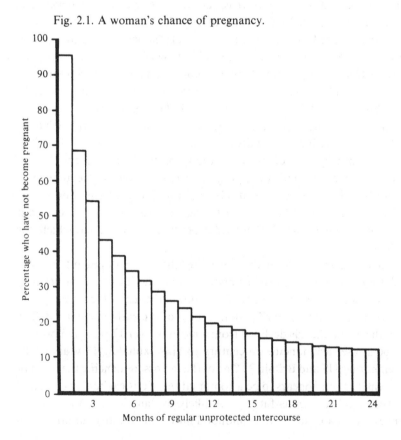

Fig. 2.1. A woman's chance of pregnancy.

pregnant on different days of the menstrual cycle is illustrated in Fig. 2.2.

In a traditional society, the greater part of a woman's fertile life is spent being either pregnant or in intervals of anovulation associated with lactation. In the modern world, contraception replaces intervals of infertility previously associated with breast-feeding and gives a measure of fertility control not previously available.[28] When a woman has a spontaneous or induced abortion, the duration of the pregnancy is shorter and ovulation usually returns within a month or six weeks. Therefore, several abortions can be fitted into the same period of a woman's fertile life as might have been occupied by a pregnancy followed by breast-feeding (Fig. 2.3).

Marriage is always a socially sanctioned event and premarital conception is condemned in most societies. In nearly all cultures an attempt is made to postpone the first pregnancy at least until marriage and to impose some limits on childbearing thereafter. In the West, the age of marriage has been an important factor in reducing overall fertility, conversely, in many traditional societies, while reproduction often begins in the teens, there are social restraints upon a grandmother continuing to bear children.[2]

Fertility can be assessed in different ways. The age-specific fertility rate

Fig. 2.2. Probability of conception by day of coitus. (Redrawn from Dixon, G. W., Schlesselman, J. J., Ory, H. W. & Blye, R. P. (1980). Ethinyl estradiol and conjugated estrogens as postcoital contraceptives. *Journal of the American Medical Association*, **244**, 1336.)

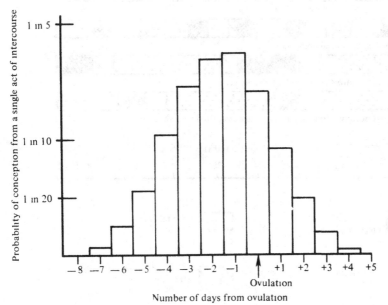

Number of days from ovulation

describes the number of births during one year to women of a given age per thousand women of that age. The total fertility rate is the addition of the age-specific fertility rates and provides a measure of the average number of live births per woman which could be expected if the current fertility pattern continued over the next 30 years or so. Louis Henry has suggested the term 'natural fertility' as being descriptive of societies where births are not subject to any deliberate control. The North American Hutterites are an Anabaptist religious sect enjoying western standards of maternal and child care but rejecting artificial birth control. The average married Hutterite woman delivers more than eight children in her reproductive life, and two-thirds have between 7 and 12 children.[8] The highest recorded average family size for a whole community is 10; this was amongst women living in rural Quebec at the time of the 1941 census. Even in the contemporary developing world, the average family size is considerably lower than this: in Egypt it is 5.3, in the Philippines it is 5.0 and in Brazil it is 4.4. Contraceptive use is commonly associated with a reduction in age-specific fertility rates among older women (Fig. 2.4).

One useful way of understanding contraceptives is to regard them as a

Fig. 2.3. Patterns of human reproduction.

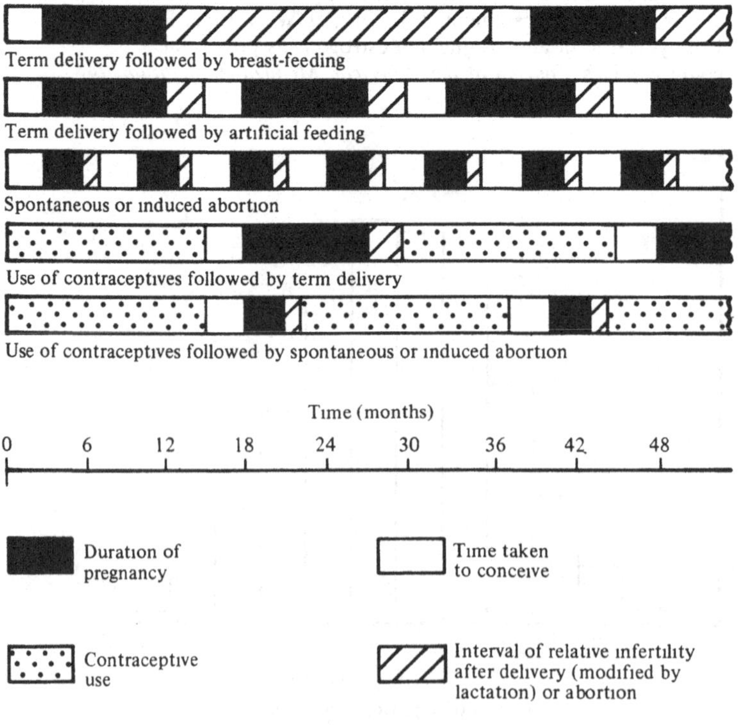

Term delivery followed by breast-feeding

Term delivery followed by artificial feeding

Spontaneous or induced abortion

Use of contraceptives followed by term delivery

Use of contraceptives followed by spontaneous or induced abortion

Time (months)

0   6   12   18   24   30   36   42   48

Duration of pregnancy

Time taken to conceive

Contraceptive use

Interval of relative infertility after delivery (modified by lactation) or abortion method of reducing the probability of conception, or, put another way, of extending the time taken to conceive. Unfortunately, even in the closing years of the twentieth century, there is no reversible method of contraception which is sufficiently predictable to allow the great majority of couples to achieve a small family. The only ways in which the fertility goals of the modern world can be achieved are through

(a) the use of contraception backed up by induced abortion;
(b) the use of voluntary sterilization as soon as a couple have had the desired number of pregnancies;
(c) the use of repeated induced abortions.

The last choice is costly in the provision of health services, less than optimal in relation to the woman's health and disagreeable to nearly all societies. In practice, contraception combined with induced abortion and

Fig. 2.4. Age-specific fertility rates. (After Potts, M. & Selman, P. (1979). *Society and Fertility*. Plymouth, England: McDonald and Evans.)

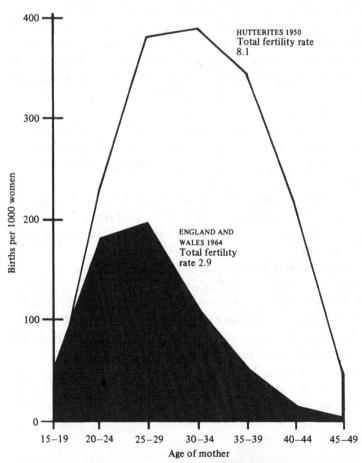

the choice of voluntary sterilization has become a worldwide phenomenon, though these choices are still not legally sanctioned and socially approved in all societies.

The demographic transition

In pre-industrial Europe, population was determined by the Malthusian checks of war, pestilence and famine. Birth-rates were commonly higher than death rates, although irregular cycles of bad harvests, epidemics and illness tended to remove excess population growth at relatively frequent intervals.[36] Wars had marginal effects except that they were often followed by famine or pestilence. This pattern existed in some developed countries until comparatively recently.

By the late nineteenth century, as a result of better diet, improved hygiene and advances in medical care, the death rate in Europe had fallen dramatically, with reductions in infant mortality leading the way.[14] The resulting imbalance produced a unique type of kinship structure. The Victorian era was the first and last time in human history in which the large surviving family was the rule. In all preceding and succeeding periods, the average couple may have produced many pregnancies, but overall an average of slightly more than two children *survived* to the next generation. Even the nineteenth-century large family in western nations did not persist for much more than one or two generations. By the early nineteenth century, marital fertility in France was well below the biological maximum and a sharp decline in birth-rates occurred throughout western Europe from 1870 onwards. In the past hundred years, mortality and fertility have fallen together to produce a new equilibrium of low birth-rates and low death rates, restoring the historic pattern of an average of two children surviving to the next generation (Fig. 2.5).

In the United States, a similar decline in fertility began slightly earlier and from an even larger family size than Europe. The crude birth-rate for white American couples was 50 per 1000 in 1830 but had fallen to less than 18 per 1000 by 1930.

The implications of this demographic revolution in family structure are clearly revealed by a comparison of English marriages of 1860 with those of 1925 (Table 2.1). Among women who remained married until the age of 45, the proportion of families with four or more children fell from 72% to 20% in the historically brief interval of 65 years, and the size of completed families dropped from six to just over two.

In contemporary Europe, North America and Japan, society has now achieved biological replacement, that is, on average each woman will be succeeded by one daughter who will reproduce in the next generation.

Table 2.1. *Changes in distribution of families by size (England and Wales)*

Number of children in family	0	1	2	3	4	5	6	7	8	Over 8
Marriages of 1860 (%)	9	5	6	8	9	10	10	10	9	24
Marriages of 1925 (%)	17	25	25	14	8	5	3	2	1	1

Source Report of Royal Commission on Population (1949). London: HMSO.

Fig. 2.5. Changing Patterns of fertility. (Modified from Bongaarts, J. (1980). *The Fertility-Inhibiting Effects of the Intermediate Fertility Variables.* Center for Population Studies Working Papers. New York: Population Council.)

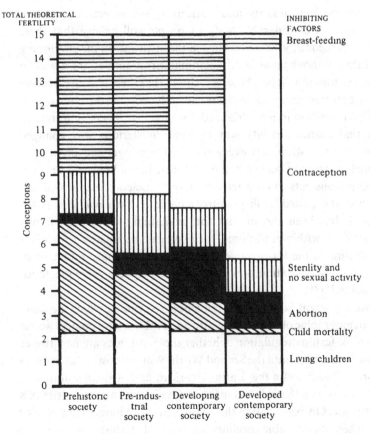

Desired family size is low (see Fig. 2.7). Allowing for natural infertility, death before reproductive age and for some individuals who never marry or who avoid having children, the actual average family size yielding biological replacement lies between 2.1 and 2.4. The challenge facing our contemporary world is to achieve a stricter limitation of birth than currently exists and to bring the whole world to a pattern of biological replacement. Looked at from the point of view of the number of children born, this task is not as formidable as is sometimes believed.

The forces driving it, and the actual mechanism of the demographic transition in the West are controversial. The greater part of the changes took place before there was any significant improvement in family planning services and at a time of complex social and economic change, so the myth has grown up that birth-rates fell because of a spread in education, improved economic standards and various other aspects of modern industrial living. A considerable body of people still believe that these changes must precede any further decline in the birth-rate in the developing world and that without them family planning programmes are a wasted investment. Historical analysis, however, shows that there was an extensive use of contraception and wide recourse to induced abortion during the demographic transition in industrialized nations.[20, 21] There is no reason to believe that marital fertility was in some mysterious way changed because of modernization, but every reason, from logic and observable fact, to conclude that the decline in the birth-rate in the West was brought about by conscious acts to limit fertility despite societal disapproval and the illegality of the limited fertility control techniques then available. In the last decade it has been shown that the availability of realistic family planning services within traditional societies can be related to a demonstrable decline in the birth-rate even in advance of those measures of education and modernization previously deemed to be a prerequisite for fertility change.[10, 26]

The most important factor which influences the rate at which a society adjusts to demographic changes is the attitude of those who control access to the means of fertility regulation, whether these attitudes are negative as was the case in the West until the Second World War, or positive as in many contemporary Asian and a few Latin American and African countries.

It used to be argued that a fall in infant mortality was a prerequisite of a falling birth-rate. On examination this hypothesis is no longer tenable. For example, when comparable declines in marital fertility occurred in Hungary in 1890 and in Ireland in 1929, the infant death rates per thousand live births were 250 and 69 respectively.[33] Data exist which suggest that those women who have most infant deaths also have most children, but this may represent nothing more than the shorter birth intervals associated with still-birth or an early infant death and the consequent failure of the mother to breast-feed and thereby avoid conception. It does not necessarily imply a deliberate pregnancy undertaken to replace a lost child.[32] It is also possible that high infant mortality may be a behavioural response to a high birthrate. The fact that in poor countries the number of deaths of girls under five years of age commonly exceeds those of boys (although biologically the male is the weaker sex) supports the hypothesis of concealed infanticide by selective neglect.

In the West, localities which were socially and economically identical saw fertility fall at different rates and at different times; for example in the Walloon parts of Belgium, marital fertility fell earlier and faster than in neighbouring Flemish areas.[17]

The retreat from parenthood

Which particular economic, social and psychological needs prompted late Victorian parents to initiate the transition from a completed family of six or eight children to the contemporary average of two? Predictably, no single factor or event provides a sufficient explanation. The Royal Commission on Population (1949) in Britain acknowledged a complex web of causes, among which social and economic change, the extension of the scientific attitude and the emancipation of women were certainly important.[31]

An outstanding contribution to historical analysis is found in Banks's *Prosperity and Parenthood* (1954)[1] in which he argued that the rising middle-class standard of living during the late nineteenth century provided the necessary impetus for adopting family limitation measures. An increase in prosperity, coupled with an expansion in the range of satisfaction regarded as essential for civilized existence, had become a reality for the Victorian middle class in western Europe and America. When this revolution of rising expectations was threatened by increases in the cost of education, domestic servants and the 'paraphernalia of gentility', a retrenchment occurred and instead of distributing the privileges more thinly amongst a larger number of children, parents chose to reduce the number of beneficiaries in an attempt to retain their standards. Undoubtedly there were other threats to the established way of life. It can thus be argued that the increasing power of the Trade Unions, the growth of feminism and, above all, the challenge to religious values and beliefs which accompanied the expansion and popularization of science, all undermined the assumptions on which middle-class prosperity were based and thereby accelerated the advance of family planning.

The process of family limitation in western societies began amongst the upper middle classes; doctors and clergymen were, according to the 1911 Census, the earliest occupational groups to limit their families, closely followed by teachers.[16] But as the economic advantages of the smaller family became apparent, broader sections of the population began to adopt the practices of those in the class immediately above them. This process of social emulation was relatively slow and was never carried to completion, but the Victorian middle-class family's choice between a third child or a carriage and pair had its equivalent in the surburban family's choice in the 1930s of a baby or a baby Austin car. The two-child family became firmly established, although the success with which individuals were able to conform to this idea depended upon their ability to overcome the barriers placed by society between them and the means to regulate their fertility.

The struggle for family planning

If the underlying motivation for family limitation is not fully understood, the means by which the process was achieved are clear; for the first time birth control techniques, formerly associated with promiscuity, became an accepted aspect of married life. The decline in the British birth-rate dates from 1877, the year of the Bradlaugh-Besant trial (Fig. 2.6), and there is little doubt that this event, and the enormous publicity which it received, was of great importance in gaining acceptance for the principle and practice of family limitation.[19]

Charles Bradlaugh, a well-known freethinker, reformer and Member of Parliament, intervened in the case of a Bristol bookseller found guilty, under the Obscene Publications Act, of selling copies of *Fruits of Philosophy*, written by the American physician Charles Knowlton.[3] Bradlaugh regarded the outcome of the case as a serious challenge to freedom of expression on a subject with which he had long been concerned. Together with Mrs Annie Besant, he reprinted the pamphlet, sold it for sixpence a copy and notified the police. Bradlaugh and Besant were charged, committed, tried, convicted and subsequently acquitted on a technicality during proceedings which lasted over many months and which were fully, often sympathetically, reported in the national and local press. The birth control controversy was thrown onto the breakfast table of the English middle classes at a time when, for reasons already outlined, they were especially receptive. The judge made it clear that he considered the prosecution ill advised and throughout the trial the defendants and witnesses made an impressive case for family planning on the grounds of improving maternal health, checking excessive population growth, reducing poverty and redressing social injustice. These arguments have changed little in the last 100 years. In his address to the jury Bradlaugh concluded: 'We want to prevent them [the poor who could now afford *Fruits of Philosophy*] bringing into the world little children to suck death, instead of life, at their mother's breast; and you tell us we are immoral. I should not say that, perhaps, you, gentlemen, may judge things differently from myself, but I know the poor. I belong to them. I was born among them . . . I plead here simply for the class to which I belong, and for the right to tell them what may redeem their poverty and alleviate their misery.'[3] Knowlton's *Fruits of Philosophy* enjoyed a new popularity, nearly 200 000 copies being sold as a result of the trial. Bradlaugh was re-elected to Parliament. Between 1879 and 1921 more than three million birth control pamphlets and leaflets were circulated in Britain, of which at least a third contained detailed contraceptive instructions.

The trial also led to the formation of the Malthusian League, which began as a defence fund set up to help to defray Bradlaugh's expenses,

Fig. 2.6. Birth- and death rates for England and Wales 1820–1980.

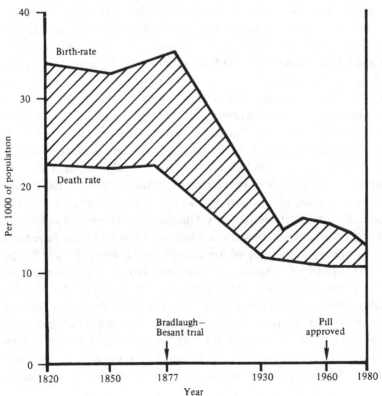

persisted as a pressure group and was later to become the forerunner of modern family planning movements. A demand for contraceptive appliances was also generated and became the subject of a flourishing, if at times dubious, postal and retail trade. Although coitus interruptus and induced abortion were probably the most important methods of fertility control, all methods of contraception now in use, with the exception of the Pill, were available by the end of the nineteenth century. A typical retail catalogue of 1896 offered, amongst other choices: Rubber Letters – 'the best, surest and most frequently used of any known appliance', Rendell Pessaries, the Mensinga Pessarie (that is, the vaginal diaphragm) and spermicides, particularly those containing quinine.[24] The cervical or stem pessary, a forerunner of the intrauterine device, first appeared in the 1880s in various forms and was patented in 1902.[6]

Precise estimates of the extent and practice of abortion are not available but it would appear to have been widespread. In London in 1898, the Chrimes brothers were sentenced to long terms of penal servitude for blackmailing large numbers of women who had applied to them for abortifacients and it was revealed at the trial that in the course of only three or four days they had obtained £800 by such sales.[20] During 1912, in an investigation of family limitation in the north of England, Ethel Elderton noted the widespread practice of self-induced abortion in almost every town and village; pharmacists, herbalists, barbers and market traders she reported, openly sold abortifacient drugs together with contraceptive appliances. One illegal abortionist interviewed by the British Medical Journal in the mid nineteenth century said she had clients who 'came back six or seven times'. She had started her trade in the early days of Queen Victoria's reign and reported herself as being 'a jokeler (jocular) person . . . and I says funny things and cheers 'em up'.[27] Mohr has analyzed the spread of abortion practices in the United States of America and quotes estimates of induced abortion as high as 1 in 5 of all pregnancies for the second half of the nineteenth century. Charges varied from $10 to $50 and some abortionists were very wealthy. Madame Restell is said to have been worth $1 million at the time of her suicide (1878), when she was finally brought to trial by Comstock, the American fanatic who did much to introduce anti-contraceptive legislation. In 1871 Ely van der Warker described abortion practices in Syracuse, New York State. He believed 'injection of water into the cavity of the womb can generally be relied on by the abortionist', and he complained that 'luxury of an abortion is now within the reach of the serving girl. An old man in the city performs this service for $10 and takes his payments in instalments'. He reviewed 21 deaths due to criminal abortion and claimed that 10 followed the use of abortifacient drugs.[27]

The extent of contraceptive use

The earliest known attempt to assess the extent of family limiation in a sample population was conducted by a subcommittee of the Fabian Society in 1905–06. The population sample was drawn 'from every section of the [British] middle class'. In answer to the question 'In your marriage have any steps been taken to render you childless or to limit the number of children?', out of 316 couples sampled 242 replied 'Yes'. Of the 120 couples who had married between 1890 and 1899, only seven had 'unlimited fertility'.[34] The survey had little statistical validity but it showed how the middle class, always the trend-setters, was behaving.

In 1946, Lewis-Faning, in a study conducted on behalf of the Royal Commission on Population, interviewed 3281 women in the general wards of selected hospitals and learnt of their contraceptive practices. All the women interviewed were in a continuing first marriage at the time of the survey and these marriages had taken place between 1910 and 1939. The data[18] (Table 2.2) provided an illustration of the increasing resort to family limitation in successive cohorts. The low figure for those using contraception during the first decade might appear to contradict the Fabian survey, but the difference is probably accounted for by the contrasting socio-economic groups represented in the two studies. In 1978 Ridley[7] and her

Table 2.2. *Changing pattern of contraceptive use (England 1910–39)*

Date of marriage	Percentage using contraception at some time during marriage
Before 1910	15
1910–19	40
1920–24	58
1925–29	61
1930–34	63
1935–39	66

Source: Lewis-Faning, E. (Ed.) (1949).
Family Limitation and its Influence on Human Fertility in the Past Fifty Years. London: HMSO.

co-workers conducted an interview of over one thousand elderly American women born in the years 1900–10, asking about family planning during their reproductive years. The survey was limited to white married women and 71% had practised contraception. On the whole, this group of women used family planning almost as much as their daughters, commonly beginning early in marriage. Those women whose childbearing years spanned the depression had had uniquely small families, 42% having one or no children. Elective sterilization was rare but 27% of women had had sterilizing operations (mostly hysterectomy) by the age of 50. The condom was used at some time by 54% of contraceptive users and coitus interruptus by 47%. Few women admitted to having had induced abortions but this aspect was probably under-reported. In Britain, during the Depression, Parish (1935) reviewed the abortion admissions to St Giles's Hospital, in East London, over the preceding 10 years.[22] These abortions were either spontaneous or illegally induced and there was no reliable way to differentiate between these two categories, but the total rose from 147 in 1924 to 293 in 1934, and over the same interval, the birth-rate in the borough declined from 18.2 to 13.2 per 1000.

In the couples surveyed by Ridley,[7] 15% or more either abstained from, or had infrequent, intercourse. There is no way of discovering if alternative and non-reproductive practices of sexual congress played a significant role in cutting down conceptions, although this is possible.

In a survey carried out in Indianapolis in 1941, 89% of American women had used contraception at some time during marriage.[35] After the Second World War an increasing proportion of couples adopted some form of family planning upon, or even before, marriage rather than at a stage when desired family size had been achieved, or exceeded. The Population Investigation Committee (PIC) Survey in Britain (1959) revealed that, of those couples married in the 1950s, 74% were using contraception, and 55% of these couples had begun the practice at marriage compared with only 36% in the 1930s.[36] Among couples married in Hull in 1965, in the longitudinal study conducted by Peel, 90% were using, had used or intended to use, some method of contraception.[25]

The English scene was comprehensively surveyed using a statistically valid sample of women under 40 who married for the first time during the winter of 1970–71. Fourteen per cent were uncertain of how many children they wanted, but over 80% of those who had decided opted for two or three, with an average preferred family size of 2.3 children[30] (Fig. 2.7).

Patterns of contraceptive choice

A large number of studies in the United States and other industrialized nations have provided information on patterns of contraceptive choice, on the success rates of different methods and on the influences which bear on the choice of method by the individual or social group. In the last 10–15 years, knowledge, attitude and practice (KAP) surveys relating to family planning have become a routine, perhaps an overdone routine, in nearly every developing country.

Patterns of contraceptive use are obviously related to the availability, or non-availability of specific methods, and are therefore highly influenced by the attitudes of those in political control and of those who provide family

Fig. 2.7. Wife's desired family size (England and Wales 1970–71). (After Peel, J. & Carr, G. (1975). *Contraception and Family Design*. London: Churchill Livingstone.

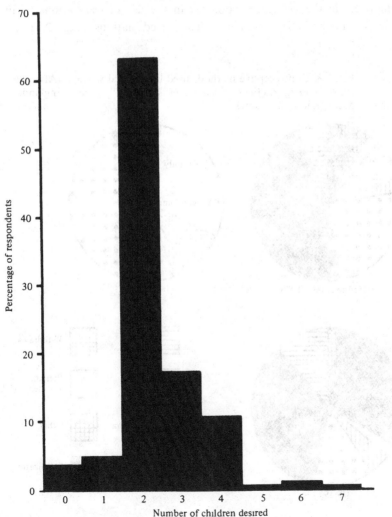

planning services. Before the widespread use of oral contraceptives and intrauterine devices, the patterns of contraceptive use in Britain and America were roughly comparable as regards condom, vaginal barrier and spermicide use. Coitus interruptus was more common in Britain than in the United States. Periodic abstinence was more popular in the United States than in Britain.

The introduction of oral contraceptives and the renaissance of interest in IUDs, together with changing attitudes towards voluntary sterilization, have brought about a marked alteration in contraceptive use in the past 10–20 years. The more modern methods of contraception usually require medical prescription, and interesting differences, which probably reflect more the differing attitudes of the family planning advisers than cultural differences in the users, are apparent in the use of the various family planning methods in different industrialized nations (Fig. 2.8). For

Fig. 2.8. Contraceptive methods used by married women. (After Potts, M. & Selman, P. (1979). *Society and Fertility*. Plymouth, England: McDonald and Evans.)

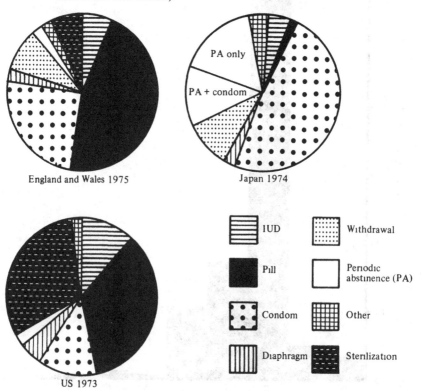

example, the USSR has a limited capacity for making oral contraceptives,
IUDs have been criticized by the leaders of the Russian medical profession,
voluntary sterilization is hardly available and condoms are of poor quality.
Not surprisingly, induced abortion is frequent. In Latvia 93 out of 100
married women over the age of 20 report at least one abortion.[5] In Eastern
Europe oral contraceptives are more readily available but voluntary
sterilization with the same frame of mind as many British and American
profession, while freely and easily providing induced abortion, regards
sterlization with the same frame of mind as many British and American
doctors felt about abortion before the law reforms of the 1960s and 1970s.
In Japan oral contraceptives are illegal and IUDs have been officially
approved only in the last few years; voluntary sterilization is performed on
as few as 30 000 women a year while condoms enjoy remarkably aggressive
and successful sales and periodic abstinence is much more widely used than
in any Catholic country (see Fig. 2.8). In the Republic of Ireland the sale of
all contraceptives was illegal until 1980, but there has never been any
legislation banning voluntary sterilization, so men were forbidden to buy
condoms but allowed to choose vasectomy! In the early 1960s, British
women who wanted a safe abortion sometimes travelled to Stockholm to
get the operation, which at that time was illegal in the UK, while more than
a decade later Swedish men who wanted a vasectomy flew to London,
because at that time the operation was illegal and not available in
Stockholm. All these variations stem not from the needs of users but from
the attitudes of providers.

Differential fertility

The adoption and selective choice of family planning practices
develops at differing rates in the various sectors of any society. To some
extent this is because doctors and other professional providers of
contraceptive services tend to communicate more readily and efficiently
with the more educated, but it is also because the expectations of, and
demands upon, family planning vary with cultural and educational factors.

When a society is opposed to financial support of fertility regulation,
then differential fertility between subgroups may persist over many decades
or even generations. Social classes IV (semi-skilled) and V (unskilled) in
Great Britain have had a significantly poorer use of contraception and a
markedly higher fertility than the more privileged groups for over 50 years.
(In Britain statistics often record social class, a fact which surprises
American readers, while in the US, records are commonly divided by race,
a method which would be unacceptable in Britain.) In Singapore, where
there is a strong government-sponsored family planning programme, the

fertility of the Chinese fell earlier than that of the Indian and Malay groups (Fig. 2.9), but the lag between the various groups was not as prolonged as in Britain. In a similar manner different ethnic groups in Fiji have also shown differences in the rate of fertility decline, but have tended towards the same low point.

One of the many paradoxes of family planning has been that those who often express the greatest political or emotional concern about differentials in fertility decline between different economic or ethnic groups tend to be the very people who most vehemently oppose the provision of subsidized family planning services by the state, which would most benefit those in greatest need. If family planning is to reach the most under-privileged then it commonly needs to be subsidized and always needs to be well advertised. It often requires a system of multiple outlets and a sympathetic attitude from the medical profession, an attitude completely different from that

Fig. 2.9. Crude birth-rates of the different ethnic groups resident in Singapore. (Redrawn from Neville, W. (1978). The birth rate in Singapore. *Population Studies*, **32**, 1.)

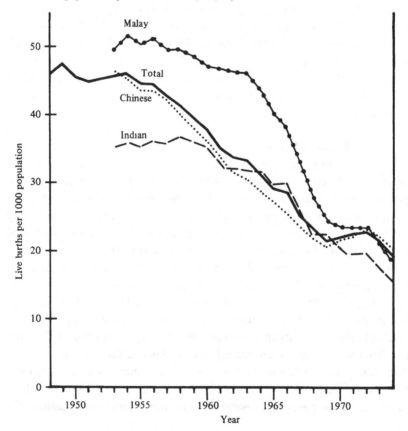

appropriate to the provision of family planning for more privileged, literate groups, who enjoy a way of life where planning for the future has been proved to bring rewards. The stereotype attitude to birth control among the poor was characterized by Rainwater in his study *And the Poor Get Children*, (1960)[29] as 'doing nothing is the easier way out'. Perhaps it merely needs to be said that amongst those where few of life's plans are fulfilled, family planning may also be more difficult to adopt.

Problems in the provision of family planning

The early birth control clinics, first established in the United States in 1916 and in England in 1921, were intended to provide for the socially least privileged portion of the population with the explicit intent of helping them to catch up on a use of contraception which the more educated had already achieved. The initial clientele in English clinics appears to have been drawn predominantly from social classes IV and V. However, by the 1960s, a disproportionate number of clients came from the upper middle and middle classes (class IIa and IIb). It was only with the setting up of domiciliary family planning services[4] and with the integration of family planning services within the National Health Service that the under-privileged at last began to catch up in their usage of contraception.

The paradox of individual approval combined with group hostility seems characteristic of the early evolution of family planning in nearly every country. As patterns of family planning change they may be encouraged or retarded by those middle-class professional groups who hold the relevant expertise and who also tend to be influential in the setting of policy and enactment of laws. The attitudes which have been documented in nineteenth-century and early twentieth-century Europe and North America found many parallels in Asia and Latin America in the 1960s and 1970s and still have their analogues in parts of Africa and the Islamic world of the 1980s. However, in the West the disparity between public and private attitudes went on for longer and ran deeper than it has in the contemporary developing world. The United States was to send Margaret Sanger to prison in 1916 and one of Marie Stopes's mobile family planning clinics was to be burnt in Britain in the 1920s, while in the US in the 1970s, arson at abortion clinics became common. Fortunately these extreme attitudes have not found a parallel in such Catholic countries as the Philippines or Brazil, nor in such Islamic countries as Pakistan or Egypt.

Conclusions

The transition from high to low fertility associated with the diffusion of voluntary fertility control appears to occur rapidly and to be an irreversible process once begun. When changes in marital fertility are reviewed in detail, in both developed and developing countries, they appear to be remarkably concentrated in time, but to take place under a variety of social and economic conditions. The differences in the timing and the rate of fertility decline are not totally determined by cultural conditions. For example, comparable declines in marital fertility began in England when it was largely industrialized (15% of the labour force in agriculture) and in Bulgaria when it was largely agrarian (70% of the labour force in agriculture).[26] Literacy was low in France and Hungary when marital fertility began to decline but high in Britain when comparable changes occurred. No single threshold of social and economic development can be defined which is an adequate predictor of fertility decline.

The perception that life is not as good as it used to be, as occurred in many developed countries in the 1870s or as was so apparent in Japan after the Second World War, or that one's neighbours are having a better life than you are, as is so apparent to those east of the European Iron Curtain, seems to be a particularly powerful pressure leading to the restriction of fertility. In the contemporary world, where inflation is a reality both for the urban poor of developing countries and for affluent nations, and where the 1980s do not promise to be such pleasant years as the 1960s or early 1970s, there is likely to be a sharp and continued decline in achieved fertility.

3

The population explosion

We are all aware that the world is already becoming overcrowded and the problem will worsen. What is not always appreciated is the time-span of population growth. There is no reliable means of estimating the total population for the long era when man was a nomadic hunter–gatherer, but 10 000 years ago, when the first walled city (Jericho) was built, perhaps 50 million people were alive. Five thousand years later, when the pyramids were under construction, the number had doubled, and over the next 2500 years, up to the time of Christ, it doubled again to a little over 200 million. The next doubling took about 1500 years and by 1850 man had achieved a total population of 1000 million. A mere 75 years later, 2000 million was reached and by 1975, only 50 years on, this had doubled again to 4000 million (Fig. 3.1). What does the future hold?

Consequences of population growth

In the previous chapter it has been shown that in western countries improved medical care reduced death rates rapidly but birth control lagged behind. The most dramatic example of differential fertility is that presented by the current gap between birth-rates in developed and developing countries.[12]

In the nineteenth century, populations of the industrialized nations rarely grew by more than 1% per annum. In the contemporary world, growth rates of 2% are common and of 3% and more are not unknown (Table 3.1). By 1980 world population stood at 4400 million. Even if the practice of family planning continues to spread, the minimum population by the year 2000 will be 5900 million, and if the world fails to meet the needs of individuals and society to regulate fertility then it will reach 6500 million. The rate of growth will be most rapid in Africa (a projected increase of 76% in 20 years), but the greatest absolute numbers will be

Table 3.1. *Population dynamics*

Country	Population in millions		Rate of natural increase (1981)	Doubling time (years)
	1980	2000		
China	957	1190	0.8	58
India	694	1040	2.1	36
Brazil	126	212	2.4	25
Bangladesh	89	153	2.6	27
Nigeria	77	149	3.2	22
Egypt	42	65	3.0	26
All developed countries	1131	1272	0.6	113

Fig. 3.1. The population explosion.

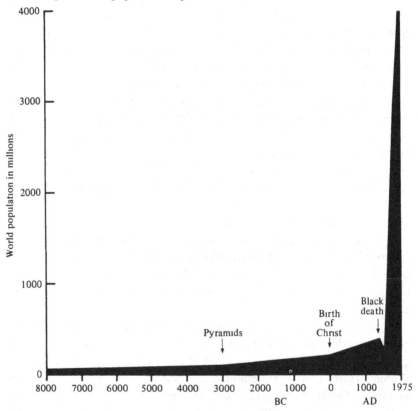

added to Asia where the population base is already so large and the population will increase by 63% by the year 2000 (Fig. 3.2).

Half of the developing world's population is now below the age of marriage (Fig. 3.3) and the imbalance between deaths and births is so great that, whatever steps are taken, global population will continue to grow until well into the twenty-first century.[3] The point at issue is whether by the year 2050 the population will stabilize at the current 'low' projection of 8.4 thousand million or whether it will reach 12.4 thousand million before growth ceases. Are there to be three people or 'only' two for every person alive now?[4] Or could there be an unprecedented rise in death rates?

Over the last hundred years, the nations of the world have become more interdependent. In the past, for better or worse, Europe could export its excess population to the Americas, to Australasia and to colonies in Asia and Africa. There are now no comparable opportunities for transfering excess population from one nation to another.

The economic implications of a population which doubles in a generation, as opposed to one that doubles in a century (Fig. 3.4), can hardly be over-emphasized.[9] The phrase *the population explosion* is a well worn one but remains meaningful. Population growth has swallowed up most of the gains made in food production at a world level in the last 20 years. Whether the economic system is capitalist or communist, high rates of population growth require high rates of investment in transport, education and health in order to do no more than stand still. The dependency burden (the combined number of young and old people in the society) is greater in a rapidly growing population than in a stable one.

Fig. 3.2. World population 1750–2150. (Redrawn from Kidron, M. & Segal, R. (1981). *State of the World Atlas.* London: Pan Press.)

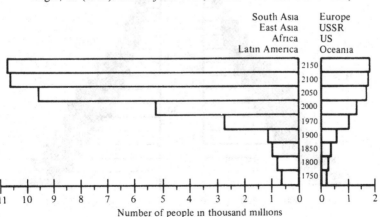

Number of people in thousand millions

Population growth has robbed the individual of otherwise achievable progress. For example, between 1955 and 1975 the gross national product of the Philippines expanded by 87% but the per capita income only rose by 20%. Even dramatic advances in technology fail to keep pace with the growth in the number of people: the high Aswan dam increased the

Fig. 3.3. World population by age and sex. (Redrawn from Barney, G. O. (1980). *The Global 2000 Report to the President of the US*. New York: Pergamon Press.)

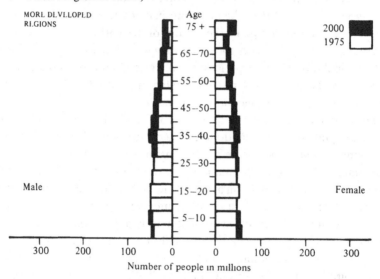

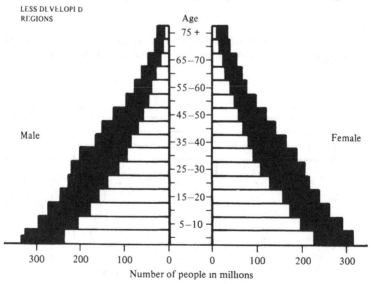

cultivable area of Egypt by 40%, but the population rose by that amount during the years it took to plan and build the dam and for Lake Nasser to fill.

The most immediate challenge arising from population growth relates to changing patterns in employment and to urbanization. Between 1970 and 1985, the number of Asians of working age will increase by 500 million. Little fertile land remains to be brought into cultivation and the world's forests are disappearing at a frightening rate. It costs many thousands of dollars to create new, non-agricultural jobs. What will the extra people do? Where will the extra people go? They have only one choice: to the towns.

The biggest migration in human history is taking place as hundreds of millions of people leave a traditional village way of life, which in many ways has changed little in over 4000 years, to enter the exploding cities of the contemporary world with their multiplying problems. In the past 15 years nearly 600 million people, approximately the population of India, have become city dwellers for the first time. By the end of the century they will be joined by another 1500 million, which is equal to the total world population in 1900. In 1950, Brazil was 64% rural; in 1970, it was 56% urban.

Urban life holds a promise which is all too rarely fulfilled. Increasing millions live in squatter areas in the meanest of shacks on the poorest of land: governments pretend they do not exist, or bulldoze down fragile

Fig. 3.4. Average family size and population growth (assuming western mortality rates).

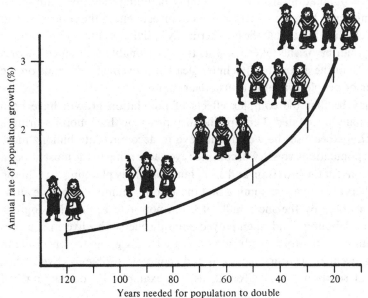

homes when they want to widen the road, or if a relative of a cabinet-minister seeks to build a new hotel. Mexico City is probably destined to contain more than 30 million people by the year 2000. Already the people speak of living in the City of the Dead. Slums develop so rapidly that they are called *colonias paracaidistad* (parachutists' neighbourhoods), because they appear to be dropped from the sky.

On the one hand, the world's wealth is spread most unevenly, and more equitable terms of trade between industrialized nations and the Third World and greater international aid would benefit rich as well as poor, opening up new markets and perhaps adding a little to national security. On the other hand, it would be naive to think the world's problems could be solved in this way, as a fully equitable distribution of the planet's wealth would provide a daily income that would do little more than, say, buy one breakfast in an international hotel for the individual from the industrialized world. The world's wealth will remain spread unevenly for the foreseeable future (Fig. 3.5); the problem is whether the gap between rich and poor can be narrowed or whether it will grow wider in future decades. A greater availability and use of family planning will be one factor determining the outcome.

In economics, every theory eventually generates a counter hypothesis. In the 1980s, at least in the United States, some development economists are challenging the need for population limitation.[10,11] Simon maintains that global energy and other physical resources are adequate to deal with sustained population growth, that family planning may give short-term economic gains because society can avoid investment in the education and care of children but that in the long term any individual contributes more to society than he or she takes from it. It is 'reasonable to assume', writes Simon, 'that the amount of [technological] improvements depends on the number of people available to use their minds'.

It may be that the complex effects of population growth have been occasionally overstated. Perhaps the new pro-growth economics bring a ray of hope because the world will have to accommodate billions more people; population growth will continue even according to the most hopeful projections for the provision and acceptance of family planning. But Simon and others are naive in assuming that the absolute number of people alone will contribute by the sheer bulk of brain power to economic progress. Farmers, labourers and unemployed slum dwellers who live in societies that cannot even afford to educate them are hardly going to contribute to solving twentieth-century technical and economic problems. Even when technical solutions can be found, as, for example, by developing leaf

43

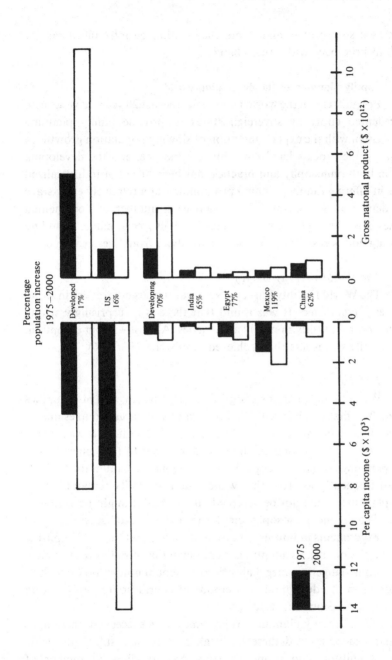

Fig. 3.5. Economic and population projections (developed and developing world and selected countries). (Redrawn from Barney, G. O. (1980). *The Global 2000 Report to the President of the US*. New York: Pergamon Press.)

protein as a source of human food, they cannot be introduced rapidly enough to keep pace with other changes.

Family planning in the developing world

Fortunately, in the world as a whole, the last 20 years have seen an unprecedented effort by sovereign states to provide family planning services, often with the explicit intention of slowing population growth. In some ways, the process has been a remarkable one, and the developing world, in both philosophy and practice, has been ahead of industrialized nations in offering family planning programmes at a relatively early stage in the demographic transition.[7] An increasing number of documented successes exist, but, inevitably, mistakes have also been made, including misleading and occasionally inappropriate advice from 'western experts'.

The World Fertility Survey

The World Fertility Survey (1970) was the largest exercise in social science ever conducted. It was found that there is a surprisingly strong desire to control fertility in nearly all societies. Almost without exception, desired family size is less than achieved family size (Fig. 3.6).

Policies

When family planning programmes first began, two philosophies emerged. The first emphasized the need to motivate target couples and to put considerable investment into education and promotion. It was widely held that certain social and economic changes had to take place before family planning would be adopted on any significant voluntary basis. It was also frequently asserted that while infant mortality remained high, family planning would not be accepted, and indeed it might be wrong to offer it. The second philosophy emphasized the role of accessibility to services: experiments in household distribution were set up and simplistic, but not unreasonable, assumptions were made that if millions of women were suffering dangerous illegal abortions, it should not be too difficult to persuade them to adopt modern methods of contraception, even before significant socio-economic development.

While not all family planning programmes have succeeded, there have been many successes and these have taken place in a sufficiently wide variety of cultural and economic situations to allow a number of generalizations to be made.[8] Ready access to contraception is important and where, as in Indonesia and China, it has been achieved on a wide scale, fertility has declined within a traditional society in advance of other changes. It does not seem to be necessary that 'threshold' progress must be made in income and education before contraception will be adopted. The hypothesis that a high rate of child survival must be secured before family planning is adopted has also been refuted by experience. Some have argued that family planning will only be acceptable in developing countries if it is linked to maternal and child care services but others have pointed out that people who seek family planning are not sick and may prefer to get their contraceptives in the same way as they obtain other low-cost domestic items. By and large, the World Health Organization (WHO) and the World Bank have pursued integrated programmes, while many private agencies, such as Profamilia in Colombia, and some governments, such as those of Bangladesh, Indonesia and Thailand, have pursued the independent, free-standing so called 'vertical' approach.

In an integrated service, family planning often gets pushed into the background by both administrators and practitioners, who must meet the daily, immediate demands of curative medicine. This is important because in many developing countries health care services are rudimentary or non-

Fig. 3.6. Desired family size and unwanted births. (Westoff, C. F., 1980). Unwanted fertility in six developing countries. In *Record of the Proceedings of the World Fertility Conference, London*, p. 707.)

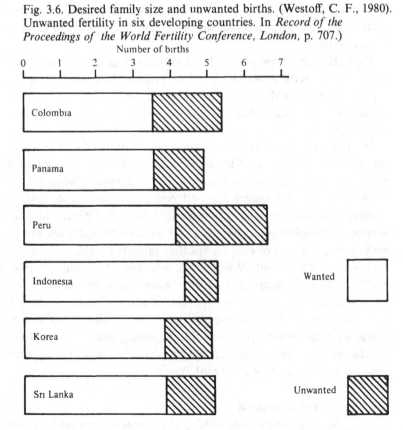

existent and emergency demands seem to justify overriding priority for tiny resources. Family planning, in its own right, has the virtue of being simple, affordable and, as the World Fertility Survey has shown, in wide demand.

In a world beset by widespread and degrading poverty, serious malnutrition, persistent chronic ill health, inadequate housing and with tens of millions unemployed and hundreds of millions of underemployed adults, any contribution to the improvement of the human situation is welcome. Family planning can be a short cut. It is often the first element of primary health care to be put in place, making a much-needed contribution to maternal and child health even before medical services are established. By the use of shops and village distributors, it is possible to get contraceptives to nearly every corner of every country.[1] When they first become available, contraceptives tend to be used primarily by older women of high parity who are exactly those at greatest risk from childbirth. The policy that health services must be created in order to make family planning available as an integrated part of health care has been shown to be less realistic, more expensive and more time consuming. It would be nice to have both, but a community-based distribution of contraceptives is a lot better than nothing at all and can be a road along which to carry other services later.

The setting up of new services has involved village distributors with one-day training. With a year or so of experience such workers can easily undertake additional duties. For example, they have already proved invaluable in the identification and treatment of intestinal parasites in children.[2]

Most exciting of all has been the concept of fertility related development introduced by Mr Mechai Viravaidya in Thailand.[12] Here, one individual with a vision and a drive no less than that of Margaret Sanger or Marie Stopes has brought knowledge and contraception services into many corners of his country. Using community rather than clinical channels of service, distribution points have been set up at the village level. These may only serve a few tens of couples but they provide a needed service with a relatively quick pay-off. When given selective additional training and relatively limited inputs, village distributors have become a source of primary health care and, most important of all, of economic development. They have become the basis for new agricultural techniques and of better markets for the farmers' products, thus bypassing some of the exploitation of the middle men, a factor which tends to hold back economic development in much of the Third World.

Variety of methods

No single method of fertility regulation is universally appealing.

As a generalization, the greater the variety of methods available, the higher the overall usage of contraception. Fortunately, in a world of over-stretched resources, different methods of family planning can be made available through different channels of distribution. The social marketing of condoms, spermicides and oral contraceptives has proved most successful. Social marketing is a step towards self-sufficiency, it uses existing channels of distribution and is totally free from the accusation of coercion.

The limitations of the reversible methods of contraception, when used over a fertile lifetime in a large community, are inescapable and there will always be a need to include voluntary sterilization and abortion amongst the range of fertility regulating methods available.

Training, skill and some type of operating-room facilities are necessary for the provision of sterilization, particularly tubal ligation. Early abortion can be done in simple circumstances by 'barefoot doctors' or midwives and, even allowing for the necessary training and back-up, should not cost more than a week's disposable income.

Channels of distribution

As with methods, so with channels of service, variety makes for easy access. Unfortunately, political restraints have often forced the organizers of family planning programmes to adopt policies which are the opposite of those most likely to meet community needs. On the whole, most communities have some forms of traditional contraception and even the poorest communities, such as those on the Indian subcontinent, have an extensive network of traditional medical practitioners. It would have been logical to make available modern methods of contraception, such as Pills and condoms, through traditional networks of distribution, and it seems likely that both would have been well received. Conversely, the virtually universal use of traditional abortion methods would be best dealt with in modern hospital facilities.

In many developing countries, private medical practice is the major source of care for the middle classes and is coveted by the poor, who often spend a considerable slice of a limited disposable income on modern medicine. The subsidy of private practitioners for such services as IUD insertion and voluntary sterilization, with the patient paying some part of the total cost and the government the rest has proved successful in the few cases where it has been tried and could be usefully extended.[5]

Over most of the developing world, traditional societies have been forced to adopt *two* innovations at the same time: namely, modern methods of contraception and the modern health care services through which they could be made available. Unfortunately, this double innovation is least efficient in those very countries and those very areas, namely the villages, which have the greatest demographic problems, the highest maternal mortality and the greatest problems of infant health and nutrition. Because it is tied to the introduction of a modern health service, something which will take a long time to reach poorly developed areas, the disadvantaged people living in such areas are being denied access to any form of family planning. Induced abortion is often the first element of fertility control to be adopted during the demographic transition, although it is usually the last to be offered in a government programme.

Family planning in the People's Republic of China

The most rapid fertility decline in any large population in the history of the world has occurred in the People's Republic of China in the last 15 years; the birth rate has plummeted from 34 per 1000 to 18 per 1000, a 47% reduction.[6] Fundamental social changes have taken place and unique concepts, such as that of the one-child family, have been developed. But underlying this success have been some of the same policies which appear to apply to all countries, that is a widespread availability of the maximum number of methods through a variety of channels, with a decentralization of decision-making and genuine community participation in the planning and execution of programmes which are enforced by strong cultural pressure upon the individual to conform.

The legal age of marriage has been raised and norms are now 24 for women and 26 for men. In Shanghai in 1979, the average age at which men married was 28 years. In some areas, contraceptive acceptance among married couples is as high as 70%. Intrauterine devices are the most widely used reversible method of contraception, although steroids, including injectables are easily available. All contraceptives are available free. Most important of all, there is ready access to abortion and voluntary sterilization. Abortion rates are high, as is inevitable in a society controlling its fertility for the first time.

Despite successes, China continues to face formidable problems. Serious crop shortages persist and an over-extended agriculture is vulnerable to small changes in seasonal rainfall. The 1980 drought is thought to have been associated with severe deprivation for 20 million people, although few, if any, actually starved to death.

The number of women reaching marriageable age will increase by more than 50% in the coming decade. China is the first country to face realistically the appalling consequences of failing to deal with rapid population growth when it arises. In absolute terms China adds 10–12 million people to its population each year and despite the current successes the population will grow to about 1200 million early in the next century. The implications for this are very different for the nation and the individual: at a national level they represent the upper limit of what a poor country, even if well organized, can support; at the individual level, it means that the current generation must average less than two children each. China has begun a series of bonuses for couples who agree to have only one child and 10 million one-child certificates had been accepted by December 1981. By 1980 in China it is thought that in some surburban areas couples had, on average, 1.5–1.7 children. In Sichuan Province (which has a population of almost 100 million, making it the world's eighth largest country if it were independent) the birth-rate fell from 40.7 to 11.2 in the decade of the 1970s. By 1980, 70% of all births were first births and 81% of those families with only one child had signed a pledge not to have any more. Currently 85% of married couples are practising family planning, a level higher than in most developed countries. In Sichuan Province alone more than 23 million IUDs have been inserted, 10 million vasectomies have been performed and over 2 million female sterilizations have been carried out over the past 10 years. Data on abortions are not so readily available but individual hospitals suggest that the ratio in relation to birth is very high indeed.

Most other developing countries have failed to recognize that when half their citizens are below the age of marriage, the achievement of a stable population, even over 20 or 30 years, requires a ferocious limitation of individual family size.

Even in China, with its strong central government and its strict community organization, it can be difficult to carry out the type of vigorous fertility regulation that the out-of-balance demographic situation demands. The national population policy has been opposed by representatives from rural areas and the army. Nevertheless, population growth has its own imperatives.

Family planning in India

While China demonstrated dramatic successes in population limitation in the 1970s, India slipped backwards and the census estimate for 1981 of 638 million people was considerably higher than had been hoped. The birth-rate was 36 per 1000 and the death rate was 14.8 per 1000. It seems likely that India will have the dubious honour of being the most populous nation in the world by the year 2000. Unlike China, India has concentrated on single-method solutions to her problem: first the use of IUDs and, later, sterilization. Unlike the 'bare-foot doctor' in China, who play an important role, their analogue in India, the traditional practitioners who are found in every town and village, have been steadfastly excluded from the programme. Traditional practitioners could have handled Pills and injectables well and selected individuals could have been taught early abortion techniques. Pills have never been offered in the government programme on a significant scale and injectables (which would probably have proved most popular) have been rejected because the Indian medical establishment has never demonstrated an understanding of the relative risks of over-fertility and contraceptive side-effects. Indian advisers have stressed the dangers and potential dangers of the Pill and of injectables, demanding the safety precautions recommended by the US Food and Drug Administration which, if they make sense at all, do so in a highly developed country with low maternal and infant morbidity and mortality but which are totally inappropriate where pregnancy is as dangerous as it is in India.

Conclusions

The global rate of population growth is thought to have fallen during the 1970s. However, the total number of people added to the world's population continues to grow year by year. Currently, the annual increase is approximately 70 million (about the population of Mexico). Even today India alone adds one million to her population each *month*: the equivalent of an extra Australia annually.

By the year 2000, global population will still be increasing and although the rate will be lower, the absolute annual addition will have grown to 100 million a year. World population will continue to grow until well into the twenty-first century and the world has little option but to adapt to a final population of between 8000 and 16 000 million. Whether this adjustment can be made without irreversible changes in the environment and without a breakdown of law and order in the exploding cities or a scrabble for diminishing natural resources between competing nations remains to be seen. The failure of the western world to develop adequate methods of contraception and adequate services in the years 1850 to 1950, and the still halting and uncertain assistance which industrialized nations provide to less privileged countries, places the world our children will inherit in real jeopardy.

At the same time, there are reasons for hope. As pointed out, if contraceptive use could be doubled in the 1980s, which is by no means an impossible task, then the final stable population which the world must accommodate in the next 100 years would be reduced by as much as 4 000 million (equal to the current world's population). The responsibility to improve methods and services is awesome.

The rural and urban poor of the Third World have shown themselves to be remarkably adaptable to twentieth-century technology and contraception; the acceptance of voluntary sterilization and the increasing use of abortion are no exception. Birth-rates are falling more rapidly in the contemporary developing world than they did during the nineteenth century demographic transition in the West (Fig. 3.7). Restraints on the more widespread use of the means of controlling fertility are sometimes due to the failure by politicians, religious leaders and social elites to be realistic about the problems of excessive fertility and to their frank political cowardice in refusing to advocate potentially unpopular but essential measures such as making voluntary sterilization available in a Moslem country or abortion in a Catholic country.

The total resources committed to family planning and population programmes in the developing world, including China, amount to approximately US $1000 million annually, with about US $450 million flowing in aid from rich to poor countries: the equivalent of seven hours' worth of global defence spending. The US, although it gives a smaller percentage of its gross national product to international assistance than

Fig. 3.7. The demographic transition in developed and less developed countries.

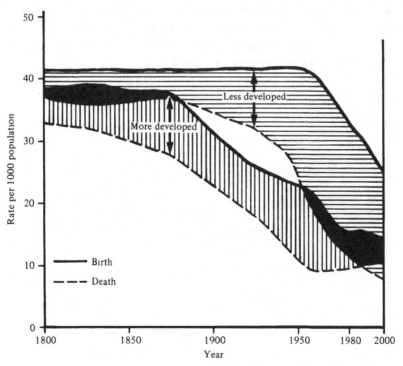

many European nations, by virtue of its wealth provides 40% of this total. In 1965, US AID gave $5 million and in 1979, $190 million. On average, it costs US $15 to provide family planning care for one couple for one year in the developing world. Currently, 75 million couples out of a total of 375 million couples of reproductive age in the developing world, again excluding China, use some form of modern family planning. By the year 2000, there will be 640 million couples and services will need to expand 20 fold to bring family planning to all the couples necessary if fertility is to fall to biological replacement levels. To do this, foreign aid programmes might have to make available each year up to $10 000 million in terms of 1980 dollars, still a trivial sum in the total world budget and approximately equivalent to the industrialized world's inventory of cosmetics. There is something piquant about a world that spends so much to increase sexual attraction in one set of countries and so little to prevent unwanted reproduction elsewhere.

But family planning programmes do not live by bread alone. In the last analysis they only succeed when there is respect for the individual, an acceptance of the fact that people make sensible decisions over their own fertility and a realization that even those who lack the privilege of education can adequately handle the technology of fertility regulation. In large part, family planning continues to be a history of tension between the consumer, where empirical observation suggests that the goals and decision-making processes of individuals adjust rapidly to family and societal needs, and the community, which often makes slow progress in the legal adjustment and policy formation necessary to provide the services the individual needs to control his or her fertility.

4

The safety and effectiveness of contraceptive methods

Background

There is little doubt that a great deal of worthless rubbish used to be sold in the name of contraception. Writing in the *Manufacturing Chemist* in 1933 Voge remarked 'Again and again we find that some product has appeared on the market, has been recalled, re-issued (possibly under another name) with the composition minimally changed. . .' One of the goals of the Birth Control Investigation Committee (BCIC), established in 1927, was an attempt to stop such unacceptable practices. The work of the committee in contraceptive testing was an early example of transatlantic scientific co-operation, in this case spurred on by the fact that the US National Committee on Maternal Health had been advised that it could not conduct any research in America because the Comstock Act might be invoked against laboratory work or the publication of research findings.[34]

The BCIC developed laboratory techniques for the assay of vaginal contraceptives, elaborated statistical formulae for the measurement of contraceptive efficacy and developed new spermicides. It established the Population Investigation Committee which continues to publish the international journal *Population Studies*. The National Committee on Maternal Health in the US was instrumental in founding the Population Council, New York, which has played, and continues to play, an invaluable role in contraceptive development, the analysis of family planning programmes and the study of social and economic factors affecting fertility regulation.

It is a measure of western society's difficulty in handling the whole topic of fertility regulation that, until 1959, the American National Institute of Health was explicitly forbidden to sponsor anything to do with contraceptive research and development.[1] In the 1960s and 1970s there was a genuine, if brief, effort to catch up with considerable expenditure on contraceptive development and evaluation, particularly in the United States.[34] However, the late 1970s saw a falling away of support[13] and there is now a possibility that the US Congress may revert to a Comstock mentality. There is an obvious worldwide need for more, rather than less, investment aimed at improving fertility regulation. Money is required for fundamental research into new and improved contraceptive techniques, for the improvement and simplification of quality control regulations for those in large-scale use, for investment in appropriate programmes of contraceptive education tailored to local needs and facilities and, perhaps most difficult of all, for the assessment of the long-term risks and benefits of use in a variety of national settings.

Quality control
Chemical spermicides
Following an extensive review of test procedures, the International Planned Parenthood Federation (IPPF) selected a method which required the partial mixing of semen and spermicide on the grounds that some co-mingling is produced during coital activity.[21] Selected dilutions of the spermicide under test are prepared using normal saline. Semen (0.2 ml) is taken from a masturbatory sample which is not more than 4 h old and meets certain specified standards of sperm density and motility. Using a magnetic mixer, the semen is mixed with 1.0 ml of saline and selected dilutions of the spermicide under test are added and mixed for 40 s at 35–37°C. After mixing, samples are examined for sperm motility under five low-power (100–150 ×) and five high-power (400–600 ×) light microscope fields. A spermicide passes the test if no active sperm are observed at 1:11 or 1:12 dilutions. The Sander-Cramer test is a similar test devised by the Ortho Company in 1940.[14, 33] A more elegant method is to test the ability of sperm that have been mixed with a spermicide to migrate across a millipore filter.

The complex mechanical and physiological events which take place during normal coitus can never be fully reproduced but post-coital tests in volunteers using a spermicide can give a general measure of whether a new entity has promise. Masters has devised a spermicide test that uses an artificial penis to artificially ejaculate semen to known quality, the women undergoing the test being previously sterilized volunteers. This is the most accurate facsimile of natural coitus available but it is difficult and expensive, and would not be acceptable in many societies.[24]

Chemical spermicides, which are used in the vagina must be non-toxic and non-irritant to the vagina as well as effective spermicides. Animal tests involve the daily application of one-fifth of the human dose into rabbit vaginae on 14 consecutive days followed by a gross microscopic examination for evidence of infection, irritation and epithelial degeneration. The rabbit vagina is as satisfactory an animal model as the monkey's.[11] The introduction of new spermicides also involves careful clinical supervision of human volunteers including the collection of material for cytological and bacteriological examination. An expert group appointed by the US Food and Drug Administration (FDA) has recently reviewed the testing of spermicides.[37]

Many contemporary spermicides rely in part for their effectiveness on the occlusion of the cervical os by means of the foam produced by the dissolution of the product within the vagina. Foaming capacity can be evaluated by adding a standard dose of spermicide to 4 ml of saline in a 100-ml graduated cylinder at 35–37°C. A satisfactory foaming tablet should disintegrate within 2 min and produce 20–40 ml of foam.

Rubber appliances

Rubber has a long-established important role in modern contraceptive practice, being used in condoms, caps and diaphragms. The properties of these appliances, as well as the effects upon them of storage, lubricants and chemical spermicides, are therefore of considerable significance.

Condoms. Many countries have devised standards for the manufacture of condoms, but these often differ in the type of physical criteria applied and in the exact measurement of performance expected.[4, 15, 30] Despite several attempts, the International Standards Organization has not been able to agree to an acceptable international standard: condom testing seems to be the subject of considerable nationalism. Comically, the shortest condom allowed under US standards would fail to pass the Hungarian standard because it would be too long. The size and thickness of condoms is commonly specified. The British Standards Institute (BSI) requires a minimum length of 160 mm (excluding the teat if provided), a minimum width of 49 mm and stipulates a maximum allowable weight of 1.7 g for a smooth condom and 1.9 g for a textured condom.[3] The standard further specified filling a sample of condoms with 300 ml of water, rolling them gently on blotting paper and looking for leaks. The product is also tested by stretching a strip of the rubber until it snaps, or by a 'bursting-strength test' when the condom is inflated with air. Even more sensitive tests for holes are commonly conducted by manufacturers and are part of the Japanese standard.

Deterioration due to storage can be an important hazard and the bursting strength is a useful measure of resistance to deterioration. The bursting-strength test requires the rubber to be generally capable of elongation to at least six times its original length and to retain two-thirds of this value after accelerated aging for 7 days at 70°C, which is the equivalent of several years' normal shelf life. The bursting strength may also be used to assess the effect of lubricants or chemical spermicides on rubber and only approved lubricants and spermicides should be recommended for use with condoms.

Samples must be taken from the factory in batches and if the sample fails, the whole batch is deemed defective. Every package sold should carry the name or trademark of the manufacturer, a batch number and the date, including the year, by which the article should be used.

Diaphragms. The major potential defects in the vaginal diaphragm are holes and flaws in the membrane, deformation of the spring and separation of the spring from the surrounding rubber. Visual examination is usually sufficient to reveal any imperfections, but since faults are likely to arise in use, women should be advised to be always on the lookout for them. They may compress the spring laterally with the forefinger and thumb and if it does not return to its original shape this may be an indication that the diaphragm is becoming ineffective. The British Standards specification makes recommendations on manufacture and describes an inflation test in which the membrane is stretched to twice its original diameter.[2] An accelerated aging test must also be conducted.

Cervical and vault caps. There is no standard test for caps other than visual inspection, although the IPPF has suggested filling the cap with water, leaving it for 15 min and inspecting for leaks.

Intrauterine devices

The plastic from which the IUDs are made must be of a high and uniform quality. Failure to achieve this has led to fragmentation of devices in utero with the consequent need for removal of the fragments. Devices need a good smooth finish, they should be manufactured within specified tolerances and the composition of the plastic should be checked by flotation in various concentrations of saline, as a test of density, and by incineration, after which analysis of the resulting ash is a measure of the various fillers. Radio-opaque barium sulphate is commonly added to allow X-ray location. Perhaps the most useful test for the devices such as the Lippes Loop is the deflection test in which the length of the device is measured before and after elongation for 20 s using a 100-g weight: the two measurements should be identical.

With the introduction of IUDs which release various hormones or metallic ions, a new range of toxicity testing and quality control is required, which approaches the complexity associated with hormonal contraceptives.

Systemically active contraceptives

The quality control for Pills and injectables (and of bacteriological sterility for parenteral medications) is essential and carried out by continually withdrawing samples from the production line for analysis which includes hormone assay and tablet strength. Additives, including colouring matter, are also scrutinized. All large pharmaceutical manufacturers in developed countries, including those in the People's Republic of China, now have good quality control. Variation in dose is usually under $\pm 3\%$, although some tableting factories in developing countries have not yet reached this standard.

The issues of effectiveness and safety, however, have not been similarly mastered.

Effectiveness
Theoretical effectiveness and use-effectiveness

The theoretical effectiveness, also known as the biological or method effectiveness, of a contraceptive method measures the pregnancy rate experienced when the method is used under ideal conditions and excludes pregnancies that are due to failure to use the method or to errors in its use. The use-effectiveness of a contraceptive method measures the pregnancy rate when the method is used under real-life conditions and includes failures due to omission of the method or to mistakes in its use. The extended use-effectiveness of a contraceptive method measures the probability of avoiding an unwanted pregnancy within a specified interval of time after adoption of that method regardless of subsequent use, that is, it includes pregnancies that may occur after cessation of use if an alternative method is not adopted.[36]

Theoretical effectiveness may be useful in helping an individual to understand the potential of a method, assuming all the rules are followed, but may be widely different from use-effectiveness for a number of reasons. In the first place, laboratory tests cannot be performed under normal physiological conditions and can therefore never be a proper basis on which to assess efficiency in real life. Secondly, physiological and behavioural idiosyncrasies may modify the efficacy of a particular method. Thirdly, the most important factor is a complex of social and psychological variables which are collectively summarized in the word 'acceptability'. Thus a method which may have a high theoretical efficiency, such as periodic abstinence, may be ineffective because most couples are unable or unwilling to use it. On the other hand, relatively inefficient and even irrational methods may survive because they are acceptable. The concept of acceptability involves a wide range of factors amongst which broad cultural influences may actually clash with the psychological motivations affecting a family or an individual. Within a particular society the most important subcultural influences include age, education and socio-economic status, all of which may affect the care, perseverance and consequent success with which a particular method is used. The failure rates for modern methods of contraception tend to be higher in developing countries (Fig. 4.1).

For a specific couple, moreover, the acceptability of a given method may depend upon the precise stage in the family building process at which it is adopted and in particular upon whether it is being used to delay a pregnancy in an incomplete family or to prevent further pregnancies in a family already regarded as complete. One of the significant findings of the second Family Growth in Metropolitan America (FGMA) study[39] was the marked improvement in efficacy of contraceptive usage as couples approached the number of children desired (Table 4.1). Older couples also had less contraceptive failures than younger ones (Fig. 4.2).

Fig. 4.1. Percentage of wives experiencing unintended pregnancy while using the specific method for one year. (Data from Laing, J. (1981). Personal communication; and Population Information Program, Series I, no. 3 (1981), Baltimore, Maryland.)

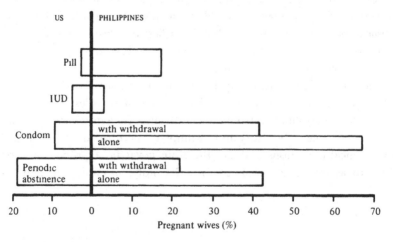

There is also a tendency for couples to adopt more efficient techniques as their families grow and theoretical effectiveness and acceptability may become interacting factors, especially in a society where the relative merits of contraceptive techniques are widely discussed. It is for this reason that an

Table 4.1 *Contraceptive failure rates per HWY for women at different stages of family building (excluding use of steroidal contraception or sterilization)*

Group of women	Number of children desired		
	2	3	4 or more
Marriage to first pregnancy	21	27	46
First to second pregnancy	8	14	16
Since second live birth	3	16	13

Source: Westoff, C. F., Potter, R. G. & Sagi, P. C. (1973). *The Third Child.* Princeton, New Jersey: Princeton University Press.

Fig. 4.2. Contraceptive failure in first year of use by age (married women, US).

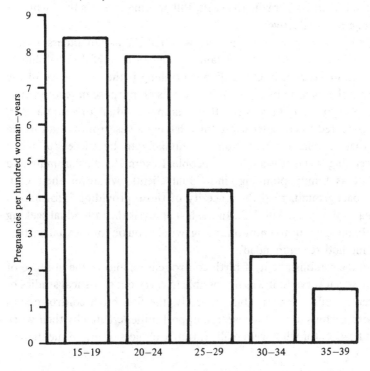

adequate evaluation of a contraceptive technique should be based on the actual reproductive behaviour of a representative group of couples known to be using that particular method.

The criteria of use-effectiveness

Part of the counselling given to an individual or a couple on contraception must involve providing information of the failure rates of the various methods. This can be difficult to give and is subject to a good deal of misunderstanding. The averages quoted in textbooks may not help in the individual case. However, there is no doubt that a ranking order of contraceptive effectiveness can be set up. Sterilization is virtually 100% reliable, with injectable contraceptives being the next most effective method. Oral contraceptives, at least in developed countries, come a close third. IUDs are not far behind the Pill in effectiveness (and generally exceed it in developing countries) while the mechanical methods such as condoms and diaphragms have a somewhat higher failure rate. Coitus interruptus and periodic abstinence have a wide range of quoted failure rates and seem to be much influenced by the socio-cultural background in which they are used.

Motivation is so important that a couple who really wish to use a diaphragm, for example, may end up with a greater success than if they are encouraged, against their will, to use the Pill or some other method which is on average more effective.

Information should be presented in a way that clients can understand. A chart giving the ranking order of failure rate can be useful in helping to make an enforced choice. Overriding everything is the confidence of the provider in the method being offered. There is no purpose in recommending a method you do not believe in. If you as an individual, or your partner, are not prepared to consider using Pills, having a vasectomy or adopting some other specific method, you are unlikely to be successful when recommending this method to other people. In something as intimate and important as family planning, individual clients, whatever their educational background, read the sincerity of those providing information with great rapidity and subtlety. In the last analysis the individual seeking family planning wants to know one thing: would you or your sexual partner use the method recommended?

Before the establishment of birth control clinics and in the absence of extensive social surveys, it was impossible to carry out statistical studies of contraceptive effectiveness. Unfortunately, the first birth control clinics were more anxious to use the research opportunities created by their work as a justification for what were really intuitive choices of technique than to attempt objective appraisals of the various methods. Thus Marie Stopes claimed a 99.4% success rate for her cervical cap but imputed an 85.5% *failure* rate to the diaphragm, which was recommended by the 'rival' clinics of the Society for the Provision of Birth Control Clinics (now the Family Planning Association).[35] In reply, Dr Norman Haire, Medical Officer of the Walworth Clinic, claimed that the diaphragm was far superior to the Stopes cap which, in his experience, failed in 88% of cases he had seen. Nevertheless both Marie Stopes and Norman Haire were in complete agreement on the almost total unreliability of every other method of birth control.

For every woman who came to the early family planning clinics because of dissatisfaction with traditional methods, there were obviously many others who continued to use such methods with relative success; the clinics were thus biased by seeing the failures associated with traditional methods. Even today, coitus interruptus still suffers unfairly from the unsubstantiated assertions of a high failure rate made by these early family planning professionals.

It took some time to develop objective criteria for measuring contraceptive effectiveness. Marie Stopes assumed, and claimed, total success for all those women who had been supplied with caps but had not returned to report a pregnancy, reasoning with domestic intuition that 'in one's own life, one complains if the milk is sour but says no word of praise or thanks to the milkman who daily delivers fresh milk'. In truth, health care professionals are well aware that dissatisfied clients do not return but seek advice elsewhere.

Determination of use-effectiveness

The use-effectiveness of a contraceptive method is defined in terms of its capacity to prevent unwanted pregnancies. It is usually expressed as the failure rate per one hundred woman-years of exposure (HWY). The basis for calculating this failure rate is known as the Pearl pregnancy rate,[26] which is expressed as Failure rate per $HWY = $ (Total accidental pregnancies $\times$ 1200)/(Total months of exposure).

In any application of this formula, the total accidental pregnancies must include every known conception whatever its outcome; the factor 1200 is, of course, the number of months in one hundred years. The total months of exposure in the denominator is obtained by deducting from the period under review all those months during which, for extrinsic reasons, conception was not possible; by convention 10 months are deducted for full-term pregnancy and four months for abortion, although these figures would have to be modified in the developing world where lactation goes on for so much longer. Necessarily such failure rates take into account only those accidental pregnancies which are known to the woman. Thus, contraceptive failures are in reality more common than is generally realized because many very early embryos abort spontaneously before pregnancy is recognized (see Chapter 13, Spontaneous abortion).

The risk of contraceptive failure within a specified number of users often falls with duration of use because of changes in the population under study. Individuals who use the method incorrectly are more likely to become pregnant and also to abandon the method. Long-term users may also include those of lower fertility. In order to overcome these problems, the life-table method of analysis has been adopted to study contraceptive effectiveness. The method takes into account all reasons for contraceptive continuation and permits the calculation of failure rates for specified intervals of use, whereas the Pearl rate pools data and gives one common measurement.[23]

Many professionals engaged in family planning have as their perspective the time between the current and the next clinic visit. Only rarely does an individual doctor or nurse work long enough in the same place to care for an individual over a significant part of their fertile life. It is easy to forget that even a method as effective as an IUD will be associated with unwanted pregnancies in between a quarter and a third of women over a decade of use. In the modern world, where most women achieve their desired family size by the late twenties, they may have to face 10–15 more years of fertile life during which fertility regulation will be required.[18, 31] Thus fertility regulation is not always very effective (Table 4.2).

Table 4.2 *Percentage of women who achieve or exceed three planned pregnancies during a reproductive life-span of 20 years[a] using an effective reversible method of contraception (IUD, diaphragm or condom)*

	%
Women with three planned pregnancies	16.0
Women with *one* additional unplanned pregnancy	33.5
Women with *two* additional unplanned pregnancies	30.0
Women with *three or more* unplanned pregnancies	20.5
Women who exceed fertility goal	84.0

[a] From marriage to the menopause and including conception and delivery of three wanted children.
Source Hulka, J. F. (1969). A mathematical study of contraceptive efficiency and unplanned pregnancy. *Americal Journal of Obstetrics and Gynecology*, **104**, 443.

Clinical trials monitor failure where the method is used under closely supervised conditions, sometimes by a self-selected group of people. Household follow-up surveys provide most data on use-effectiveness and extended use-effectiveness, particularly about over-the-counter and traditional methods of contraception.

Clinical studies usually include only volunteers (and to this extent are atypical) and are confined to specific, commonly clinic-recommended methods. Failure rates in over-the-counter methods such as condoms and spermicides are much more difficult to determine than those of the medically prescribed methods such as IUD and diaphragms. Demographic studies are retrospective and thus subject to error through faulty recall whereas clinical trials are concurrent or prospective but, however adequately supervised, are subject to loss through failure to follow up every user.

A number of important points should be observed when designing and interpreting use-effectiveness trials. A minimum of 600 months of exposure is usually considered necessary before reasonable conclusions can be reached and the sample of users should represent a compromise between a large number with short exposure and a small sample with longer exposure.[27] It is also essential that couples taking part in any trials should be as representative as possible, especially of the different stages of family building. Social class, length of education and age are other important factors in determining contraceptive success. An effort should be made to exclude the use of two methods at once, such as spermicides with IUDs, unless this is a deliberate subject of investigation.

In their discussion of contraceptive failure rate, some authors have attempted to distinguish between 'patient failure' and 'method failure'. It will be obvious, from the nature of use-effectiveness studies, that such a distinction is not permissible: from the point of view of use-effectiveness a patient failure is also a method failure. The continuation rate of a contraceptive method measures the attrition amongst users due to pregnancy, those stopping the method because of unacceptable, or perceived, side-effects and discontinuation for any other cause such as marital separation or the death of a partner.

Use-effectiveness and continuation rate data, particularly of the sort that would demonstrate trends over time and would be ideal for the management of national family planning programmes or the individual clinic, are often lacking. However, useful numerator analysis can be conducted by following trends amongst users, such as the age and parity of women attending a clinic or receiving services from a national family planning programme.[31]

Contraception is not an exact science and it is easy to misuse data on effectiveness of particular techniques. Failure rates should not be quoted as exact measurements nor be given to potential users as firm guides as to how such methods may be expected to work for them. What can be established is a ranking order with Pills being more effective than IUDs and these in turn being less liable to failure than condoms or barrier methods. There is, however, considerable overlap and careful condom users may in fact do better than poor Pill users. In the Third World completely different ranking orders may apply because of different cultural acceptability (see Fig. 4.1).

In the complete absence of birth control practices, but taking into account natural fertility and infertile intervals, the pregnancy rate would probably be about 40 per HWY.[16] This corresponds to 10–12 live-born children in 25 years of marriage.

The failure rate per HWY is perhaps more meaningful to a lay enquirer if it is interpreted as four times the number of accidental pregnancies to be expected in 25 years of marriage.

Safety
Pre-marketing testing

The introduction of a new drug or device into medicine is necessarily a complex problem, although it is only in recent years that an attempt has been made by the state to regulate the process. The US FDA was established in 1927 and considerably strengthened in 1938 because 70–100 people had died after a small manufacturer had illicitly mixed sulfanilamide with diethylene glycolantifreeze. In the early 1960s the use of thalidomide (it is not generally known that 2.5 million doses were distributed in the US) once again drew public attention to the problem of drug regulations. Congressmen Kefauver and Harris developed additional legislation, passed in 1962, which began with a concern over drug pricing but, propelled by a full awareness of the thalidomide catastrophe, ended in dealing with general aspects of safety.[32]

Currently in the United States a manufacturer or institution developing a new drug must obtain an Investigation of a New Drug (IND) for each of three phases of chemical trial and then, if the findings are satisfactory, apply for a New Drug Application (NDA). Phase 1 clinical trials usually involve a small number of carefully screened volunteers who use the drug in question for perhaps 10 days. Under FDA legislation such studies must be preceded by at least 90 days of tests in rats, dogs and monkeys. Phase 2 clinical trials involve between 50 and 100 subjects who use the drug for several months and must be preceded by one year of animal tests in three species. They are designed to give a rough impression of efficacy and a crude impression of side-effects. More extended, Phase 3 clinical trials may involve a thousand or more users and give a better measure of efficacy. They can be expected to uncover any serious short-term effects.

In order for NDA to be granted for a contraceptive, evidence must be provided from two-year toxicity studies in three species of experimental mammal and of the initiation of seven-year chronic studies in dogs and ten-year studies of primates at several dose levels. There are, however, many limitations to such studies. Florey (1898–1968) has pointed out that if penicillin had first been tested on guinea-pigs, it would have been rejected as too toxic for human trials. There are numerous differences in drug action between species and these are especially marked in the case of reproduction.

Tests for carcinogenicity

As long as we remain ignorant of the cause and control of cancer, it will be impossible to predict with certainty the effect of exogenous substances on the incidence of cancer. Some in vitro tests exist for substances such as shale oil, and animal studies have proved reasonably consistent in the case of frankly mutagenic compounds.

Spermicides, plastics and other materials used in IUDs can be tested for their cancer potential. However, in the case of contraceptive hormones a much more complex situation obtains.[6, 40] Not only is it likely that a long latent period may exist between the use of exogenous hormones and any effect on the incidence of cancer, but the absolute dose, the degree of supression of the woman's own ovarian activity, the ratio of oestrogen to progestogen and the duration of exposure may all be significant. In addition, steroids could have a different effect if taken early in the development of cancer from that produced if they are taken when the same cancer is established. Finally, there is no reason why the use of contraceptive hormones might not protect against cancer at one site, or at one stage of the evolution of a particular tumour, while increasing the risk at another site, or even of the same cancer at a different stage of development.

Animal tests can be useful but extrapolation has a number of difficulties in the case of hormones. Age, sex, the stage of reproductive cycle, the number of pregnancies before and after the experimental treatment, the route of administration, metabolic pathways and clearance of endogenous hormone production are all relevant. Studies must always include control animals and it must be appreciated that some species are prone to cancer without dying out in their natural environment. For example, some strains of mice are sensitive to the 'milk factor' carrying mammary cancer from one generation to another. In the Committee on the Safety of Medicines study[6] some 99% of some untreated control groups of rats developed mammary tumours and it was common for up to one quarter of control rodents to develop lung and liver tumours. Most beagle bitches develop mammary tumours if they live long enough.

Rodents, dogs and monkeys have all been used in testing contraceptive steroids. Rats and mice have been given 2–400 times the weight equivalent contraceptive dose for 80–100 weeks. Pituitary and mammary tumours occur at high doses but, in the words of the British Committee on the Safety of Medicines, 'although a carcinogenic effect can be produced when such preparations are used in such high doses throughout the life-span in certain strains of rat and mouse, this evidence cannot be interpreted as constituting a carcinogenic hazard to women using these preparations as oral contraceptives'.[6]

The use of beagle dogs has become a mandatory part of contraceptive steroid testing in the US, but has been criticized by the WHO and abandoned in Britain. Beside the obvious species differences which exist between discontinuous seasonal breeders and humans, who are continuous breeders, beagle dogs handle ovarian steroids in a markedly different way from women. Beagle dogs on depomedroxyprogesterone acetate develop acromegalic changes but no such alteration occurs in human users. The bitch uterus undergoes marked proliferation in response to progestogens, while in women it becomes atrophic. Beagles often develop pyometra and in long-term studies are routinely hysterectomized.[38] Primates probably provide a more suitable model for human use, but only small numbers can be studied for long intervals, so high doses of up to 50 times the human level are given. While such a strategy makes sense in the case of studying carcinogens like tobacco, it is more difficult to interpret the results in the case of hormones, where it is not even known if natural ovarian hormones given at up to 50 times the normal level might not be carcinogenic in long-term use.

Animal experiments are useful and need to be conducted, but should be taken as a systematic way of asking questions that may need special attention in human use. Dramatic and well-publicized decisions about contraceptive use based on animal tests for carcinogenicity may not be in the best interests of medicine. For example, the progestogen chlormadinone, which was amongst the most potent ever synthesized, was withdrawn in Britain and the US in the early 1970s because its use in high doses in beagle bitches resulted in benign mammary tumours. Chlormadinone remains off the market today, even though Britain has stopped recommending beagle dogs as an animal model. Similarly seven- and ten-year animal tests of depomedroxyprogesterone acetate have not led to the withdrawal of the drug as a therapy for endometrial cancer but have caused its non-approval as a contraceptive in the US. Several other injectable contraceptives are currently under extended animal test and seem more likely to merit medical approval. A paradoxical situation is arising where the public, and a good many physicians, seem to have greater faith in something where tests are incomplete and there has been no adverse publicity than in a more thoroughly understood compound where some flaws may have become known.

Post-marketing surveillance

The history of oral contraceptives, and to some extent of IUDs, has been the accumulation of important knowledge *following* widespread use. There seems to be every reason to assume that this generalization will apply to all new drug development and the rational response would probably be to cut back current requirements for the introduction of a new drug and improve post-marketing surveillance. Conditional approval for a new drug, analogous to the Federal Aviation Authority's Certificate of Airworthiness, might be more realistic because, logically, the true proof of safety can only come after prolonged and widespread use.

Great Britain and a few other countries have a system of voluntary recording of adverse side-effects by physicians. Such procedures can raise questions and uncover trends but are of limited usefulness, as physicians rarely report more than 15% of significant events.[19] In practice, most knowledge about rare adverse side-effects has been gained from specially designed epidemiological studies. The safest and cheapest type of study to conduct is the case-control retrospective study. In order that a retrospective study may be set up, there must be a suspicion that a drug causes side-effects. This suspicion should be based either on clinical impression, as happened in the case of thromboembolism and the Pill, or on questions raised by animal studies such as those experimental studies on monkeys which led to the follow-up of vasectomized men for subsequent cardiovascular disease. Starting with the disease under suspicion, individuals who have had the disease are examined and divided into those using, and those not using the method in question. Then a control group is established from among, say, victims of road traffic accidents where there is no likely correlation between the method and the condition, and the users and non-users of the method are again separated. The total number of cases to be gathered depends upon the prevalence of the method within the society, not on how rare or common the disease happens to be. If very few people use a method, or if nearly everybody uses it, case-control studies are more difficult to conduct (Table 4.3).[7]

Retrospective disease studies of this type have built-in difficulties. There may be a bias in diagnosis because of the awareness of doctors of the suspected correlation between the disease and the method. Also, it may be difficult to determine the number of users of the method in the population from which the sample has been taken. Retrospective studies can give a measure of the increased risk associated with a method but cannot measure an absolute rate. They can measure a protective effect of a method if one is suspected, but unpredictable effects may well go undetected.

A prospective study of a contraceptive method can pick up unpredictable as well as suspected good and bad side-effects. Such a study can measure the absolute rate of the disease under question in the community.

Table 4.3. *Minimal samples required to detect differences in disease rates between contraceptive users and non-users*[a]

Prospective studies

Disease	Duration of study (years)	Incidence of disease (per 100 000 controls per year)	Sample size
Cancer of the breast	1	22	85 000
Cancer of the endometrium	1	3	600 000
Cancer of the cervix	10	56	35 000
Diabetes		200	9 000

Retrospective study

Proportion of women who have ever used the method		Sample size
0.25	Incidence of disease in controls	120
0.50	not relevant	110
0.90		340

[a] Results which are statistically significant at the 0.05 level are assumed and in the case of prospective studies the study is designed to detect a doubling of the disease rate. Prospective studies lasting longer would require correspondingly smaller samples. Retrospective studies measure a *relative risk* not a *rate*.

The methodology is relatively easy to understand but the investment in time and money to achieve a result is inevitably many times greater than for a retrospective study. A number of controls and users of a method must be matched and followed for a specified length of time which depends on the prevalence of the disease to be studied, the statistical power expected in the final observation, the assumed change in the incidence of the disease consequent on the use of the method, and the length of time for which the study is planned to run (see Table 4.3).

In practice, it is exceptionally difficult to follow tens of thousands of contraceptive users over a number of years. Modern populations are often mobile, divorce, remarriage and changes of name and status are common, and medical care is expensive and may be sought from a variety of outlets making the linkage of an individual's needs from different sources difficult, and sometimes impossible. The United Kingdom, with its system of general practice has proved the best base for conducting prospective studies and that of the Royal College of General Practitioners on oral contraceptives is probably the most successful yet carried out. In America, health insurance schemes, such as the Kaiser Permanente in California have provided an appropriate base for certain epidemiological studies (see Chapter 10).

It is essential to distinguish between the *relative risk* of a disease in users of a contraceptive technique and the *attributable risk*, which indicates the number of people (per 1000 or 100 000) who are at risk to suffer from the condition. It is an important distinction because the relative risk may be high, as in the case of Pill use and liver hepatoma, but the disease is exceptionally rare so that the attributable risk remains low. The risk of hepatoma following Pill use is clinically far less important than that of pelvic inflammatory disease following IUD use because in the latter, although the relative risk is small the disease itself is common. In some conditions, such as cardiovascular disease, the attributable risk amongst non-users begins to rise steeply towards the end of the fertile years, so when Pill use exerts it small relative risk the age of the user becomes of great significance in determining the attributable risk.

There may be a strong statistical relation between the number of telegraph poles in the community and the frequency of heart attacks but there is no plausible explanation of any biological relation. There may be a deficiency, or an excess, of women with diabetes using the Pill but this could reflect prescription practices rather than any causal relation between the drug and the disease. Pitfalls in epidemiology are many: some are obvious and some more subtle. Questions must be asked about the matching of controls and cases. For example, women who use the Pill may have different lifestyles, including such things as exposure to sunlight, which may be relevant to the incidence of melanomas, or different sexual practices, which can be relevant to the incidence of pelvic inflammatory disease or cervical cancer.

In judging the usefulness of a study the following simple questions should be asked. What is the strength of the statistical relation? Is there an appropriate temporal relation between the use of the method and the observed effects? Is there any relation between the dose and the severity of the condition? Is there any relation between the duration of use and the occurrence of the condition? Is the relation a specific one? And finally, is it biologically plausible and consistent with other clinical data?

In the last analysis epidemiological studies depend on the accuracy of disease diagnosis. Unfortunately, medicine is a less exact science than is sometimes thought. Studies in New York,[22] Great Britain[25] and Japan[17] have all found something under 50% agreement between ante-mortem and post-mortem diagnosis and a 1980 study in the US[12] found that the cause of death listed by the pathologist was among those identified clinically as contributing to the death in 72% of cases, and discovered that cardiovascular diseases were overrepresented in ante-mortem diagnoses. Clearly physicians are alert to certain diseases, which therefore get overdiagnosed. Once a condition has been associated with a possible contraceptive side-effect it may well be reported where it does not truly exist. This is especially the case in conditions which are difficult to diagnose such as deep vein thrombosis. Epidemiological studies do not prove causal relations, they suggest areas of concern.

In developing countries, where diagnostic skills are unequal, where there are many informal and unregistered sources of medical advice and where the prevalence of contraceptive use is often low, epidemiological studies are even more difficult to conduct. However, the WHO has launched some case-control studies which should provide important information about the use of steroids in Asia. The International Fertility Research Program (IFRP) is exploring the risks and benefits of contraceptive use in Third World populations by studying deaths due to all causes among women of the fertile age-group and, at the same time, recording contraceptive use.[20]

On the one hand, it has been said that if you torture the data enough they will scream; on the other hand, it has been said that a study does not have to be perfect to be useful. Unfortunately, epidemiological studies have become the focus of media attention and instant interpretation which is often misinterpretation. There may be epidemiological observations on methods of contraception which have produced a great deal of important information and an increasing number of studies are likely to be conducted which will undoubtedly contribute further to the responsible management of an ever-widening range of fertility regulation methods. However, if these studies are to be used to the benefit of people, they must be interpreted soberly, with understanding and wisdom. The findings must be kept in perspective and reassuring results given as much publicity as alarming ones.

Private considerations and public perspectives

There is no single answer to the problem of assessing the effectiveness and safety of contraceptives, nor indeed of any other drugs. There may be several, often conflicting answers from animal studies, clinical trials and from epidemiological surveys. Ultimately the assessment depends on the perspective of the individual, whether user, professional adviser or administrator, who has to make a decision.[28, 29]

Rare serious complications can occur with almost any drug but where the drug in question is effective in the treatment of serious illness we all approve its clinical use and such use, even if it results in occasional deaths, would not attract media coverage. On the other hand, the very rare occurrence of the toxic shock syndrome (only 55 cases were reported up to 1981[5]) received excessive exposure on the mass media worldwide even though there was no negligence by manufacturers or doctors! Many millions of women must have been worried and apprehensive to a degree in no way justified by the facts. Society, as expressed through the media, accepts danger from drugs in the treatment of disease but not from everyday medicaments of ordinary living. Contraceptives are regarded as such and their side-effects are newsworthy.

All methods of fertility regulation have drawbacks and in recent years, each one, from periodic abstinence to abortion, has accumulated documentation of either genuine or suspected adverse side-effects. Family planning providers often rate effectiveness as the most important attribute of the contraceptive, although users may be more interested in acceptability. This emphasis of effectiveness partly stems from a reluctance to deal with the problems of unwanted pregnancy through the provision of induced abortion. (The history of oral contraceptive development would undoubtedly have been more successful if the early clinical trials could have been conducted with lower doses of hormones and with the back-up possibility of induced abortion in the case of failure.) The biologist sees man as a mammal subjected to the special stresses of civilized living and to some extent this wide view encompasses the narrower disciplines of pathology, epidemiology and clinical medicine. Epidemiologists deal in probabilities, but administrators, like individuals deciding on contraceptive methods, must make 'yes' or 'no' decisions. They must react not only to real and perceived physical risks of fertility regulation methods but also to political and logistic effects.

Ultimately, all administrative decisions assessing the balance of the risks and the benefits of contraception involve judgement. Even for the expert committee member, the WHO or the US Congressman on the Hill, decisions about contraceptive risks and benefits are not made in a wholly rational manner after deliberation about accurate, complete data. In fact, such decisions always contain an element of intuitive reasoning, based on past personal experience, and the data never are complete and conclusive, but always to some extent inadequate and conflicting. Drug regulatory authorities must respond to many different pressures and currently the US FDA in particular is trapped: it is asked to prove the safety of a drug before it is marketed, but logically such a task is impossible. In the last analysis, every new drug is an experiment on our own species. All that can be done is to establish a testing system which takes all reasonable and prudent steps to reduce foreseeable risks: the unknown is, of its nature, unpredictable and there will always be a hazard when new chemical entities or new devices are introduced for protracted use as in contraception.

In 1970 Djerassi estimated that it would take up to 10 years and cost between ten and twenty million dollars to introduce a new method of contraception and he suggested that requirements had become unrealistically strict and were inhibiting the introduction of new drugs and in particular the development of new contraceptives.[9] History has shown this prediction to be true and today the cost of introducing a new drug can be as high as US $50 million.[10] Experience may yet show that the investment is not cost effective. Perhaps testing before marketing should be simplified and post-market surveillance improved.

By contrast surgery remains an area of unregulated individualism where personal judgements, unsupported by factual data, are happily accepted by patients and public alike as an adequate basis for dangerous therapies. For example, alternative routines of obstetric management or options in the surgery of breast cancer need to be subjected to randomized trials just as much as does drug therapy.[8]

In the end it is the perspective of the individual consumer that is of overriding importance. The man waiting for his vasectomy, or the woman taking the Pill, may see decisions concerning fertility regulation very differently from the epidemiologist, the biologist or the administrator. In developing countries with inadequate resources should the Pill be freely available without prescription? The politician sees the need but fears the responsibility for the serious clinical complications which must inevitably, though rarely, occur. Unfortunately epidemiologists have not yet conducted a randomized trial comparing the relative risks of unsupervised Pill usage against those of being subjected to an unskilled village abortion. The biologist cannot quantify the emotional trauma associated with attempting to bring up five children with love and dignity on a dollar a day and then compare this with the husband's potential risk of developing anti-sperm antibodies 10 years after the vasectomy which would have avoided two or three of the children. It is difficult for a committee of medical administrators sitting in an air-conditioned room in a capital city deciding what tasks should be delegated to medical auxiliaries, to really understand what it means to be in labour for four days attended by a traditional midwife or to be delivered of a dead baby and left with a fistula between vagina and bladder. Assessing the safety and effectiveness of fertility regulation is indeed a complex process demanding wisdom and compassion as well as scientific observation and accurate statistics.

5

Traditional methods

Modern methods of family planning only account for one part of the control which individuals exercise over their fertility. An appreciation of the other variables is important in understanding achieved family size, setting national policies, in particular in developing countries, and, above all, in advising the individual man or woman who is seeking contraceptive advice.

Abstinence is an important variable in achieved fertility in nearly all societies. In the western world most individuals still abstain from intercourse for a proportion of time between puberty and marriage. Even where sexual relations before marriage are common and accepted, they rarely extend back to the early teens and coital frequencies are usually less than within marriage. The later the age of marriage, the higher the percentage of unmarried individuals, many of whom abstain from intercourse partially or totally. Raising the age of marriage is important in many third world countires, such as Pakistan, which have national family planning programmes. In China couples are subjected to very strong cultural pressure to delay marriage. For example, in Guandong province in the mid 1970s, the mean age of marriage was 21 for women and 24.8 for men. In Shanghai the mean for both sexes combined (1975–79) was 27.9 years.[16]

Certain groups, such as Catholic priests or Buddhist monks, are formally forbidden to have sexual congress. Amongst some Hindus, celibacy within marriage is admired and sleeping with one's wife only a few times in a lifetime (while probably excessively rare) is still an ideal which some groups regard as likely to be associated with exceptionally healthy offspring. In mediaeval Europe, as in part of contemporary India, sexual abstinence was expected at the time of religious festivals. The mediaeval Church frowned on intercourse on Fridays, Saturdays and Sundays, on Saint days and during Lent. Some Orthodox Brahmins are only expected to approach their wives on Fridays. Many contemporary societies, for example those in parts of Africa, Indonesia and Bangladesh, refrain from intercourse for long intervals during lactation.

In differing cultures the pressure which society exerts upon sexual behaviour varies in response to the local circumstances. In the western world celibacy used to be expected of the young unmarried because if pregnancy occurred there would be inadequate financial and social support for the child. Since the advent of effective contraception the cultural mores are still against pregnancy but not necessarily against sex. In other parts of the world, such as West Africa, breast-feeding is essential to infant survival, and if the mother does become pregnant while lactating her milk will dry up; there are therefore strong cultural prohibitions against sex whilst breast-feeding. For example, among the Yaruba a generation ago, postpartum abstinence lasted three years and even today averages 27 months for rural residents. Social pressures support the taboo and women who break it are called 'animal-like' or 'sex-crazed' and are ostracized. Relatives may even take the children away if they think the parents are having intercourse too soon.

Coitus interruptus
Use

Coitus interruptus is an ancient, probably the earliest, form of birth control. It is well known in most parts of the world under a variety of names and euphemisms which reflect its widespread usage. However, although 'withdrawal', 'coitus incompletus' and 'being careful' are virtually international terms, local idioms such as 'getting off at Cottingham instead of going through to Beverley' (a term used in Hull, England, but having many regional equivalents) can mislead survey interviewers unless they have been adequately briefed. Such factors lead to a general underestimation of the method's popularity.

The Genesis passage concerning coitus interruptus is one of the oldest references in history and the only explicit mention of contraception in the Bible: (Genesis 38.8–10)

> Then Judah said to Onan, Go to your brother's wife and perform your duty as brother-in-law and raise up seed for your brother. Onan knew that the descendants would not be his own, so whenever he had relations with this wife, he let (the seed) be lost on the ground.

The text has been subject to volumes of exegesis but it remains unclear whether Onan's sin was coitus interruptus, disobedience to his father or lack of family duty.

Later Jewish writers referred to the practice with a charming phrase, 'threshing inside and winnowing outside'. St Augustine, who lived as a Manichee for 11 years, faithful to the same wife and having only one child, probably practised the method. Indeed this may account for his hysterical condemnation of it when he became converted to Christianity.[13]

The prophet Mohammed adopted a more liberal attitude towards al-azl, as coitus interruptus is called in the Koran.[14] In the Tradition of the Prophet it is written:

> A man said, 'O Prophet of God! I have a slave girl and I practise coitus interruptus with her. I dislike her becoming pregnant, yet I have the desires of men. The Jews believe that coitus interruptus constitutes killing a life in miniature form.' The Prophet replied, 'The Jews are liars. If God wishes to create it, you can never change it.'

Hollingsworth studied nearly 2000 members of British ducal families[9] and found that family size varied from 3.7 for those born between 1330 and 1479 to 5.6 for those born between 1730 and 1779. This suggests the use of varying but effective methods of fertility control, of which coitus interruptus was almost certainly the most important. Similarly, in France in the eighteenth century, the fertility of the aristocracy was considerably lower than that of the peasantry: the use of coitus interruptus is again suggested.[8] Wrigley has pointed out how the demographic transition in the West 'was achieved largely by "pre-industrial" methods, by coitus interruptus and the procuring of abortions, both means which have been available to society centuries previously'.[25]

In the fifteenth century, St Bernardine bemoaned the fact that in Sienna, 'of 1,000 marriages, I believe 999 are the Devil's'. She was implying the use of coitus interruptus, although the accuracy of this early Knowledge, Attitude and Practices (KAP) survey is unknown. What is certain is that coitus interruptus played a significant role in the demographic transition and remained a major, and commonly the primary, method of contraception until the second half of the twentieth century. In a study of 3300 marriages carried out by the Royal Commission on Population in England in 1947, it was affirmed that amongst recently married couples with contraceptive experience 43% used withdrawal as the sole method of birth control, the proportion rising to 65% in social class V.[11]

Withdrawal was always less popular in the United States, and whereas in Britain in the 1960s 4% of professional couples and 19% of semi-skilled couples used the method, in the US less than 5% of all couples adopted it.[5] However, an analysis of 12 American surveys conducted between 1917 and 1934 and covering 25 000 couples showed that two-thirds of these admitted to having used withdrawal at some time.[12]

Studies in contemporary developing societies reveal a similar pattern.

For example, withdrawal was used, at least on some occasions, by 60% of Jamaican couples, 54% of couples in Puerto Rico[22] and 67% of couples in Hungary[17] as late as the 1960s. The method was used by fully 42% of a sample of doctors in Uttar Pradesh and by 45% of upper-class Hindus in Calcutta.[20] In Turkey in the 1960s, the proportion of couples reporting the use of coitus interruptus increased from 14.5 to 25.2%, while the proportion of those using oral contraceptives only rose from 1.1 to 2.3%, demonstrating both the demographic significance of coitus interruptus and the ways in which it is often used by those adopting the practice of family planning for the first time.[18]

Amongst those professionally engaged in family planning, coitus interruptus is often overlooked, omitted from programme strategy and still commonly condemned or ridiculed. Perhaps its neglect is due to the fact that it has no manufacturers to advertise its virtues and no clinics to press its claim. The method costs nothing, cannot be left at home when the couple go away at the weekend, requires no prescription and does not predispose to weight gain or cause menorrhagia. Its use has been associated with some of the lowest birth-rates in history, as in Eastern Europe after the Second World War. It is obviously acceptable to many users, if not to those who provide family planning services. A study in 1956[4] of 750 women from the Birmingham Family Planning Association (FPA) Clinic who gave up the recommended clinic method found that 58% *chose* coitus interruptus as an alternative and the investigator commented: 'Dependence on coitus interruptus is so widespread that many women think of it not as a contraceptive but rather as a normal part of sexual intercourse. In a number of instances, the husband had become so accustomed to withdrawal that he was unable to give up the practice when the wife wore a cap.'

Reliability

Testimony of the above kind stands in sharp contrast to the aesthetic biases which most middle-class commentators have revealed in discussing coitus interruptus. All too often this bias has encouraged condemnation of the practice not merely on hygienic grounds but also on grounds of unreliability and psychological hazards. The high failure rates alleged by the early clinic personnel have been noted (in Chapter 4) and these have been quoted and re-quoted by two generations of writers with the result that withdrawal has become synonymous with ineffective contraceptive usage. Yet the evidence contradicts this view. As long ago as 1949 the Royal Commission on Population reported that 'no difference has been found between users of appliances and users of non-appliance methods as regards the average number of children'. Amongst those relying on non-appliance methods of all kinds (of which withdrawal was, of course, the most popular) the pregnancy rate was 8 per 100 years of exposure. In a survey in Princeton the overall pregnancy rate for those couples practising withdrawal was 17 per hundred woman-years (HWY) compared with 14 for the condom and diaphragm and 38 for the 'safe period'.[23] The Indianapolis study revealed a failure rate of only 10 compared with an average rate of 12 for all other methods, and amongst high-income couples the rate was precisely the same as for the diaphragm.[18] In Calcutta an extensive survey revealed that pregnancy rates were lower at each occupational level for those employing withdrawal than for those using other traditional methods.[6]

It is commonly suggested that withdrawal is unreliable because pre-ejaculatory loss of fluid from the penis may contain sperm. The origin of this hypothesis goes back to Abraham Stone who, in 1931, was puzzled as to why coitus interruptus ever failed at all.[21] He 'asked several of (his) medical friends who (had) miscroscopes' to examine pre-orgasmic secretion for sperm. He finally collected 24 slides from 18 individuals. Two showed many sperm, two contained a few and one an occasional sperm. Stone rightly reported that the figures were 'insignificant for a definite conclusion'. Today, the physiology of fertilization is more clearly understood and many biologists would consider the risk of fertilization to be minimal unless a high concentration of sperm is present in the tubes. To obtain this, many millions must be deposited in the vagina. In addition, the sperm in the pre-ejaculatory fluid will have been stored at body temperature since the last ejaculation and are therefore unlikely to have retained their fertilizing ability. Nevertheless, the myth that such sperm make coitus interruptus unreliable is copied uncritically from one textbook to another.

Safety
The only recorded mortality from the use of coitus interruptus is that of Onan, for whatever his sin was, it 'did displease Yahweh [God], who killed him'.

A number of psychological and physical complications of coitus interruptus have been suggested, but no significant adverse effects have ever been demonstrated. The supposed psychological drawbacks of the method and the consequences of possible lack of satisfaction for the woman have been listed frequently but in a survey of nearly 2000 British women questioned in 1967–68 by Cartwright, among 311 who had discontinued the use of the method, 60% did so because they thought it was unreliable, only 31% because they found it unpleasant to use and a mere 4%

because they believed it harmful to health.[2] By contrast, among 381 former condom users, 54% abandoned the method because they found it unpleasant to use.[3] If a couple love one another, there seems every reason to assume that they can have a sexually satisfying life and use coitus interruptus if this is what they choose.

The side-effects ascribed to coitus interruptus, as with many other contraceptive methods, go back to a moral condemnation of the method and sometimes what is really being condemned is contraception itself. In 1878, Dr Rugh, addressing the Obstetric Section of the British Medical Association on the subject of contraception, stated that 'the moral and physical evils likely to follow . . . affects the whole population'. He claimed that 'conjugal onanism' caused metritis, leucorrhoea, 'ovarian dropsy', sterility, nymphomania, nervous prostration, mental decay, galloping cancer and suicide. Even pioneers of family planning, such as Marie Stopes, condemned coitus interruptus as 'harmful to the nerves as well as unsafe'.

Evaluation

Coitus interruptus is like a bicycle or a buffalo cart; there are better methods of transport and better methods of contraception, but for a great many people it represents a practical solution to an everyday problem. Instead of criticizing the method, it should be capitalized upon and as and when those who use it feel the need, they will move on to more modern methods. To change the metaphor, coitus interruptus is a type of primary education from which many individuals in the West have graduated but which may still play an essential role in the spread of family planning in the developing world.

Coitus reservatus

A technique that is closely related to coitus interruptus but which calls for a greater degree of male constraint is known as coitus reservatus, male continence, magnetation or karezza. In this case there is no ejaculation either within or outside the vagina; instead the man avoids a too-close approach to orgasm and allows detumescence to take place slowly over a prolonged period. Frequently mentioned in the erotic literature of most cultures, it is best known as the prescribed practice of the Oneida Community, a voluntary colony, established by John Humphrey Noyes near New York in 1869, which was devoted to perfectionism in eugenic selection, sexual relations and the production of silver-plated tableware.

Noyes claimed coitus reservatus allowed complete, or even multiple, orgasm to the female partner. Male self-control was to be assisted by spiritual contemplation; as a secular alternative one of Kingsley Amis's heroes has more recently recommended the conjugation of Latin verbs.

In the Orient, and particularly in Chinese cultures, there is a long-established mythology that the loss of semen at ejaculation has a weakening and unhealthy effect. There is a strong tradition which recommends coitus reservatus for men over about the age of 45, and here sociology may be underscoring a biological need to restrain fertility at about the time the man's partner is approaching the menopause.

Because this practice, unlike coitus interruptus, involves no ejaculation, it is a method to which the Catholic Church takes no particular objection.

Douching

Within the spectrum of family planning techniques used by those married at and around the time of the Second World War in the United States, douching seems to have occupied the place that coitus interruptus then had in Europe. Twenty-eight per cent of women married between 1935 and 1955 used the method at some time, although a third claimed to have used it for 'vaginal cleanliness only'. By contrast, in the English Population Investigation Committee survey in 1959, only 3% of women reported vaginal douching. Vinegar, salt and in some developing countries, Coca Cola, are among the substances used in douches. Apart from the fact that it is not effective, douching interrupts the relaxation which normally follows intercourse and the appropriate apparatus is an embarrassment in most households.

Comic and curious

Attempts to control human fertility are legion. Some are amusing, but others, by going to extreme and sometimes painful efforts, are a testimony to the near universal need to restrict family size.

'Holding back'

It is still a commonly held belief that female orgasm involves a discharge comparable to male ejaculation and on this erroneous notion has been erected the theory that by 'holding back' from orgasm a woman may avoid impregnation. The idea is completely mistaken; Kinsey revealed that a large number of women never achieve orgasm, or do so only once or twice in their lives,[10] but this does not prevent them becoming pregnant.

Coitus saxonicus

Coitus saxonicus consists of normal unprotected coitus up to the point of ejaculation when the man exerts pressure on his perineum so as to cause reflux ejaculation into the bladder. No external ejaculation takes place and the sperm are passed with the next urination. It appears to be a method most suitable to blacksmiths, though the erotic literature recommends the female partner should be trained to do the pressing. It has recently been revived as the Diamond Method in the US and the promotional literature even carries a US patent application number. Its use has been associated with haematuria. It seems unlikely that coitus saxonicus will ever appeal to more than, choosing the appropriate adjective, a handful of men.

Non-vaginal intercourse

Every time ejaculation occurs outside the vagina in biological and social terms it is also a contraceptive act. Sometimes there is a deliberate intention to avoid pregnancy, as in petting among young people and coitus interfemora. At other times variations in coital practice may be the result of pressures and desires far removed from fertility control, as applies to most homosexual relationships.

A Planned Parenthood clinic in America, which during a rebuilding episode innocently hung the notice, FAMILY PLANNING–USE REAR ENTRANCE, demonstrated how easy it is to overlook such alternative patterns of sexual congress. Fellatio and anal intercourse appear to occur in many societies. Although not included in routine KAP surveys, it nevertheless seems reasonable to assume that at least in some cases, and probably especially among older couples, they may be explicitly adopted as a means of preventing unwanted pregnancy. The Moche culture of approximately AD 1600 in Peru produced quantities of ceramics illustrating all aspects of sexual behaviour. One series of figures illustrates couples engaging in anal intercourse when in bed with a young child (Fig. 5.1), and Kauffmann Doig has interpreted this as a specifically contraceptive act, commenting that the Conquistador reported that vaginal intercourse was avoided during lactation 'as it was bad for the milk'.

Miscellaneous

Numberous bizarre surgical and mechanical practices have been devised in attempts to control fertility. In 1925 Haendly devised a plastic surgical procedure which divided the vagina longitudinally, one channel being intended for coitus for pleasure and one, having access to the cervix, for pregnancy.[7] It is not clear how the appropriate entrance was found at moments of passion.

Among the more unusual mechanical methods of contraception was an 'internal contraceptive' sold in England in the 1960s. It consisted of a short nylon stem with a small latex sac. The whole apparatus was to be inserted into the male urethra so that on ejaculation the semen would be forced into the sac which extended from the stem. It was said to have been developed after 'painstaking [sic] research'. The dangers of infection and urethral damage are obvious.

By contrast, the ideas of scrotal hyperthermia and ultrasonic destruction of sperm have a reasonable basis in physiology, but would require ingenuity in application and have never been made to work on any scale.

In all mammals, except the whale and the elephant, the testes are placed outside the abdomen, at least during the breeding season.[24] There are numerous examples of raised scrotal temperature leading to infertility. The anatomy of the testicular vessels is such that they act as a heat exchanger and a varicocele, which disrupts this function, may impair fertility. Merino sheep fail to breed in the hotter parts of Australia and amongst men in the State of Maharashtra in India who, by custom, wear tight scrotal suspenders, subfertility is common.[1, 15] Experiments have been conducted to raise the scrotal temperature artificially and Robinson & Rock showed that a jockstrap with a disposable paper lining worn during working hours for several weeks caused a 75% reduction in sperm count.[19] However, the method has always been associated with a good deal of discomfort and it has never been possible to turn it into a practical method of family planning.

Attempts have been made to destroy testicular sperm by placing the testicles in a water-bath and exposing them to ultrasound. There appears to

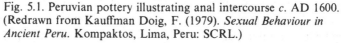

Fig. 5.1. Peruvian pottery illustrating anal intercourse *c.* AD 1600. (Redrawn from Kauffman Doig, F. (1979). *Sexual Behaviour in Ancient Peru*. Kompaktos, Lima, Peru: SCRL.)

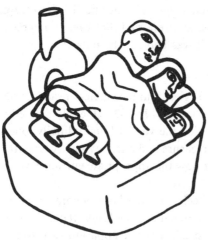

be cellular damage, but the possibility of damage to scrotal cells and to the testes is obvious.

An ancient form of surgery with possible contraceptive implications is subincision or *mica* as practised by Australian native peoples. In some tribes, as part of a puberty ceremony, an artificial hypospadias was created by cutting through the perineum to the urethra.[12] The man then both micturated and ejaculated through the artificial opening unless he closed it – like playing a flute. If the intention was contraceptive then it was unique in that fertility was abolished unless deliberately turned on at a specific intercourse.

Conclusions

Family planning is not an invention of the twentieth century. The 24–48-month separation of births which most couples seek and which epidemiology shows to present least risk to the mother and her baby was achieved naturally by breast-feeding when human beings lived in small mobile bands of hunters and food gatherers.

As the pattern and duration of breast-feeding falls, so contraception becomes increasingly important. Seen in this context, coitus interruptus in particular becomes a reasonable choice, at least for pregnancy spacing.

The wide range of unusual and sometimes harmful methods that have been attempted shows the lengths people went to in trying to regulate fertility even before the twentieth-century population explosion. Those who counsel the individual and those who set policies in birth and family planning should understand the importance of traditional methods in many societies. It is better to build on the foundations that selected traditional methods such as coitus interruptus provide than to criticize, misunderstand and sometimes destroy valuable and acceptable factors that are used in the quest to control human fertility.

6

Contraception and lactation

Lactation is nature's contraception, but of all aspects of human reproduction it is amongst the most complex and is certainly subject to the greatest variations as the result of subtle changes in behaviour. The relation between lactation and modern contraception is important and an understanding of pregnancy spacing due to lactation gives a deeper insight into several aspects of family planning.

Physiology

In all mammals which breed throughout the year, a lactation-controlled mechanism exists to ensure the optimal spacing of pregnancies. In some animals, such as mice, ovulation and fertilization take place but the implanting blastocyst remains dormant in the uterus, while in others, such as man, ovulation is suppressed.

Man is the only primate in which the breasts undergo major anatomical development at puberty.[27] Breast enlargement is, in fact, one of the first signs of puberty in girls and full adult breast size can be achieved before the first ovulation occurs. Perhaps this early development occurs because, exclusively among humans, the breasts have come to be regarded as erotic. Most of the pre-pregnancy growth is stromal and size is not a good predictor of function, although the further development which always occurs during pregnancy is correlated with lactational ability. Breast size changes of up to 20% occur during the menstrual cycle. The cyclical volume change is much reduced in women taking the Pill. In humans, only brief exposure to conjugated oestrogens is necessary to establish milk secretion. Unlike those from other species, human breast cells in tissue culture do not require hormones to maintain their normal morphology. Lactation may occur without a term delivery, as in the case of milk secretion following abortion, and milk secretion has occurred in men with pituitary tumours that secrete large amounts of prolactin.[31]

Normal lactation is initiated by the disappearance of the placental steroids. During established lactation, the secretion of pituitary gonado-trophins and prolactin remains under neurogenic control from the breast. Afferent nerve stimulation influences hypothalamic function, prolactin levels and, to some extent, luteinizing hormone (LH) secretion. Both the duration and intensity of sucking are important.[21] The paramount significance of nerve stimuli from the nipple is illustrated by the documen-ted fact that some nulliparous women who massage their breasts prior to the adoption of a child have actually fed the infant.

The hormonal changes associated with lactation can vary in the course of minutes, yet may be part of an overall pattern that extends over a year or more. Suckling is associated with a 12- to 18-fold rise in serum prolactin levels, but considerable differences in the levels of circulating prolactin are to be found in breast-feeding women in different countries with different lifestyles.[4] Women who breast-feed on demand have higher prolactin levels, because nipple stimulation is more frequent and prolonged, than those who feed according to some arbitrary schedule. Factors that affect the degree of nipple stimulation include whether or not the baby sleeps with the mother and suckles at night, and also patterns of supplementary feeding. All the factors are significant in determining the length of postpartum amenorrhoea. The nomadic hunting, food-gathering !Kung peoples of South Africa average 44 months between successive live births. They carry their babies over long distances and nurse them briefly but frequently, often four times or more each hour. Suckling is less frequent in !Kung women who adopt a more settled pattern of life, and shorter birth intervals occur (Table 6.1).[18]

The baby of a malnourished mother may have to suck harder and longer to get the milk that it needs and this in turn may lead to more complete suppression of ovulation. It is possible that a woman must regain a certain minimum weight to height ratio before ovulation returns.[7] However, the single most important factor determining the return of ovulation is almost certainly supplementary feeding. Longitudinal studies

Table 6.1. *Mean birth intervals for !Kung women (1963–73)*

Lifestyle	Mean birth interval (months)
Nomadic	44.1
More settled	36.1

of breast-feeding women suggest that ovulation practically never returns before some supplementary feeding is begun.[8] Each month of breast-feeding adds approximately 0.3–0.6 months to the duration of anovulation.[20]

As long as ovulation is suppressed lactation is a totally effective method of contraception with no untoward side-effects. The role of lactation as a contraceptive is explicitly recognized in many traditional societies.[25] In Ghana, the first six months after delivery are described as a good time for sexual relations. However, in some other communities, as in much of Indonesia and many other Asian societies, lactation is often also associated with long intervals of abstinence. When ovulation does return, there is some evidence that the initial luteal phases of the cycle may not be adequate to support implantation. Up to 1 in five women become pregnant at the first ovulation during lactation, before menstruation returns.

Breast-feeding and artificial feeding

In the western world, and some developing countries, for example North East Brazil, women begin supplementary feeding relatively early in lactation. Among British women who do not breast-feed, basal body temperature and endometrial biopsy studies have shown that ovulation can occasionally occur as early as the twenty-ninth day postpartum. It has also been shown that among breast-feeding women who give milk supplements early, ovulation may only be postponed for two or three months.[2] These modest differences between lactating and non-lactating women are in marked contrast to the long intervals of anovulation found in many developing countries. In countries where supplementary feeding begins later, there are many groups where ovulation is suppressed for 12–24 months postpartum (Fig. 6.1). In Bangladesh, traditional patterns of breast-feeding space pregnancies at 30 months or more.

Wet-nurses and artificial feeding have a long history, at least in western society.[15, 17] In the contemporary western world, bottle-feeding has largely replaced breast-feeding to the extent that many doctors and health workers no longer understand the basic elements of breast-feeding. As long as milk is removed from the breast, secretion will take place. The complaint that a woman has insufficient milk to feed her infant is sometimes a tragic misdiagnosis by the mother and those around her. In fact she may have so much milk that the infant finds it difficult to grasp or to release itself from the engorged breast.

There are many advantages of breast-feeding,[11, 34] ranging from reduced infection in the child to possible alterations in the behaviour of the mother. There is a lower incidence of respiratory and diarrhoeal diseases in breast-fed infants than in those who are bottle-fed[3] (Fig. 6.2). Maternal milk contains a unique immunoglobulin of the IgA type and in the neonate at any rate, this is not destroyed by the infant's gastrointestinal enzymes and therefore transfers some of the mother's protective immunity directly to her child. Nowadays, it is well recognized that colostrum is rich in such

Fig. 6.1. Duration of lactation and postpartum amenorrhoea. The percentage of infants who were breast-fed is shown in parentheses. (Data from McCann, M. F. & Laskin, L. S. (1981). Breast-feeding, fertility and family planning. *Population Reports*, Series **J**, 527.)

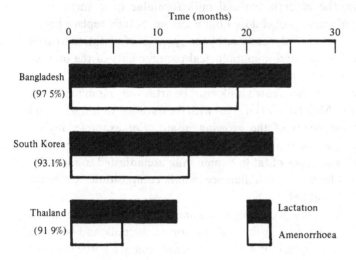

Fig. 6.2. Effect of rooming-in policy on neonatal infection in Baguio Hospital, Philippines. (Modified from Relucio- Clavano, N. (1981). *Assignment Children*, **55/56**, 139.)

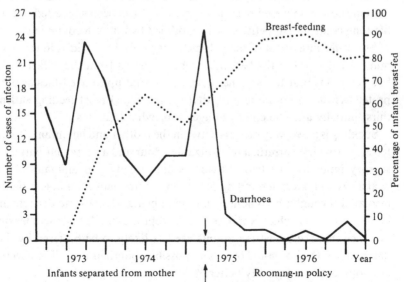

antibodies but less well known that in fact all human milk contains them together with significant numbers of maternal white cells which may also act to prevent gut and upper respiratory tract infections in the child. This protection which the mother shares with her infant is tailored to meet the profile of diseases found in her particular home.[32] Women often lay down body fat before and during pregnancy and then lose it when lactating: the western woman's complaint that she gained weight during each pregnancy is often an admission that she did not breast-feed.

Undoubtedly, the modern artificial milk formulae have successfully nourished tens of millions of children but it can never fully replace breast milk which has been uniquely modified by long periods of evolution to meet the multiple nutritional and immunological requirements of the infants. Human milk contains relatively little protein (1–2%W/V) and large amounts of lactose, whereas cow's milk must be artificially modified to suit the infant's needs. Milk content changes with the duration of lactation and is adjusted to the needs of the growing infant. For example, myelin accounts for 25% of the brain weight and 95% of it is accumulated after birth. The levels and types of fat in human milk are adjusted to meet this growth pattern. There is even a difference in milk composition if an infant has been born prematurely.

Bottle-fed infants may grow larger and more quickly than breast-fed infants owing to differences in the composition of the milk and because, from an infant's point of view, it is easier to get milk out of a bottle than out of the breast. Bottle-fed babies accumulate more fat than breast-fed ones and it is possible that some adult diseases, such as those of the cardiovascular system, are more common in those who were bottle-fed than in those who were breast-fed babies.[22] It has been suggested that the life-long control of appetite may be modified by bottle-feeding: in the case of breast-feeding, most of the volume of the milk is provided in the first 5 min of suckling, but the last milk to be extracted from the breast by the baby contains four to five times as much fat and up to five times as much protein as the more dilute milk that comes first. Breast-feeding satisfies thirst initially and the child's hunger somewhat later.

Suckling is a two-way process between the mother and her infant. Breast-feeding provides warmth, a recognizable odour and a particular pattern of sensory input for the two individuals concerned.[28] In animals such as goats, strong maternal bonding occurs soon after delivery and is probably mediated through pheromones. In human beings, there is no discrete and limited time over which a mother will accept her child, but there is some evidence that the breast-fed infants are less likely to be battered by their parents than the bottle-fed ones, and possible that their overall intellectual development is marginally better.[26]

The role of the medical profession in breast-feeding has been one of over-emphatic advice based on insufficient evidence. The rigid schedules of breast- and bottle-feeding which were recommended in the first half of this century can be traced to a mechanical and inappropriate interpretation of an infant's needs. Advice on weaning and patterns of breast-feeding has varied widely over the last few hundred years and appears to have reflected society's attitude towards the role of the child in the family rather than any understanding of the physiology and nutritional facts of lactation. Contemporary obstetric practices often separate the infant from the mother immediately after delivery and many hospitals, particularly in the developing world, still do not room-in babies with their mother. A new-born infant can be put to the breast immediately after delivery. Stimulation of the nipple increases the output of oxytocin, which in turn will lead to uterine contractions and expulsion of the placenta. The advice given by the medical profession has been a contributing factor to the rapid decline of breast-feeding throughout the world and is even more reprehensible than aggressive advertising by milk manufacturers.

The main effects of abandoning breast-feeding are on the child. In the developing world, protein–calorie malnutrition affects 10–20 million children. While plain lack of food is the basic cause, in many cases bottle-fed children are at greatest risk; the high cost of artificial milk (US $200 to $300 for one year) encourages the mother to over-dilute it. Infection from dirty water and unhygienic conditions gives rise to diarrhoea and further nutritional strain in an already hungry child. In societies which are tending to emulate the western countries an early effect is often a reduction in the length of time for which infants are breast-fed and it is becoming apparent that in some poor countries, such as Egypt, a small but measurable rise in infant mortality occurs. It is most marked in the least educated.[10] It cannot be over-emphasized that the poorer the society, the more economical it is to feed the mother with simple, cheap foods such as rice and a little dried fish rather than the infant with expensive artificial milk.[33]

The epidemiology of breast-feeding

As in other areas dealing with human reproduction, such as the adoption of contraception, societies often act in a homogeneous way, adopting new conventions rapidly and virtually universally. The social support of breast-feeding, which traditional societies normally provide, can be replaced too quickly with new perceptions which equate the lactating woman with a cow and see bottle-feeding as a desired aspect of modern technology. In Sardinia, mothers over 40 report that they breast-feed their infants for at least nine months, many of them doing so for two to two and a half years, while mothers under 30 often limit breast-feeding to three months. A fear of adverse effects on physical appearance, changing patterns of female employment and mass media advertisements, and ill-advised medical practices have all influenced this change. Initially, older women may urge their daughters to breast-feed, but once they see that a bottle-fed child gains weight rapidly, their criticism often ceases.

In western countries, breast-feeding in public is rarely seen. In Victorian times modesty in this respect was considered an attribute of civilization, and the embarrassment lingers on. Many women find the embarrassment either to themselves or to others of breast-feeding on demand to be an important factor in favour of an early change to bottle-feeding.

Today, in most of the developed world, lactational amenorrhoea is a trivial variable in overall fertility. In one study in the United Kingdom only 50% of the women breast-fed for as long as two months and a further 44% were giving solid food by the second month. In the US breast-feeding reached an all-time low in 1972 with only 22% of women ever breast-feeding. The number today has risen to 30–40% of women at least trying for a few weeks or months.[8] In the developing world, however, lactational amenorrhoea often remains the most important single item determining child spacing. Rosa estimated in the early 1970s that 35 million annual couple-years of contraceptive protection were provided by breast-feeding in developing countries, while artificial techniques provided only 27 million years. In subSahara Africa, the contrast is even more dramatic with 10 million years of protection being offered by breast-feeding compared with only 250 000 years of protection by modern methods of contraception: so in this region breast-feeding is 40 times as important as family planning programmes. However, the present decades are ones of rapid change: in Taiwan the percentage of women that breast-feed has fallen from 93 in 1966 to 50 in 1980 and the average duration of lactation has fallen from 14.6 to 8.8 months; in rural Thailand it fell from 22.4 months in 1969 to 17.5 months in 1979.

The fact that breast-feeding remains an important element in the control of fertility in traditional societies, that it has particular nutritional advantages in a poor society and that it confers extra protection against infection should make those interested in international family planning eager to prevent the premature and unnecessary adoption of bottle-feeding in the developing world. At the same time, every effort should be made to ensure the availability and distribution of contraceptive methods in traditional societies. Those who adopt bottle-feeding are usually also those most ready to use contraception. An understanding of the importance of lactation in fertility control in developing countries leads to an appreciation that contraception everywhere plays two separate roles: (a) it substitutes for the protection against pregnancy provided by lactational amenorrhoea in former days and (b) it provides a new measure of control over fertility that did not previously exist. In industrialized nations, contraception has replaced breast-feeding as the principle means of spacing pregnancies but, in fact, the average interval between birth (as opposed to final achieved family size) does not differ very much between, say, Britain or America and those countries such as Bangladesh or Indonesia where lactation is the main factor responsible for spacing pregnancies.

From the demographic point of view, an exceptionally serious situation can arise if breast-feeding is abandoned too rapidly, and, at the same time, contraception is adopted too slowly. This is exactly what appears to be happening in urban areas of West Africa, parts of Pakistan, Malaysia and even among Eskimos, where the total fertility has risen to uniquely high levels. Bongaarts estimates that if patterns of breast-feeding were altered so as to reduce postpartum amenorrhoea from 18 to 9 months, then fertility in parts of Africa would rise by 35%[9] (Table 6.2).

We need sound epidemiological data on the duration of lactation and the average length of lactational amenorrhoea for a number of societies. Efforts should be made to determine which socio-economic groups behave in the most homogeneous way so that the best advice can be given with regard to the time when postpartum contraception should be started.

Lactation and modern methods of contraception

For each country, or subgroup within the country, a balance will exist between the resumption of contraception and the interval between delivery and the resumption of ovulation: in other words, if couples start

Table 6.2. *The extra use of contraception needed to hold fertility at current levels if duration of breast-feeding falls*

Country	Total fertility rate	Mean duration of postpartum amenorrhoea (months)	Percentage of fertile women using contraception		
				Future use if postpartum amenorrhoea falls to	
			Current	6 months	2 months
Kenya	7.7	10.7	7	24	38
Bangladesh	6.4	18.5	9	43	54
Colombia	5.3	7.2	37	41	52
Costa Rica	4.0	5.3	59	–	66

Source Jain, A. K. & Bongaarts, J. (1981). Breast-feeding: patterns, correlates, and fertility effects. *Studies in Family Planning*, **12**, 79.

contraception too soon after delivery, some may give up the contraceptive before they even finish breast-feeding, while if they wait too long, they may fall pregnant before they get around to using a modern method. Potter has evaluated alternative strategies for starting contraception in Bangladesh using known data on fertility, contraceptive continuation rates and the duration of amenorrhoea, and the probability distribution associated with ovulation occurring during the first menstrual cycle after delivery.[24] In situations in which contraceptive continuation rates are poor and breast-feeding prolonged, the adoption of contraception immediately after delivery adds little to the average birth interval (Table 6.3). The optimum strategy is to wait until menstruation returns, although approximately 7% of women will become pregnant before they can implement this strategy. In the Bangladesh situation, if all women begin contraception at six months postpartum, then fewer than 1 in 200 women will become pregnant before they start contraception. However, women will, on the average, still be faced with seven months of overlap between contraceptive practice and lactational amenorrhoea.

Breast-feeding alters the profile of advantages and disadvantages of nearly every method of artificial contraception.

Coitus interruptus, condoms and vaginal methods

Coitus interruptus and condoms provide adequate protection of the breast-feeding woman. It is interesting that in Yucatan, Mexico, one of the reasons given for the husband being present when delivery takes place

Table 6.3. *Contraception and ovulation in breast-feeding women*

Contraception begun	Women becoming pregnant before using contraception (%)	Contraception/ ovulation overlap (mean months)[a]	Mean months of additional contraception added
Postpartum	0.0	8.7	10.25
Six months	1.4	7.1	11.30
After menses return	7.0	0.0	15.25

Assumptions: fertility equal to 0.1; contraceptive effectiveness equal to 0.95; continuation rate equal to 50% at 3 years; period of anovulation equal to 23 months.
[a] This is the number of months when the woman is simultaneously protected by the contraceptive chosen and the suppression of ovulation due to lactation.
Source: Potts, M. & Whitehorn, E. (1980). Contraception and the lactating woman. In *Research Frontiers on Fertility Regulation*, ed. G. I. Zatuchni, M. H. Labbock & J. J. Sciarra. Hagerstown, Maryland: Harper and Row.

at home is that by being aware of the pains of delivery, he is more likely to practice coitus interruptus thereafter.[12] The condom and female barrier methods are satisfactory methods of contraception in many situations and, because there are no systemic side-effects, can be used during lactation, which is not inhibited.

Intrauterine devices. Conventional IUDs, inserted immediately postpartum, have a high expulsion rate, especially in young, low-parity women. The expulsion rate is lower if insertion is delayed for as little as 4 days to 1 week postpartum, but then the rate of perforations rises.[19, 29] In Singapore, there were 0.9 perforations per 1000 IUD insertions performed one week after delivery but 11.8 perforations per 1000 insertions performed 4–6 weeks postpartum.

The clinical impression is that devices inserted during lactational amenorrhoea are reasonably well tolerated. Some bleeding may occur following insertion, but the menorrhagia commonly associated with IUDs may be less troublesome during lactation.

To avoid the problems of expulsion and perforation, investigators for Family Health International (formerly the International Fertility Research Program, IFRP) are testing the use of IUDs with small biodegradable projections. Care must be taken to place the IUD at the fundus immediately after delivery of the placenta and the projections appear to hold the IUD in the optimum position during the critical weeks of involution.

Periodic abstinence. Calendar rhythm is inapplicable until regular menstruation has returned. Temperature, symptothermic and ovulation methods have been advocated, but there are no statistical data on the reliability of these methods postpartum.

Steroidal contraceptives
The mother. The pharmacology of drugs which affect lactation is complex because the sites for potential action are numerous. A compound may inhibit the initiation of lactation, affect milk output, alter the lipid, carbohydrate, and other content of milk and, finally, hasten or postpone the time of weaning. The variety of these effects, combined with the individuality of each episode of lactation, no doubt accounts for some of the confusion and contradiction found in the literature describing oral contraceptive use during lactation. The formulation of the Pill has changed markedly in the past two decades, but much of the literature refers to the high-oestrogen dose Pills that are now rarely used.

Oestrogen alone and in high dosage inhibits the initiation of lactation and, until the danger of deep vein thrombosis with exogenous oestrogens was recognized, was much used for this purpose. With modern low-oestrogen Pills, this effect is rare and women taking a contraceptive pill actually have higher daytime prolactin levels than breast-feeding women who are not using the method. Galactorrhoea is a known, but rare, complication of Pill use. Progestogens are generally believed to have no direct effect on lactation. It should be noted that some progestogens (the 19-norsteroids) used in oral contraceptives are partly metabolized to oestrogen and Pills containing high dosages of 19-norsteroids should probably be avoided during lactation.

In a double-blind trial of a placebo and norethisterone (1 mg) with mestranol (0.05 mg), begun the day after birth and continued for eight days, lactation was not inhibited, but the percentage of babies with supplementary feeds was higher in the user groups (12%) than in the controls (3.5%).[13] No difference in the growth of the babies was demonstrated. In one of the careful studies on lactation carried out by Kamal's group in Egypt, it was found that 81% of women had stopped breast-feeding by 6 months postpartum, when a combined pill (norgestrel 500 μg and ethinyl oestradiol 50 μg) was taken, compared with only 62% in the previous pregnancy.[14] In Chile, Guiloff and colleagues found that the mean duration of lactation was shortened in women on the Pill.[6] However, the pattern of lactation may be changing with time for reasons un-associated with the Pill and all these studies involved Pills with higher oestrogen content than would be used today. Measurement of weight gain among fully breast-fed babies found no difference between the babies of mothers not using oral contraceptives and those of mothers using combined oral contraceptives containing 30 μg of oestrogen.[1]

Progestogens, given either as progestogen-only pills or as injectables such as Depo-Provera (depomedroxyprogesterone acetate) and Deladrox-one (dihydroxyprogesterone), do not adversely affect any parameter of lactation, even when given within 2 h of delivery and some studies suggest that women using them experience heavier lactation. Progestogen-only pills could be much more widely used in countries where breast-feeding is common and prolonged.

When considering appropriate contraception in the developing world, it must be remembered that unintended conception in a lactation woman may be associated with a reduction in milk production which can be life-threatening to the infant, so that in some situations, even if oral contraceptives can be demonstrated to have a mild adverse effect on lactation, they remain a sound choice.

The baby. It is known that less than 1% of the maternal dose of oral contraceptives is excreted in the milk.[23] The neonate is particularly vulnerable to exogenous steroids for several reasons: the binding capacity of the plasma is small, the liver is less able to conjugate and to oxidize drugs and the kidneys are immature so that excretion is inefficient. The capacity to metabolize drugs, particularly with regard to detoxification in the liver, improves rapidly after birth. It is interesting to note that the suckling infant is exposed to endogenous maternal steroids and that cow's milk contains more steroids than does milk from women who are taking Pills or accepting injectable contraception. Only the injection of Depo-Provera immediately postpartum presents any theoretical problems.

Voluntary sterilization

Female sterilization involves significant physical trauma and, in many cases, is associated with general anaesthesia, which can effect the neuro-endocrine control of lactation. A single study of lactation following minilaparotomy found that the procedure had no adverse effects if performed on the day of delivery, but did result in a temporary reduction in milk yield when performed 4–6 days postpartum.[5] The effect of female sterilization on the initiation of breast-feeding warrants investigation.

The choice of vasectomy would seem particularly attractive to some couples during lactational amenorrhoea. If done at, say, three months in a society where breast-feeding lasts for over a year, the couple can feel reasonably secure that the most recently delivered baby has a good chance of survival and that the man is almost certain to become sperm-free before ovulation returns to the woman.

Induced abortion

Induced abortion is an important means of fertility control in all societies. The woman who becomes pregnant during lactational amenorrhoea may not recognize her pregnancy as early as does the menstruating woman. This is important because the risks of abortion are strongly linked with the duration of gestation at the time of the operation.

Conclusions

An understanding of the role of lactation in fertility control and its outstanding significance in traditional societies, and of the pattern of advantages and disadvantages of modern methods of contraception is important for those who work in any aspect of family planning. However, much of our understanding is relatively recent. More research is genuinely needed and some exciting opportunities and novel methods of contraception may yet exist in this field. Oral contraceptives imitate the suppression of ovulation which occurs during pregnancy, but without the presence of the baby. Will it ever be possible to devise a hormonal method of contraception which will imitate the suppression of ovulation which occurs during lactation, but without the milk?

In this respect it has already been shown that thyroid-releasing hormones enhance prolactin production and limited clinical trials have been conducted using the exogenous hormone to increase milk volume.[30]

Not only has scientific knowledge about the physiology and epidemiology of lactation and their relation to fertility been slow to accumulate, but the response of health administrators to the important role lactation plays in fertility control has been even slower. It should be realized that the use of artificial milk formulae may not only be a strain on poor communities but also an element in the balance of payments of developing countries, as the raw materials needed for its manufacture are primarily products of temperate farming. In recent years, a great deal of attention has been focused on the role of multinational corporations in the aggressive promotion of bottle-feeding in the developing countries. Much of the criticism of their activity is justified but they are only one part of a complex series of interactions in which the role of the health providers is also of great importance. Theologians have been slower still to respond to current changes in breast-feeding habits. Yet in the iconography of the Catholic Church, Mary never feeds the infant Jesus artificially, and the Koran states: 'Mothers shall give suck to their offspring for two whole years (11.233).'

Those who are involved in family planning should also be committed to active policies for ensuring that bottle-feeding is only adopted in defined and necessary situations. They must unite with paediatricians in opposition to aggressive promotion of bottle-feeding, particularly to women in poor communities, and should help obstetricians and paediatricians to set their own houses in order to ensure that when the mother is delivered she finds herself in an environment that gives her the maximum opportunity to breast-feed her new-born infant. At present, women who deliver in a hospital or health centre in a developing country often breast-feed less well than those who deliver at home.[16] Variations in hospital policy concerning placing the neonate in a separate nursery or rooming-in the baby with the mother in the lying-in ward have a dramatic impact on the incidence of breast-feeding (see Fig. 6.2). Realistic contraceptive advice must be available to all couples before the protection that breast-feeding provides ends, whether that is after a few weeks, or a year or more.

7

Periodic abstinence

History

Attempts to avoid conception by varying the timing of intercourse have been undertaken in most societies about which we have historical or anthropological knowledge. The most common of these involve the avoidance of intercourse before, during or after menstruation and variations of this practice have been reported from the Greek physician Soranus, through the Indian cultures of New Mexico, to the Nandi of East Africa.[16]

As early as 1843, Raciborski in Paris noted that women who married soon after menstruation usually conceived in the first cycle after marriage, while if the wedding occurred later in the cycle they often had another period before pregnancy occurred, but the false association of bleeding with ovulation persisted.[43]

In 1853, the Bishop of Amiens asked the Sacred Penitentiary how to deal with those amongst his flock who were confining intercourse to the *tempus ageneseos* and was advised not to interfere, so long as they did nothing to impede conception.

St Augustine, who did so much to create the Catholic ethics of marriage, had specifically condemned periodic abstinence and, very significantly, Noonan remarks: 'In the history of the thought of theologians on contraception, it is, no doubt, piquant that the first pronouncement on contraception by the most influential theologian teaching on such matters should be a vigorous attack on the one method of avoiding procreation now accepted by twentieth-century Catholic theologians as morally lawful.'[37] Nevertheless, periodic abstinence was accepted in a Vatican statement of 1880, alluded to in the encyclical *Casti Connubii* (1930) and finally reaffirmed in *Humanae Vitae* (1968). What is truly important about the Catholic Church's endorsement of periodic abstinence is that at least the need for, and legality of, contraception is formally recognized.

Accumulating knowledge on human ovulation, resulting from observations made at human operations, and increasing information on menstrual physiology at last provided the basis for an accurate description of the infertile period by Knaus (1929)[27] in Austria and Ogino (1939) in Japan.[39] They proposed contraceptive regimes based on the assumption that ovulation occurs on or around the fourteenth day prior to the next menstruation. The Ogino–Knaus theory was enthusiastically taken up by Roman Catholic doctors in the 1930s and a flood of books appeared expounding the 'non-contraceptive method of birth regulation'. One of these, *The Rhythm of Sterility and Fertility in Women*,[29] gave rise to the popular name 'the rhythm method'.

Although usually associated with Roman Catholicism, periodic abstinence is more prevalent in Japan than anywhere else. As in other countries, its use is often combined with withdrawal or condom at the time of maximum fertility (see Fig. 2.8). By 1955, one-fifth of all American couples practising birth control had used the method[9] at some time and in the 1959 Population Investigation Committee survey in England, 16% of informants had used it.[41] However, with the advent of more effective methods, there was a rapid decline in its use so that by 1970 this figure was only 6.7%.[28] Paradoxically, the technique was abandoned more rapidly by Roman Catholics than by non-Catholics. Periodic abstinence is not a majority method of family planning anywhere in the developing world although in Korea, the Philippines and Sri Lanka its use reaches significant levels.

As with other methods of contraception, failures may end in induced abortion. A study in Colombia found that before the rhythm method was adopted, 13% of pregnancies ended in spontaneous or induced abortions, while the figure rose to 35% for pregnancies occurring after adoption of the method.[19] 'I still use the principles of rhythm', said a Filipino informant, 'sometimes if she is delayed, there are prescriptions . . .'[28]

Patterns of periodic abstinence
The ovary normally expels one ovum per cycle and this is available for fertilization for approximately 24 h. Sperm, once they have entered the uterus, can remain viable for approximately 48 h and thus there is a maximum period of three days in each cycle during which conception should be possible.

In practice, the gametes may live for longer, ovulation may be multiple and in rare cases it is possible that it occurs in response to intercourse rather than spontaneously. Above all, ovulation is an internal event with few outward and visible signs that it is about to occur.[8, 34]

Calendar rhythm

In most women menstrual irregularities occur spontaneously and these variations are most marked at the extremes of fertile life. This is particularly unfortunate in that an unplanned pregnancy is likely to be least acceptable and also maximally dangerous at just these times.[47] Another cause of menstrual irregularity is stress, particularly when of emotional origin.

Allowing for possible irregularity and taking into account the viability of eggs and sperm, for those using calendar rhythm, abstinence is normally recommended between the eleventh and seventeenth (or eighteenth) days of the cycle counting the first day of menstruation as day 1. If a record of cycles is kept over a period of six months and 18 is subtracted from the number of days in the shortest cycle and 11 from the number of days in the longest cycle, then a rough estimate of the 'safe period' can be made. If all else fails, the joints of the fingers can be used as a permanent calendar, but this is not recommended (Fig. 7.1)!

Fig. 7.1. A handy guide to the safe period.

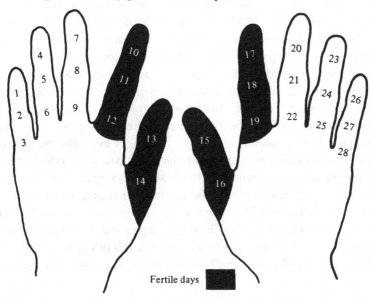

Fertile days

The temperature method

In 1868 a British physician, W. Squire, reported that women showed a small sustained rise in basal body temperature in the second half of the menstrual cycle.[44] In 1905, van de Velde associated these changes with ovulation[49] but it was not until 1947 that Ferin, a priest, the son of a doctor and the second of 11 children, recommended the recording of temperature change as a way of securing greater accuracy in the use of the rhythm method.

The rise in temperature to be recorded is small ($0.3–0.5°C$ or $0.5–1.0°F$) and it may occur either abruptly or slowly. Body temperature must be recorded daily, it is easily overridden by mild fevers and if taken orally, the woman must be at rest and not smoke or drink prior to the recording: until the 1950s it was the official teaching of some enthusiasts that it was best to 'gently insert the clinical thermometer into the rectum as you are lying in bed. It should be left in position for THREE minutes by the clock and then removed and read immediately.'[31] Needless to say the method proved difficult to teach and interpret. In poor countries, the cost of clinical thermometers, which are easily broken, was another additional barrier to success.

Cervical mucus method

Monthly changes in the quantity and consistency of cervical mucus were noticed in the mid nineteenth century but only associated with ovulation by Seguy in the 1930s.[42] In 1964 an Australian husband and wife team, Drs John & Evelyn Billings, began to teach the recognition of changes in cervical mucus as a predictor of ovulation.[2, 3]

Following menstruation, there may be a 'few dry days' then, as oestrogen levels rise, a cloudy yellow or white sticky discharge is observed. Immediately before ovulation, the consistency of the mucus changes from thick to fluid and becomes clear and slippery, resembling egg white and producing a lubricative sensation. These changes normally persist for about three days and then, as progesterone levels rise, the cervical mucus decreases in amount and becomes cloudy and sticky again. The mucus is secreted by glands opening into the cervical canal and at the time of ovulation the output rises from approximately 20–60 ml a day to as much as 700 ml. The extra excretion is mainly water but the glycogen and mannose contents increase. The main effect is a fall in viscosity while the pH of the secretion changes from 7 to 8.5. These changes assist the passage of sperm.

In theory, if coitus is limited to the post-ovulatory interval, the method should be applicable to all women irrespective of menstrual irregularities. Intercourse itself confuses the reading of cervical mucus and coital frequency may have to be limited even on the infertile days.

A proportion of women find the mucus signs easy to identify and some well-taught and carefully monitored groups have used the method with low failure rates.[25, 30]

The Sympto-thermic method
It is possible to adopt a belt and braces approach and combine recognition of changes in the cervical mucus with the recording of basal body temperature.[32] The extra information can reduce the failure rate.

Extent of use
The ovulation method has become the choice of organized Catholic groups and, as with any method of family planning, the enthusiasm of the teacher of the method is important. Good teaching aids and well-tested routines have been evolved. Some programmes define a learning interval during which total abstinence is demanded and if pregnancy occurs, it is sometimes omitted and not counted as a 'method failure' in published papers. Claims made for the technique should be carefully scrutinized.

Couple-to-couple dissemination of the method has occurred, particularly with the organized training group SERENA in Canada. A few small-scale programmes have been launched in developed countries. L'action Familiale in Haiti visits clients twice a week during the first month of the instruction and weekly for five months thereafter. In India, couples are taught on four separate visits to learn the method and are then visited every week or every other week until they are fully familiar with it. The cost of teaching the method has varied from US $2 to US $120,[7] although once the technique has been learned, there is no recurrent expenditure as there is with other reversible methods of family planning.

In overall perspective, the teaching techniques which have been evolved to disseminate this difficult and demanding technique and ways of organizing couple-to-couple assistance are of interest and genuine value to anyone involved in family planning services. What emerges is that where a group or society is strongly motivated, fertility control can be achieved even though the use-effectiveness of the method may be low.

Periodic abstinence appears to be most acceptable in cultures with a tradition of sexual abstinence, such as those in parts of India. Elsewhere, the need for daily digital examination of the cervix is unacceptable and in other cultures, for instance those in much of South America, recruitment has been of more than usual difficulty. In Colombia, for example, over a $2\frac{1}{2}$-year period 20 000 home visits were made. Eighteen thousand people attended lectures and 61 000 pamphlets were distributed but only 1240 couples agreed to participate in a trial of the method. Half of these were excluded because they did not meet study requirements and after 15 months only 168 were still using the method.[35] By contrast, oral contraceptives continued to gain in popularity in the same community.

Side-effects

The self-discipline required for the correct use of periodic abstinence is unlikely to impair a healthy marriage although it may exclude a certain amount of rightful pleasure. Some couples have reported the method to be beneficial in sexual adjustment. On the other hand, a poor marriage, especially between individuals who find it difficult to plan ahead, can be wrecked by the frustrations and failures of the method. It has also been argued that a method which requires a woman to acquire daily awareness of her own fertility also continuously draws her attention to the act of coitus, and the conflict which exists between her husband's desire and her fear of pregnancy. This perhaps accounts for the high drop-out rate often associated with the method. One clinic in Mexico City abandoned the use of periodic abstinence when several women had been beaten up by their husbands for refusing intercourse on fertile days.

Three medical complications of periodic abstinence deserve consideration. In experimental animals, there is convincing evidence that, when fertilization involves aged gametes, the abnormality rate in the offspring is raised considerably.[4, 45, 50] The systemic disjunction of the time of ovulation and time of coitus involved in periodic abstinence could have the same effect in human beings.[5, 10, 13, 33, 36, 51] However, the key animal observations involve animals such as rabbits which ovulate on coitus and it could be argued that spontaneous ovulators, such as *Homo sapiens*, may be at little or no risk for congenital abnormalities induced in this way. The high incidence of anencephaly and spina bifida in Catholic populations has been attributed to the use of periodic abstinence but may be due to genetic variations, or some other factor.[21] One case-controlled retrospective study of Dutch women with congenitally abnormal children reported a higher than average prevalence of the use of the rhythm method.[20, 21, 22, 23] A prospective study in the US did not confirm this suspicion[38] and studies on coital frequency have not demonstrated any correlation between possible delayed fertilization and the outcome of pregnancy.[48] The problem of birth defects, like many in fertility planning, remains without a definitive answer. Planned Parenthood in America currently informs potential users about

Use-effectiveness

all known and possible adverse reactions and warns couples about possible congenital abnormalities that could arise as a result of using the method.[1]

The second possible side-effect is abnormal implantation of the blastocyst. Iffy has suggested that some ectopic pregnancies occur when implantation occurs late in the cycle and fails to inhibit the next period, with consequent displacement of the ovum to an abnormal location.[17] It is reasonable to assume that failures of periodic abstinence will fall into this group. Iffy supports this hypothesis by the fact that spontaneous ectopic pregnancies only occur in animals which menstruate and by the statistical analysis of embryonic and fetal size in tubal pregnancies and other types of abnormal implantation, such as placenta previa.[18] When women with previously abnormal babies and examples of pathological implantation confine intercourse to the middle of the cycle, it appears to reduce the risk of recurrence.

Thirdly, if fertilization is associated with intercourse sometime before or after a predicted time of ovulation then the spontaneous abortion rate may be higher.[12]

There is sufficient animal, clinical and epidemiological evidence to raise suspicion about one or more of these three possible categories of side-effects but insufficient evidence to force a broad-policy condemnation. However, even a reasonable suggestion of serious disease outcome among users of periodic abstinence could cloud any advocacy of the method as 'natural family planning'.

Use-effectiveness

Unfortunately, the studies available on periodic abstinence are nearly always more limited in scope than those for IUDs and oral contraceptives, but some generalizations can be made. Hartman found a Pearl rate of 30 per calendar rhythm[15] and Tietze, Poliakoff & Rock found one of 14.4 per HWY.[46] Marshall followed 3545 menstrual cycles in women using basal body temperature and recorded 57 pregnancies, a Pearl rate of 19.3,[31] but Guy & Guy in Mauritius found a rate of 8.0 in 16 735 cycles.[14] Among married women aged 15–44 who conceived an unplanned pregnancy during the first year of contraceptive use in the United States (1970–76), the highest failure rate (18.8 per HWY) was associated with periodic abstinence; it exceeded even that of spermicides (17.7) and was twice that of condoms (9.6)[11] (see Fig.4.1).

The use-effectiveness of the ovulation method in a multicentre trial in the US of 1139 couples, who were followed over a minimum of 24 months, was 0.91 when calculated by both the Pearl formula and the more useful life-table technique. However, more than 3800 couples had to be recruited to secure the 1139 who finally entered the trial and only 39% of these couples were still using the method at 24 months. More importantly, use-effectiveness was low, with 16% of the couples, as calculated by life-table analysis, being pregnant at 12 months and 23% at 24 months.[26] Multi-centre international trials by the WHO have given equally disappointing results. Five per cent of women became pregnant during the teaching phase.[52]

Many couples combine some form of periodic abstinence with additional protection during the fertile interval. When this was done in the US multicentre trials of the ovulation method, failure rates dropped to approximately 7 per HWY.

In reviewing the use-effectiveness of the method, most authors overlook the fact that the interval of exposure of users of periodic abstinence to the risk of pregnancy is considerably reduced compared with other methods.[6]

Evaluation

The ability to monitor changes in basal body temperature or cervical mucus, or to predict ovulation from the calendar, provides the basis of fertility awareness. When this knowledge is combined with periodic abstinence it is the basis of a contraceptive technique. The ovulation method in particular is a useful addition to family planning choices. Uniquely among contraceptive methods, an awareness of the bodily changes which accompany ovulation can be of value to those who wish to conceive. The self-knowledge that the method requires of the couple is said by some who have worked with the technique to enhance the psycho-social life of the couple.

Unfortunately, the ovulation method in particular has become a banner under which a small but very vocal group have assembled to preach the method as the sole solution to all fertility regulation problems.[24] They have the same passionate intensity which characterized Marie Stopes's efforts to popularize vaginal barrier methods. The World Organization Ovulation Method Billings (WOOMB) advocates exclusive use of the method, claiming it to be natural, criticizing all other methods as dangerous and disowning any overlapping use with mechanical methods. Unplanned pregnancies, which are frequently encountered, are said to result from a deliberate misuse of the method and can be an expression of an unconscious desire to conceive. 'The so-called unwanted child', writes Poltawska in the *International Review of Natural Family Planning*, 'should be understood as God's gift to *men*' (emphasis added).[40]

For some, perhaps a relatively large number of people, the ovulation method and other types of fertility awareness provide one of several valid family planning choices. Looked at in this light, the ovulation method is a useful method. Like a condom, its observed use-effectiveness varies widely but can reach low levels amongst selected couples. Like the IUD, the method has undergone technical improvements in the last decade and may be open to more. Like those using the diaphragm, users often prove to be those with the privilege of above-average education and economic opportunity. Like those using other reversible methods of contraception, some users are more likely to resort to abortion if the method fails than if they had never used the method at all. As with the use of Depo-Provera, which can cause benign breast tumours in beagle bitches, the deliberate mating of animals at other than fertile times leads to an increased incidence of fetal abnormalities. Unlike steroidal contraceptives, periodic abstinence has never been tested on animals at 50 times the equivalent human dose!

In a detached view, periodic abstinence should be rated like most other contraceptives as acceptable and valuable for some and worse than useless for others. It seems unlikely, however, that there will ever be consensus on whether sexual intercourse deliberately undertaken at times of biological infertility is theologically, philosophically and morally in any way different from sexual intercourse undertaken at times of fertility with condoms, or from sexual intercourse undertaken at times of artificially induced infertility as with the Pill. The strength of the sincere belief of the few that there is genuine difference perhaps reflects the fact that most rational people as well as many moral theologians are unable to find any serious asymmetry between the rapid death of a sperm in a condom and a slow death in an eggless tube.

8

The condom

History

In the folklore of contraception, the invention of the condom is attributed to a Dr Condom, who was reputedly a physician at the court of Charles II. The story, as commonly related,[6] suggests that the king, who had become alarmed at the numbers of his illegitimate offspring, subsequently knighted the doctor in recognition of this unique contribution to monarchical welfare.

It is certain, however, that the device was well known before the reign of Charles II (1660–85) and it is doubtful whether any such person as Condom ever existed. More probably, the term which first appeared in print in 1717 as 'condum' was derived from the Latin (*condus*: a receptacle) as a euphemism for an article already widely known. There are, indeed, a score of terms by which the device has been known at various times, and it is significant that whilst the French refer to it as 'la capote anglaise' we have reciprocated with the term 'French letter', 'letter' being a fairly recent corruption of the word 'envelope'.

The earliest published description of the condom is that of the Italian physician Fallopio who, in 1564, recommended a linen sheath, moistened with a lotion, to be used as a protection against venereal infection. In 1597 Hercule Saxonia described a similar device made from some kind of fabric soaked in a solution of inorganic salts and subsequently allowed to dry. The condom was still regarded primarily as a prophylactic a century later when Mme Sevigne, in a much-quoted letter to her daughter the Comtesse de Grignan, describes a sheath made from gold-beaters' skin as 'armour against love, gossamer against infection'.

By the eighteenth century the condom, 'preservative', 'machine' or 'armour', as it was variously described, had achieved some popularity for its contraceptive as well as its prophylactic function and it was widely praised in the erotic poetry of the period. In his *London Journal* Boswell tells how, on 19 May 1763, he 'picked up a strong young jolly damsel, led her to Westminster Bridge and there, in armour complete, did I enjoy her upon this noble edifice'.[8] From the mid eighteenth century there is evidence of a flourishing trade in London, largely in the hands of Mrs Perkins and Mrs Philips, whose advertisements gained a wide circulation and contained the invitation:

> To guard yourself from shame or fear,
> Votaries to Venus hasten here,
> None in my ware e'er found a flaw,
> Self-preservation's nature's law.

Mrs Philips, in a handbill dated 1796,[19] boasted 35 years' experience and claimed to supply 'apothecaries, chemists and druggists' as well as 'ambassadors, foreigners, gentlemen and captains of ships going abroad' with 'any quantity of the best goods in England on the shortest notice and at the lowest price'.

The condoms of this period were apparently made from the caeca of sheep or other animals and there is an illustration, in a publication of 1744,[33] which shows men and women seated at a table engaged in their manufacture. In 1952 a locked box was discovered in the muniment room of an English country mansion and when opened it was found to contain a quantity of these early condoms in three different sizes, double-wrapped in packets of eight. Dated between 1790 and 1810 they were made of some animal membrane and were 190 mm long, 60 mm in diameter and 0.038 mm thick.[12]

Skin condoms were expensive and obviously beyond the means of the growing number of couples who, by the latter part of the nineteenth century, were beginning to practice family limitation. It was fortuitous, therefore, that the vulcanization of rubber, first carried out by Hancock & Goodyear in 1844, could be applied to the manufacture of condoms, and from the 1870s this device entered a new phase of popularity.

Methods of manufacture

The vulcanization of rubber revolutionized the world's transport and its impact on sexual relations and the contraceptive habits of western society has been equally significant. The replacement of the skin sheath by the rubber condom in the late nineteenth century made available an inexpensive, hygienic and reliable method of contraception at the precise time when family limitation was beginning to be regarded as an essential aspect of married life, and the condom figures very prominently in the contraceptive catalogues of the 1890s.

The earliest rubber condoms were moulded from sheet crepe and carried a seam along their entire length. By the end of the nineteenth century, this defect had been overcome and seamless condoms were being produced by dipping hollow glass formers into a solution of crepe rubber. The earliest teat-ended products appeared under the trade name Dreadnought in 1901.

The next major technological improvement was the development, in the early 1930s, of the latex process. Glass formers were dipped directly into liquid latex (the sap of the rubber tree suspended in water and stablized with ammonia and antioxidants) and curing was achieved by redipping the formers in hot water.[36]

The rapid expansion of both domestic and world markets during the last 50 years has stimulated further refinements in the basic latex process.[23] The modern condom plant is a typical automated system which employs a minimum of staff.[32] Machines may be over 100 m long and consist of a conveyor moving at about 15 m per min over latex tanks, heated air chambers and hot water baths. The open ends of condoms are beaded on while still on the former by a set of brushes which roll down the still-liquid latex prior to vulcanization in heated air chambers. After further drying the finished product is rolled, by means of nylon brushes, off the former which is then scrupulously cleansed before re-entering the latex on the next circuit.

The modern condom factory can produce hundreds of millions of condoms in a year and production is concentrated in relatively few countries. The Japanese manufacturers have set the pace in making ever-thinner products and in pioneering the addition of colour in 1949.[21] However, other manufacturers have been quick to compete, and British and American producers now market thin, high-quality, coloured condoms as well as the plain varieties. By adhering to almost surgical standards of cleanliness, it is possible to exclude particles of dust which would result in flaws.

Condoms may be either dry or lubricated. The idea of pre-lubrication developed in the United States where condoms were marketed in sealed capsules containing glycerine and glycol. In the 1960s silicones began to be added to the final packaging prior to sealing and lubricated condoms now command a major share of nearly all markets, although the Indian Government programme continues to use unlubricated products.

In 1975 spermicidally lubricated condoms were introduced into the British market.[30] Trials had shown that they were acceptable to potential users and provided an additional sense of reassurance; however, it is a fact of epidemiology that ordinary condoms have such a low failure rate that it would require tens of thousands of cycles of study to demonstrate whether spermicidally lubricated condoms are associated with an even lower failure rate than non-spermicidally lubricated ones. Their distribution, therefore, is one of several decisions in family planning based upon common sense and it is unlikely it will ever be confirmed or refuted by clinical trial. Spermicidally lubricated condoms only received preliminary US FDA approval in 1982.

Condoms are made in two main sizes: western and Asian. When American-manufactured condoms were first supplied to Thailand, the numbers of complaints about sheaths slipping off almost reached the level of a diplomatic incident between the two countries. Subsequent measurement of erect penile size in Bangkok massage parlours found that the average Asian penis was 5.14 inches (13.1 cm) long and 4.34 inches (11.0 cm) in circumference,[11] while Kinsey reported comparable measurements of 6.0 inches (15.2 cm) and 5.0 inches (12.5 cm) for Caucasian males. In Japan, condom size was selected by paying individuals to make an agar cast of the erect organ.

It appears to have been the practice of manufacturers from the earliest days to apply some sort of testing procedure to their products and in the first decades of the present century the more reputable firms carried out inflation tests on each item before despatch. (Contemporary National Standards are noted in Chapter 4.) In 1951 automated machinery was adapted to the electronic testing of each individual condom in Great Britain in what was virtually an extension of the production process. This routine is based on the fact that rubber is a poor conductor of electricity. The condoms are drawn by hand on to a second series of metal formers and the loaded formers are then immersed in ionized water which is contained in a metal tank. When both tank and former are electrically charged, pinholes and even weak patches in the rubber are detected and defective items are automatically removed from the production line for destruction. It should be noted that whether water tests and/or electronic tests are used, the purpose of detecting holes is not to identify those few condoms which might allow the escape of a few sperm (which would be insufficient a deposit in the vagina to achieve fertilization) but to monitor the presence of flaws and thus the overall quality and strength.

When produced in bulk for international distribution, condoms can be manufactured for a few dollars a gross. Electronic testing processes and sophisticated packaging, which appeal to richer markets, add significantly to costs. Traditionally, condoms have been items with a high mark-up at the point of purchase and trials have shown that, given the same quality of condom, many consumers will purchase the more expensive one on the supposition that it should be safer and more pleasant to use.

A few skin condoms manufactured from the caeca from lambs are still marketed. They are individually encapsulated in glycol and are claimed to be superior to latex by ensuring greater sensitivity, the animal membrane being a better conductor of heat than rubber and the device more loosely fitted over the major part of its length. At three or four times the price of the best quality latex product, they are clearly intended as luxury items. Trials have been conducted with plastic condoms, which are also good heat conductors and loose fitting. Like disposable gloves they are stamped from ethylene ethyl acrylate sheets and two pieces are heat-sealed together with a rubber ring sealed in the open end. However, large-scale manufacture has never been attempted even though a cheap, tough, potentially reusable product could be produced and might be useful in the developing world.

Extent of contemporary use

In the 1960s the condom was the most widely used contraceptive device in Britain and many other western societies. Among 1340 couples married in the period 1930–49 who were interviewed in the course of the Population Investigation Committee study in 1959, 48% had used condoms at some time during marriage and 36% were current users.[26] Similarly, in the Family Growth in Metropolitan America study in 1957, 31% of the 1165 white couples interviewed were using the condom as the sole method of birth control.[39] Approximately 50–70% of adult American males have used condoms at some time. A survey of high-school students in 1975 found that half of white students, a quarter of black, and one-fifth of Hispanic students had used a condom at last intercourse.[14] The method is often adopted by blue-collar workers and it is interesting that in the United States condom use among white couples fell in the 1970s but rose from 7.1% to 9.9% among the black community and black women questioned postpartum reported the use of condoms by their partners three times as often as white women.[20] There has also been good acceptance in domiciliary family planning services in Britain.[28]

The highest prevalence of use (see Fig. 2.8), the largest total sales and some of the most imaginative condom sales techniques are to be found in Japan. By 1972, 5.7 million gross, or enough condoms if placed end to end to stretch half-way to the moon, were being manufactured in Japan, approximately 20% of which were exported. Japan does not permit the use of oral contraceptives, although steroids are sold for so-called therapeutic reasons, and voluntary sterilization is only permitted 'when the mother has several children and there is fear of deterioration in health'.[13] Poor communication between the spouses on sex, a male-dominated society, a conservative medical profession and well-established (and profitable) abortion services all maintain the status quo in contraceptive use, although given wider options there is reasonable evidence that couples might chose a broader range of methods, as in the West. Midwives now sell condoms, but there are no family planning clinics.[9, 31]

In some developing countries, the condom has proved a remarkably useful addition to family planning choices, seeming to gain its greatest use in those countries where the male is the dominant partner within the marriage, as in Muslim societies.[24] Deys has suggested that contraceptive choice within the marriage partnership partly depends upon the sociology of the relationship.[10] In those families where the marriage roles are strictly divided, the husband is the wage-earner and the wife looks after the home and brings up the children, then condoms, coitus interruptus and vasectomy are predictable choices. In those families where husband and wife take joint decisions, where the wife often seeks employment outside the home and where the husband may play a significant role in the care of the children, then the Pill, diaphragm and tubal ligation are more likely to be used. Conversely, Bauman & Udry (1972) found a strong correlation between an individual's sense of powerlessness in relation to their environment and failure to use contraception consistently.[5]

Marketing

The major virtue of the condom, of course, is precisely that it is easily available from non-clinical sources and can be used without medical supervision. The marketing of condoms in both developed and developing countries is important not only in itself but also because it teaches some general lessons about family planning.

Satisfactory marketing depends upon having the right product of the right type in the right place.[2, 18, 32] In Britain pharmacies and barbers' shops are the major outlets, accounting for two-thirds of the trade. The sale through hairdressers is particularly appropriate as a place where men go at approximately the frequency they need to buy condoms and the phrase 'Is there anything else, Sir?' familiar to every Briton who has ever had his hair cut, could well become a slogan for the whole of family planning: it removes the possible embarrassment of asking for a contraceptive and allows the potential consumer a polite 'No thanks' or a grateful 'Yes, please'.

Although condoms are commercially available under many trade names, in a variety of colours and packs and at widely varying prices, the pre-lubricated latex product dominates western and Japanese markets. Condoms are invariably rolled and hermetically sealed in aluminium sachets and are usually retailed in packs of three. In nearly all situations the predominant market is directly to men, but in the 1950s and 1960s the

Japanese Family Planning Association pioneered the sale of condoms by women to women. In contemporary Japan, approximately 20% of condoms are sold in this way, largely through highly organized teams of door-to-door sales ladies, who can make up to US $800 a month in commissions.[9] Special packages have been devised to appeal to the feminine market, some imitating boxes of sweets and even packages of tea! In Poland, during an episode of bureaucratic mismanagement, condoms were packaged in the butter cartons from the local dairy industry. Unfortunately, sales have sometimes been promoted by denigrating alternative methods such as the use of an IUD.

Most of the condoms sold in Great Britain are teat ended but this is an essentially national idiosyncrasy. Consumers in the rest of Europe and the US usually prefer plain-ended varieties. In Kenya, red condoms proved the most popular choice and in Japan black condoms are the most frequently purchased of the coloured variety: presumably an element of contrast attracts. Condoms are sold under a variety of trade names from Abdulla to 777, and including such amphibologues as Golden Carriage, Patrician, Waverley Pearl and Rameses. In Malay they are called sarongs. In Britain approximately 20% of condoms are sold through mail-order houses, sex shops and surgical stores. Mail order has the advantage of anonymity and has been widely used in the West and explored in some developing countries which have adequate and honest postal services, such as Sri Lanka. Mail order is a significant source of supply of condoms to college campuses in the United States.

Vending machines, at such sites as petrol filling stations, are another satisfactory outlet where condoms can be supplied conveniently and anonymously at any hour of the day or night. The limitation of vending machines is that they can invite vandalism, not all countries have suitable coins to activate such machines and in some situations contraceptive vending machines are forbidden by local regulations or custom. Unscrupulous vendors rapidly discover that this particular product is the single one where the customer does not complain if the machine swallows his money and fails to produce the required item!

Unfortunately, very few family planning programmes in industrialized nations run by governmental or charitable agencies have attempted to promote condoms systematically. One, in South Carolina, US, distributed condoms through appropriate community outlets and was associated with a 3.2% decline in the illegitimacy rate, while in control areas in the same state, over the same years (1972–75), the rate rose.[22] A free distribution of condoms in a test area in North Carolina was associated with a 19% decline in the teenage fertility rate over four years, while in non-project areas the rate remained unchanged.[3] Pharmacists Planning Services, Inc. in California organizes an annual National Condom Week which starts on Washington's birthday and runs to St Valentine's day. In addition to street music and posters for family planning, the organizers run a contest for condom couplets, for example:

> Use a condom and you will learn
> No deposit, no return

Unfortunately, codes of advertising practice still hold back condom marketing in the West. It is illegal to advertise contraceptives on commercial television in Britain (see Chapter 15, Contraceptives and the law).

In developing countries, social marketing programmes have developed some names such as *Kinga* and *Preethi* (which means friend in Ceylonese). In Bangladesh, Population Services International now sell over 5 million condoms a month. There has been a careful selection of the brand names (e.g. Raja), appropriate advertising, distribution through a number of channels and adjustment of the price to suit an extremely poor society.[7, 24]

The Nirodh programme in India was the first effort at the social marketing of condoms. It used nearly 100 000 retail outlets but the programme never sat happily within a government structure and the approval of advertisements, pricing and even the production of the condoms themselves were all at times influenced by political as well as commercial considerations. Nevertheless some lively advertisements, such as 'Men! The Power to prevent births is in your hands' were created.

Until the 1960s, washable reusable sheaths were sold in Britain; these were manufactured from thicker latex and intended for repeated use. No systematic effort has been made to market a similar product in the developing world although it might well prove attractive in some societies. Certainly, amongst the poor few things are thrown away and some ingenious recycling of parts of condoms has been invented by Third World rural populations: it is easy to separate the rubber ring from the rest of the condom, and this can be used for a variety of purposes, including braiding your woman's hair; the problem then remains of what to do with the remainder of the sheath, but here again a solution has been found, namely keep it available in your pocket because it makes an excellent tourniquet in case of poisonous snake bites!

The condom can become a memorably appropriate symbol for family planning in general. In Thailand, lectures on family planning are commonly accompanied by condom blowing contests to find the man with the strongest lungs who can burst his condom first. This apparently adolescent activity has a deeper meaning: it uses humour to reassure everyone in the audience that contraceptives are a necessary and acceptable article in daily (or perhaps nightly) living and that the condom is a well-made and pleasant-to-handle product. In Sweden and Thailand 'Proud Pete' (Fig. 8.1) has become not only an advertising symbol for the condom, but also an unambigious instructor in its use.

Effectiveness

Those who choose to use condoms do not normally seek professional advice and help. It is not surprising, therefore, that studies on use-effectiveness are less plentiful and less reliable than for methods where expert supervision is mandatory. Even where we do have studies, it is always possible that clinic attenders are a self-selected group and may not be truly representative of condom users in general.

In Britain, Fisher followed a group of users attending a family planning clinic in Oxford between 1935 and 1950 and reported a Pearl rate of 7.5 per hundred woman-years (HWY).[15] The Indianapolis study followed up middle and upper income US couples over a fertile lifetime and found a

Fig. 8.1. Swedish condom promotion.

Proud Pete

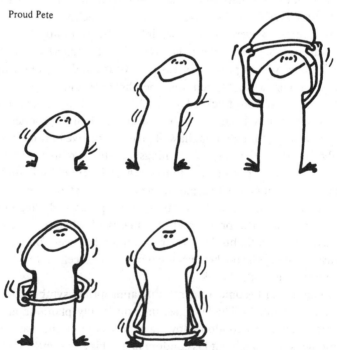

Pearl rate of 6 per HWY.[38] Perhaps the most useful study was that of Peel on 312 newly married couples in Hull followed over five years in which condom users overall had a failure rate of 3.9 per HWY and consistent users a rate as low as 1.6 per HWY.[29] Vessey found a failure rate of 4.0 per HWY among a selected population of family planning clinic users.[17] In the US, Westoff's follow-up of over 1000 couples after the birth of a second child found a condom failure rate as low as 2.6 per HWY,[34, 37] and in the US National Survey of Family Growth (1970–73), 6.6% of the sample of women aged 15–44 experienced a contraceptive failure in the first year of condom use. The comparable percentages for IUDs and diaphragms were 2.9 and 10.3 respectively.[35]

As with many methods of contraception, failure rates recorded in developing countries are somewhat higher, but the condom retains the same ranking of contraceptive effectiveness as in the West, where it is as good as or better than a diaphragm and cream and can approach that of an IUD.

The choice of the condom

The persisting popularity of condoms largely derives from the fact that they can be bought without prescription and if necessary from sources other than pharmacies. For individuals wishing to pursue their sex lives in complete privacy, the condom is often an effective, easy, acceptable and sensible choice.

In addition, the condom has some particular advantages for certain groups. It is an ideal method for couples whose acts of intercourse are sporadic or unpredictable: for a woman who may, for example, only see her sea-faring husband twice a year the condom would appear to be both satisfactory and economical. Similarly, the unmarried, for whom inter-course may be isolated and spontaneous, will usually find the condom a satisfactory receptacle for wild oats. The condom can be useful in cases of premature ejaculation, when it may be effective in prolonging coitus, and in cases in which immediately successful protection against conception is psychologically important to one or both partners.

Condoms reduce the possibility of venereal infection and this includes cases of vaginal trichomoniasis and moniliasis, where there is a likelihood of reinfection by the male.[4] Unfortunately, condoms appear to be least used by those who are most likely to have numerous sexual partners. Nevertheless, an effect can be shown: in Sweden in 1970, 34 million condoms were imported and there were nearly 39 000 reported cases of gonorrhoea (Fig. 8.2). Two years later, after a vigorous promotional campaign by the RFSU (the Swedish Family Planning Association), 55.6

million condoms were imported and the number of reported cases of gonorrhoea fell by over 7000. The programme was backed up by informative but amusing advertising.[1] Among condom users at a London clinic, the diagnosis of gonorrhoea was significantly less common than among non-users. However, there was no difference in the rate of non-specific urethritis between users and non-users.

The condom is the one form of contraception which is virtually without contraindications or side-effects. A search of the literature over more than 30 years reveals only one reported case of alleged side-effects.[25] The condom is commonly said to reduce sensitivity, but it would be no less accurate and a good deal more positive to say that it can prolong sexual intercourse. Family planning organizations, because of their predominantly female orientation, have tended to underrate condoms. Doctors recognize their high acceptability and effectiveness. They may also wish to recommend the condom as an interim method or as an alternative technique for couples who wish to share the responsibility for birth control.

Condoms have been associated with death, but only in non-contraceptive situations. Some professional smugglers attempting to carry drugs into the United States filled condoms with heroin and swallowed them hoping to collect their contraband when they passed the frontier and it passed the rectum. In two cases the condoms burst and the smugglers died from rapid intestinal absorption of the drug. Heinrich Himmler is thought

Fig. 8.2. Gonorrhoeal cases in thousands and condom imports in millions (Sweden). (Redrawn from Ajax, L. (1974). How to market a non-medical contraceptive: a case study from Sweden. In *The Condom: Increasing Utilization in the United States*, ed. M. H. Redford, G. W. Duncan & D. J. Prager. San Francisco: San Francisco Press.)

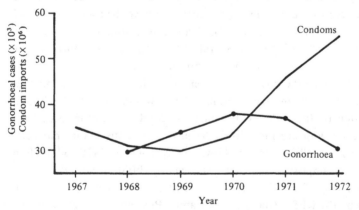

to have committed suicide prior to the Nuremburg trials by hiding cyanide in a condom.

One case-control study purports to demonstrate a strong correlation between the use of condoms earlier in married life and the subsequent development of cancer of the breast. The study is statistically sound but breaks a basic rule of epidemiology in that it lacks biological plausibility (see Chapter 4), and the explanation of the correlation almost certainly lies in some unseen variable related to lifestyle or some other factor.[16] Sadly, condoms do seem to pose dangers to other species. The thin part of a condom biodegrades before the ring at the end. The Marine laboratory of the Department of Agriculture and Fisheries for Scotland has reported on large numbers of fish ringed with rubber bands 3.6 cm in diameter.[27]

Use and care

The condom is less open to misuse than most other forms of contraception because of its simplicity, but its efficacy can nevertheless be enhanced by simple instructions, and, since most failures result from carelessness in use rather than from defects in the product, professional interest and intervention is undoubtedly justified.

No attempt should be made to stretch or inflate a condom prior to use and it should be kept away from long fingernails. There is no need, despite repeated statements that have been made to the contrary, for the condom to be worn during foreplay, although it is essential that the condom is placed in position well before ejaculation takes place. The remote possibility of sperm being present in the pre-ejaculatory fluid is discussed in Chapter 5. The condom should be unrolled on to the erect penis (a task which the woman as well as the man may learn to perform), care being taken to ensure that the air is expelled from the teat, or in the case of the plain-ended article, that a portion of the closed end is deflated and left free. Withdrawal should be carefully undertaken with the open end firmly held to ensure that the condom does not slip off after detumescence has occurred.

In the cases where contraceptive failure would be disastrous it should be recommended that the condom is used in conjunction with a vaginal spermicide: either a pessary or spermicidal gel. It is reasonable to assume that this would reduce the risk of pregnancy if a mechanical failure should occur and it would also assist in lubrication. The most essential feature, however, is that the condom should be worn on every occasion. Most experienced observers would probably agree that the majority of condom failures are user failures rather than method failures, the device simply not being used on the relevant occasion. This is a particularly important feature because many couples have used the alternation of condom and safe period and partial use of the latter (particularly if wrongly calculated) will increase the apparent failure rate. A modification of this risky technique is that withdrawal is used at times when the couple have believed or have calculated that the risk of pregnancy is low, and a condom is worn only during the accepted fertile period (see Fig. 4.1).

Evaluation

The condom is traditionally outside the sphere of clinical concern and has therefore often been regarded as a 'merely commercial' and, by some perverse logic, unreliable form of contraception. When, during the 1950s, representative data became available from the first retrospective studies of wide sections of the population it became clear that the condom had a remarkably high use-effectiveness rate. Perhaps the greatest disadvantage of a condom is that it was not a method of contraception invented on the West Coast of America in the 1960s. It might then have been vigorously promoted as an effective, economical, easy-to-use method that does not require the advice of a third party to use effectively. In addition, the condom is an excellent treatment for premature ejaculation and, in normal intercourse, can lead to prolonged erection and greater satisfaction. The complaint that it is disruptive to the sex act can be cancelled by the suggestion that the condom, particularly if it is of high quality and coloured, can be an adjunct to the erotic aspects of coitus.

9

Vaginal contraceptives: chemical and barrier

Given even an elementary knowledge of the physiology of reproduction, the occlusion of the cervix and the use of chemicals in the vagina appear obvious methods of contraception. There is a large literature relating to historical and pre-literate societies in which a variety of gums, leaves, fruits and seed-pods were adopted for this purpose.[11, 16] Casanova[5] is said to have used half a lemon, squeezed of its contents, and inserted over the cervix; the residual citric acid, mildly spermicidal, would undoubtedly have provided additional protection. During the Second World War, Marie Stopes listed a number of what she called 'good domestic methods', including a bath sponge cut to shape, a powder puff dipped in olive oil and even a child's rubber ball cut in half.[36]

Spermicides

Egyptian papyri of 1850 BC offer written instructions for vaginal contraceptives made with honey and natron (naturally occurring sodium carbonate) and for various other irrigating, plugging and gummy substances to insert into the vagina before coitus. In 1885 Walter Rendell, an English pharmacist, produced quinine pessaries[25] but not until the 1920s was science really mobilized in the search for effective spermicides.

With the resurgence in the 1970s of vaginal contraception the place of spermicides has had to be reassessed.[9, 17, 27, 34, 37] It should be said that they are safe, with no proven systemic effects nor serious local reaction; freely available from commercial sources worldwide; convenient, particularly to couples who have intercourse infrequently and need unplanned immediate protection; acceptable to many women who might not otherwise use family planning and protective to some degree against venereal disease.

Mode of action

Morphologically and biochemically, sperm are some of the most intensively studied cells in biology. Numerous interlocking events take place between the processes of maturation in the testes, ejaculation, transport through the female reproductive tract and fertilization, the latter process being very complex.[2, 21]

Sperm are dependent on a variety of biochemical processes both for normal functioning after ejaculation and for penetrating the corona radiata and zona pellucida of the ovum. It is known that sperm must undergo capacitation in the female reproductive tract before fertilization can occur. The nature of the process, which may take approximately 7 h in humans, is not fully understood, but does involve morphological changes in the acrosome of the sperm and can be reversed by re-exposing the sperm to seminal plasma.[2] The acrosome is derived from the Golgi apparatus and can be regarded as a lysosome rich in enzymes. Among these, hyaluronidase probably functions to assist in the separation of the cumulus oophorus cells, acrosin probably helps the penetration of the sperm through the zona pellucida and the corona penetrating enzyme, which is poorly defined, probably assists in penetration past the corona radiata. Yet, despite the depth of understanding, the complexity of the processes concerned and the manifest need for improved contraceptives, relatively few chemical entities have reached human use as spermicidal agents. In fact, the number of such products on the market actually declined in the 1960s and 1970s.

Currently available local contraceptive agents are either spermiostatic or spermicidal.[12] They fall into three main groups: electrolytes, enzyme inhibitors[45] including sulphydryl-binding substances and surface-active agents. Electrolytes disrupt sperm osmotically, but like mercury, lead salts, arsenites and selenites are of little practical use. Several organometallic compounds were formerly available in the United States, but have now been withdrawn from use. Surface-acting substances (such as nonylphenoxypolyethoxyethanol) probably act by altering the permeability of the cell membrane and indirectly exposing it to osmotic disruption,[32] although other actions are also possible. Surface-active agents represent the most commonly used type of over-the-counter contraceptive agents available on the market today.

Recent work has shown that β-adrenergic-receptor blocking drugs, much used in the treatment of hypertension, are spermicidal in very low concentrations and these drugs are under active investigation for contraceptive use.

Types available and patterns of use

Spermicides may be formulated as suppositories or pessaries (when the active compound is prepared in gelatine or cocoa-butter), jellies, creams or pastes. Foam and aerosol preparations have gained popularity since the Second World War. In Europe a water-soluble plastic film (C-film) has been used as a vehicle for spermicide.[29]

In most developed countries, 3% or less of the population use spermicides, although in Japan the level reaches 6% of currently married fertile women.[6]

Diaphragms and cervical caps

History

The earliest commercial surgical caps had to wait the development of crepe, and later, vulcanized rubber. The first medical reference occurs in the German literature where, in 1838, Dr F. A. Wilde[44] describes the use of a cautschuk-pessarium as a 'comfortable and effective' method of birth control. In 1867 an identical article was described and illustrated in the Lancet as a form of treatment for 'anteflexion and anteversion of the uterus', but the occlusive cap was not referred to again in the English birth control literature until 1887 when Allbutt published his famous manual *The Wife's Handbook*; an action for which he was struck off the medical register (See Chapter 1). By this time the name of Mensinga,[23] the pseudonym of a Flensburg physician whose real name was Hesse, had become associated with the device, largely through publicity given to it by the Dutch Neo-Malthusians. The development of vulcanized rubber had enabled Hesse to produce a thinner and more pliable device incorporating a flat watchspring in the rim. The diaphragm lay diagonally across the vaginal canal, occluding both the cervix and the upper part of the vagina.

In Britain and the US the early birth control clinics followed the Dutch example in adopting the cap as a basic technique. It was both appropriate to the female clientele which they hoped to attract and, combined with the use of spermicidal cream, offered a highly effective method. Margaret Sanger was taught the method by Rutgers in Holland but the Comstock laws (Chapter 1) prevented official importation into the United States. In 1920 Holland Rantos began a US manufacture.

The two branches of the British clinic movement adopted different and 'rival' varieties of the technique, which provided the basis for a long and acrimonious disagreement. Marie Stopes's clinic advocated a high-domed cervical cap in combination with greasy suppositories. The Society for the Provision of Birth Control Clinics (SPBCC, later the Family Planning

Association (FPA)) favoured the spring-rim vaginal diaphragm together with a spermicidal jelly and subsequent douching. Marie Stopes alleged that the diaphragm caused distension of the vaginal muscles while the SPBCC replied that the cervical cap produced erosion of the cervix. Neither side produced any scientific observations to support their assertions.

Diaphragms and caps were to family planning what the steam locomotive was to transportation: they were the first in the field, brought emancipation to millions and for a long time had no rivals. Ultimately, they were overtaken by a new technology, in this case oral contraceptives. They still have a band of zealous supporters and, when the newer technology is under criticism, wide publicity is given to the possibility of returning to caps and diaphragms, although in real life they are unlikely to regain really widespread popularity.

Use

The diaphragm reached the peak of its popularity around 1959, which was the year in which the Population Investigation Committee reported its use by approximately 12% of those British couples who were practising contraception[26] while in the US the National Fertility Study of 1965 found a figure of 10%. In a survey of women attending 315 British FPA clinics in 1960, it was found that over 95% were offered the diaphragm. Cervical caps were available but were rarely used.[18] In the US Planned Parenthood Survey in 1961, 64% of women coming to clinics were found to be using the diaphragm but cervical caps were not even available.

Use of the diaphragms and caps plummeted with the advent of the Pill and by 1973 only 5% of contraceptive users in England and Wales adopted the method while in the US the comparable figure in 1973 was 2.7%.[6] As a technique, it was always more likely to be used by school teachers than by shop assistants and was commonly claimed to interfere with 'love-making' and to be 'messy'. However, even in 1973, the US clinics found that for women who chose the method, more than 80% were still using it after one year.

The United States, characteristically, has the widest swings in contraceptive fashion. A much-publicized upsurge in the use of barrier methods occurred in the late 1970s,[28] but in absolute terms the number of users still remains small and is mainly limited to younger women who represent a generation not personally familiar with the drawbacks and limitations of barrier methods but vulnerable to the adverse publicity surrounding Pills and IUDs.

In contemporary America, the Federal Drug Authority (FDA) has come to play a Comstock role and in 1980, approximately 150 years after their invention, categorized caps as 'investigational devices' and placed them with other 'probably harmful' contraceptives.[10] To date the use of the cap has been so miniscule that there is not sufficient American data to fulfil the requirements of registration. Some feminist groups smuggle them into the country.

Diaphragms have been little used in family planning programmes in developing countries, partly because the motivation to accept the method may be weak and the privacy to install it and a place to store it difficult to find, but possibly also because there are too few people to train others in its use. In the Philippines and Colombia well under 1% of contraceptive users adopted the method, and in Africa and the Middle East prevalence is too low to measure.[43]

The woman who is going to learn to use a diaphragm or cap must have two qualities, and they are not necessarily related. She must have the intelligence to understand and carry out the correct insertion of the cap and she must have the self-discipline to use it on every occasion she has intercourse. In addition she must not find exploration of her own anatomy distasteful. A woman who has had children is usually more ready to accept the cap than her nulliparous sister.

Types available
Several types of diaphragms and caps (Fig. 9.1) are available in Europe through pharmacies and clinics. Products should be stamped with the date of manufacture as they have a finite storage life. All the

Fig. 9.1. Vaginal barriers.

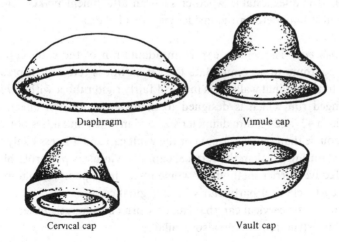

Diaphragm   Vimule cap

Cervical cap   Vault cap

intravaginal barrier methods, diaphragms or caps, require the additional use of a spermicidal cream or jelly.

The diaphragm (Dutch cap). The diaphragm is by far the commonest form of occlusive device and for most women it is the easiest to fit and reuse. It is made from fine latex in the form of a thin dome mounted on a thick rim containing a metal spring. The flat spring type is more rigid and stronger than the coil spring variety and provides a less easily distorted, more easily inserted device. Claims have been made that one or other type of spring is especially suited to some particular pelvic anatomy but firm evidence is lacking and supplier preference appears to be the most significant factor influencing choice. Diaphragms are manufactured in a series of sizes from 45 mm diameter to 105 mm diameter. The height of the dome varies from maker to maker.

The vault cap. The vault cap is a firm hemispherical rubber or plastic cap which fits in the vaginal vault and covers the cervix like a dome. It is held in position by suction. The centre is relatively thin but the rim is much thicker and provides the elasticity which maintains sufficient suction to hold it in place. There is no metal spring in the rim. The vault cap is made in sizes of 45, 48 and 51 mm diameter.

Cervical caps (check pessaries). Cervical caps (check pessaries) are thimble-shaped rubber caps with thick bases and are designed to fit snugly over the cervix. They are manufactured in three or four sizes from 22 to 31 mm diameter. Some cervical caps have a thread attached to the rim to assist removal. It is questionable whether such an attachment makes removal easier and it may deform the inside contour of the cap.

The vimule cap. The vimule cap is an adaptation of the vault cap with formed contours to accommodate the cervix but is retained in place by suction to the vaginal walls. It is made of fairly rigid rubber with a thicker and flanged rim which is designed to increase the suction effect. It is available in 42- and 55-mm diameter sizes. Many men find it less obtrusive in intercourse than the diaphragm or the vault cap and it is less likely to be displaced during sex than the cervical cap. The vimule cap is probably the most effective barrier method for women who have poor vaginal muscle tone. a cystocele or a particularly long vaginal cervix.

A rigid plastic cervical cap that can be worn continuously except at the time of menstruation is now also available.

Recent developments. While the vaginal diaphragm is usually regarded as a vehicle for holding a spermicide in the path of the ejaculate, Stim has experimented with the use of a thick diaphragm without spermicide. A 60-mm diaphragm is given to all women, who are instructed to leave the contraceptive in place day and night checking it only occasionally.[35] This may have been the way in which diaphragms were first used in the nineteenth century but additional clinical studies are certainly necessary to check the validity of this simplification.

Family Health International has completed research on a disposable polyurethane vaginal sponge incorporating the spermicide nonoxynol-9. Called *Today*, it has received US FDA approval as a non-prescription item. The sponge should be inserted up to 24 h before coitus and may be left in place, or reused on one or two occasions. A comparative trial of the contraceptive sponge and diaphragm among women who had not previously used a barrier method found a 12 month cumulative life-table pregnancy rate of 16.1 and 12.0 respectively. In an attempt to apply modern technology to the old problem of barrier contraception, experiments are being conducted in which an individual mould is made of the cervix and a latex cap formed to the cervical contours of the individual user, exactly as was first done by Frederick Wilde.

Fitting

Initially, occlusive diaphragms and caps must be fitted by a trained person, but the fitter need not be a physician. Experience shows that nurses and paramedical workers are likely to have greater commitment and far more time to teach and encourage the woman to overcome problems and difficulties and to understand the essential principles underlying effective use. Ever since Marie Stopes established her first clinics in the 1920s, nurses in Great Britain have been more involved in fitting vaginal barrier devices than have doctors. Today non-physicians are being trained as instructors in countries as diverse as Japan, Hong Kong, Thailand, Kenya, Tunisia, Colombia and Jamaica.[43]

The fitting of a vaginal barrier device requires at least two appointments. At the second appointment the woman should attend with the device in place so that its fit can be checked under realistic conditions. Sometimes, under such relaxed conditions, a larger sized diaphragm is needed than was first assessed.

At her first attendance every woman should be examined, either lying on her back or in the left lateral position. A speculum is passed as part of the normal pelvic examination and, when appropriate, a smear is taken. The length and position of the cervix is noted and the tone of the perineal muscles and vaginal wall are determined. The choice of the diaphragm or cap is determined mainly by the findings on pelvic examination. The criteria for using a diaphragm are:

(a) There is no major degree of uterine prolapse.

(b) There is good vaginal tone, no marked cystocele and a defined depression or 'shelf' in the lower, anterior vaginal wall behind the symphysis pubis.

(c) The woman is able to feel her own cervix.

The cervical cap and vimule cap can be used only if:

(a) The cervix is readily accessible to the woman.

(b) The cervix is long enough to hold the cap.

(c) The cervix is not severely distorted, eroded or lacerated.

The vault cap may be the choice of the woman herself but more often it is used where a diaphragm or cervical cap proves difficult. It is useful in the woman who has some degree of prolapse or poor vaginal tone, making a diaphragm difficult to fit, or if the cervix is torn or too short for a cervical cap. In fact, the vault cap is contraindicated if the cervix is too long as it will hold the rim of the cap away from the vaginal vault, making it impossible to establish the necessary degree of suction. The vimule cap may then be suitable.

Fitting a diaphragm. A diaphragm which is too small may slip out of place leaving the cervix partially uncovered, while one which is too large may buckle and be uncomfortable to the woman and to her sexual partner. A good fit implies that the diaphragm fits snugly between the back of the symphysis pubis and the posterior vaginal fornix, that the cervix is covered and that the rim of the diaphragm is in close contact with the lateral vaginal walls. The woman is taught to put an adequate amount of spermicide on the dome (or on both sides) and around the rim, to insert the diaphragm properly, checking that the cervix is completely covered, and to remove, cleanse and powder the diaphragm after each use so as to care for it properly.

When a woman goes to have a diaphragm fitted, the length of the vagina from the posterior aspect of the symphysis pubis to the posterior fornix is assessed. An appropriate size of diaphragm is selected, the rim is compressed between the thumb and forefinger of the right hand and the diaphragm inserted into the vagina in such a way that the tip is passed along the posterior vaginal wall so that the rim comes to lie in the posterior fornix. The proximal edge of the rim is then pushed up behind the symphysis pubis.

The flat spring type of diaphragm is more easily inserted than the coil spring type and is more readily placed in the posterior fornix. It is usual to insert the diaphragm dome uppermost. When correctly positioned, the cervix can be felt through the dome of the diaphragm and one finger can just be inserted between the rim of the diaphragm and the symphysis pubis. The woman should not now be aware of the presence of the diaphragm. It is often helpful for the instructor to place the diaphragm in the wrong position deliberately so that the entire device is anterior to the cervix; the woman will then notice some discomfort and find that she can easily feel the rim with her fingers. This rim is hooked down from behind the symphysis pubis to remove the diaphragm.

The woman can be taught to insert the diaphragm in one of three positions: lying on her back with her knees drawn up, standing with one foot raised on a chair or toilet seat, or squatting. It is worth enquiring whether the woman uses vaginal tampons as inserting the device is very similar. Most women find the standing position with one leg raised the simplest. The woman is shown how to compress the diaphragm over the first finger by pressure with the middle finger and thumb. She is then shown how to hold the labia apart with her left hand and insert the diaphragm along the posterior wall of the vagina as far as it will go while keeping it below and behind the cervix; the anterior rim is then tucked up behind the symphysis pubis. In the standing position the diaphragm is inserted almost horizontally and in the lying position almost vertically. It is important to make sure that the woman understands that the anatomical axis of the vagina is upwards and backwards. The lay concept of the vagina is often of a passage placed vertically in the trunk like the lift-shaft in a skyscraper. Unless this idea is corrected the patient will find it difficult to insert the diaphragm and she is liable to place it anterior to the cervix. Some manufacturers supply an introducer, but, although like the invention of the knife and fork it can make the procedure which is being undertaken easier and more attractive, accidents are more likely to occur and all introducers are potentially more damaging to the diaphragm than is the finger.

When any vaginal contraceptive is first fitted the user should be told to practise inserting and removing it and then to leave the appliance in place for several hours at a time to make sure that it does not move out of position if she empties her bladder or has her bowels open. A practice cap or diaphragm can be used without a spermicide or lubricant cream but it must not be relied upon as an effective contraceptive.

In learning to fit her diaphragm it is essential that the woman should be able to feel and recognize her own cervix. To the woman who is not familiar with her own cervix, it can usefully be described as feeling 'like the tip of your nose'. If the cervix is too remote to feel easily, or the woman has fingers which seem too short, or if she has a strong dislike of feeling inside her own vagina, and if there are still reasons why the method is thought suitable, then it may be sufficient for the patient to make sure that the anterior rim of the device is comfortably placed behind the symphysis pubis instead of trying to feel for the cervix.

Fitting cervical, vault and vimule caps. The fitting and use of the cervical cap, vault cap and vimule cap follow similar lines to those for the diaphragm but the techniques are harder to master. It has been demonstrated[39] that inability to learn the technique of use and a fear that the device was inadequate were significant reasons for discontinuing the use of cervical caps in a trial series.

Caps are more rigid than diaphragms and are held in place mainly by suction. The user must be shown how to manoeuvre the cap into position over the cervix. When in use the caps should be about one-third filled with contraceptive cream but the woman must be told not to use too much cream as this will make it difficult to obtain the correct degree of suction. Extra spermicide may be added from an applicator or inserted as a pessary though this is not usually considered necessary.

The cap can be removed by the fingers or by a thread if one is attached. When properly fitted it should be quite difficult to remove.

Care and regular use of vaginal barrier contraceptives

Careful teaching about the use and care of a cap or diaphragm is as important as correct fitting. The user should be reminded that sperm remain capable of fertilizing the egg for many hours after they have been placed in the vagina. The necessity to use the device at every intercourse needs re-emphasizing and the instructor as well as the women herself must be prepared to make some assessment of how well the method is likely to be used in the long run. Every woman has to decide upon her 'strategy' in using her contraceptive. If she decides to insert it only when sex has already been suggested or the first overtures played, she runs the risk of either being swept along on the tide of sexual passion and failing to insert it at all or else calling a halt to the proceedings whilst she finds and fits her cap only to find that sexual ardour on one side or the other has cooled so that in fact the device is no longer needed. If she plans to insert her cap at bedtime whenever she feels it will be needed, she may overestimate her partner's desires and when no overtures are made may then feel frustrated and foolish. When sex is frequent, most women prefer to put the cap in every night as a routine action like brushing their teeth; in this way a woman is prepared for sex, but if it does not occur, she is not frustrated.

The use of a spermicidal cream is essential. Three or four inches (about 7–10 cm) of cream (about a teaspoonful) should be squeezed on to the dome as with other methods of contraception. Unambigious instructions are essential and the user's comprehension should be checked. A Wyoming woman instructed to use a diaphragm and jelly produced a purple, discoloured device when she returned pregnant and was found to have been using grape comfiture from the breakfast table as her jelly.

The device can be put in place up to 2 h before having intercourse. If it is put in close to the time of coitus it is important that it should be inserted before any sexual play takes place. The appliance must remain in place for a minimum of 6 h after intercourse and it can remain in place much longer. In practice it is usually inserted on going to bed and taken out next morning. If the cap has been inserted more than, say, 4 h before intercourse or if a second intercourse takes place more than an hour after the first, spermicidal cream should be added with an applicator or inserted in pessary form. A pessary is less satisfactory as it takes time to melt at body temperature, and should be inserted about 10 min before coitus, which is not always convenient.

The choice of spermicidal cream or gel is important. Any product approved by the International Planned Parenthood Federation, the FPA or Planned Parenthood will be reliable and will not damage rubber though in some cases slight discoloration may occur. The woman should be offered as wide a choice as possible because aesthetically intangible factors such as smell and colour as well as consistency may be favoured by one woman but repel another. The degree of self-lubrication experienced by each woman when sexually aroused will greatly influence her informed choice; one woman may feel the need for extra lubrication and choose a cream which another woman would find messy and reject in favour of a thick gel.

After use the appliance should be washed in warm water. Excess heat should be avoided; if soap is used it should be a mild, unscented variety and antiseptic solutions are unnecessary, potentially damaging to the rubber and should not be used. The device should be dried, dusted with talcum powder and replaced in its container. The user should learn to examine her own cap; at intervals it should be held up in front of a good light or filled with water to see if there are thin patches or holes. Flaws are most likely to develop near the rim of a diaphragm and if the rubber in this region becomes puckered the diaphragm needs changing. The dome should not be stretched and the woman who doesn't work in the kitchen and has long fingernails should be warned about piercing the rubber during handling. Diaphragms are not expensive and should be changed at least once per year; a new one can be bought in any pharmacy and size-standardization is reliable.

A woman beginning regular intercourse should be seen after about three months because she may then need a larger size of device. Regular users should visit their adviser annually but should be encouraged to return more often if they so wish. Women should also be seen after a pregnancy, after any pelvic operation or if they have experienced a substantial change in weight (10 lb (4.5 kg) or more). At all times there should be a willingness to answer questions and give explanations. For example, a woman may need reassurance that the appliance cannot get lost inside her, or that it will not cause infection. Some women believe that the vagina is a germ-free place and it may be useful to point out the other unsterile things that are normally placed in it. A woman may need to be told that if menstruation occurs with an appliance in place it will not do her any harm. If the woman is in the habit of douching, she should be told not to do this until the cap has been removed, and that this should not be done for a minimum of 6 h after last intercourse.

Effectiveness
Spermicides
There have been very few clinical trials of spermicides alone. Those which have been conducted show failure rates varying between 2 per hundred woman-years (HWY) and 25 per HWY.[17] More useful data are obtained from trials which compare various different methods of contraception in the same group of users. Tietze[39] and Lewitt found a pregnancy rate of 28.3 per HWY from a foam, 36.8 per HWY for jellies and creams used alone and 17.9 per HWY for diaphragms and spermicides used in the same clinics.[40]

When one considers the failure rate of spermicides used alone the motivation of the user is of paramount importance because user failure is clearly likely to be an important factor. As with the reported failure rates for condoms, risk-taking and failure to use the method with every act of intercourse explain many failures.

Foaming tablets, such as Neo Sampoon, which are compact, easy to use and resist a humid atmosphere, have found some popularity in countries such as Egypt and Bangladesh. In the latter they were associated with a pregnancy rate of 6.4 per HWY and continuation rate of approximately 70% at 12 months.[3]

Vaginal barriers
The failure rate of vaginal barriers used with a spermicide is closely related to the degree of motivation shown by the woman using it. This is

best demonstrated by the increasing effectiveness with which these methods are used within marriages as the couple approach, or exceed, what they regard as the ideal size of family. Vessey & Wiggins (1974) measured the failure rate of the diaphragm and showed that this decreased with duration of use (Table 9.1).[41, 42] The study, which was limited to married women over the age of 25 (71 000 months of exposure), gave a pregnancy rate of 2.4 per HWY. However, some other studies have given Pearl formula rates ranging from 6 to 19.6 per HWY for the diaphragm. The few studies reported from developing countries give consistently high failure rates of approximately 1 in 5 women becoming pregnant each year.[43]

Side-effects

Spermicides

Spermicides can cause local irritation but problems always resolve with discontinuation of use. Most chemicals placed in the vagina enter the systemic circulation[31] but spermicides have never been demonstrated to give rise to any adverse effects.

Jick and colleagues followed up 763 deliveries in white women in the US who had used a spermicide in the 10 months prior to conception.[14] The prevalence of major congenital abnormalities (2.2%) was slightly higher than in births to nearly 4000 women in a control group (1%). However, the data did not provide proof that the women were actually using the spermicide at the time of conception but merely that they had had a prescription for such a contraceptive during the preceding months. In addition, there was no specific type of congenital abnormality as usually occurs with a teratogenic agent. In the absence of substantiated evidence of the harmful effect of the use of spermicides no clinical action needs to be taken although no doubt additional epidemiological studies will be conducted in the future.

Table 9.1. *Use of the Diaphragm: practice makes perfect*

Duration of use (months)	Pregnancy rate (per HWY)
5–23	4.2
24–29	3.7
60 or more	1.4

Sexually transmitted diseases

In vitro tests demonstrate that the surface-active agents such as nonoxynol-9 are highly effective against *Neisseria gonorrhoea, Trichomonas vaginalis, Candida albicans* and herpes.[8] To date relatively little effort has been made to confirm these findings in clinical practice but a double-blind study using pessaries of phenylmercuric acetate, nonoxynol-9 and a placebo in 78 women exposed to the risk of gonorrhoea found a statistically significant reduction in the incidence of the disease amongst users of the two spermicides.[30] In a Louisiana clinic 10.6% of women using oral contraceptives, 9.5% of IUD users and 1.7% of cap users had a positive culture for gonorrhoea.[4]

The effectiveness of vaginal contraceptive pessaries (containing 0.4 mg phenylmercuric acetate) in protecting against gonococcal reinfection in women attending venereal disease clinics in the Florida towns of Orlando and Tampa was assessed in a prospective controlled trial, and the value of such vaginal chemoprophylaxis was clearly established[7] (Fig. 9.2). Other studies confirm this trend.[1]

Epidemiologists have suggested that if only 25% of individuals at risk of gonorrhoea used a contraceptive that was 25% effective against gonorrhoea, then the disease would be virtually eliminated within a few years.[19]

Fig. 9.2. Reduction in gonococcal reinfection in women using contraceptive pessaries of phenylmercuric acetate (Florida, US). (From Cole, C. H., Lacher, T. G., Bailey, J. C. & Fairclough, D. L. (1980). *British Journal of Venereal Diseases*, **56**, 3͡4.)

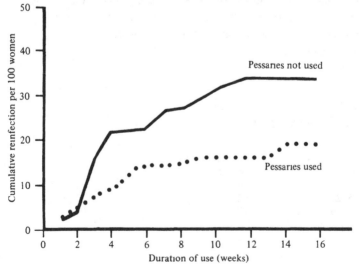

It is more difficult and expensive to study the spread of herpes infection than of gonorrhoea, but if the same protection could be achieved as occurred with gonorrhoea in Tampa, it would be even more important in view of the life-long and so far incurable nature of herpes and the possible association with carcinoma of the cervix. The partial protection offered by spermicides might also extend to Kaposi's syndrome. These findings have important public implications for the gay community and efforts are being made to market a sexual lubricant containing nonoxynol-9. A chemopro-phylactic lubricant or jelly might reduce syphilis and other infections in homosexual men, who are currently the main reservoir of this disease.

Pelvic inflammatory disease and toxic shock syndrome
Women who use barrier methods have a decreased risk of being admitted to hospital with pelvic inflammatory disease (Table 9.2).[15]

Isolated cases of toxic shock have been reported among diaphragm users,[20] but overall the use of barrier methods and a spermicide appears to lessen the risk of this exceptionally rare condition even further.[33]

Cervical cancer
The long-term use of barrier methods may reduce the risk of cervical cancer (Table 9.3).[13] Melamed at New York Planned Parenthood showed that approximately four cases of carcinoma-in-situ were diagnosed in diaphragm users every year while among Pill users there were 7–9 cases.[22] However, it is uncertain how many other variables may have been involved in the differences even though other studies have shown a similar trend.[13, 38]

Evaluation
Spermicides used alone, or with barrier contraceptive devices, not only act as contraceptives but also have a prophylactic effect against

Table 9.2. *Contrasting contraceptive practices of non-pregnant women admitted to hospital with pelvic inflammatory disease (PID) and a control group admitted for other reasons*

Declared contraceptive method	Women with PID ($n = 306$)	Control group ($n = 1175$)	Relative risk (95% confidence limits)
Spermicide	4.2%	6.0%	0.7 (0.4–1.4)
Diaphragm	4.6%	12.4%	0.4 (0.2–0.7)
Condom	10.5%	18.1%	0.6 (0.4–0.9)

sexually transmitted diseases in both sexes, and pelvic inflammatory disease decreases in women. The development and promotion of spermicides as prophylactic agents against these diseases is a recent development that shows great promise. The over-the-counter availability of spermicides in all countries fills an important need. In the US alone more than a million sexually active teenagers use no form of birth control and when shyness, fear of their parents being told or lack of access to other methods prevails, spermicides can play a significant role.

The diaphragm and cap, like the condom, are entirely harmless methods of birth control and have no medical side-effects. Compared with the condom they have the advantage of being fitted and removed remote from intercourse, but are more complicated to use. They leave the control of pregnancy entirely in the hands of the woman and are reasonably effective when carefully used. It is to be hoped that a device which fits all women will be developed for over-the-counter sale.

For some couples barrier methods are a very suitable method of spacing a family. For certain older couples who have completed their family and where early safe abortion is available and acceptable, vaginal barrier devices can be a first choice. Non-acceptance of this method may be associated with a complex of sexual taboos, such as a reluctance for a wife to be seen nude by her husband, a sense of shame at breast-feeding before others and a strong desire to check genital play in infants. To extend the last example, 9 out of 10 wives of unskilled labourers are disturbed if their children 'play with themselves' and will smack the child or try to stop the habit in some other way, whereas only a quarter of the wives of professional men try to prevent such activities.[24] It is not difficult to see that this type of attitude may be associated with a refusal on the part of the mother to use a cap, or may cause her to use it badly and inconsistently.

Sometimes clinic personnel are more enthusiastic about the diaphragm than are potential users. An anatomically perfect fit is of no value if the

Table 9.3. *Relative risk of contraceptive users developing severe cervical dysplasia*

Duration of use (years)	Barrier method (condoms or diaphragms)	Oral contraceptives
None	1.0	1.0
Less than 5	0.9	1.1
5–9	0.4	3.6
More than 10	0.2	4.0

woman has neither the inclination nor the opportunity to use the method every time she has intercourse. Objective discussion of the risk and benefits of oral contraceptives and IUD may disclose that the real reason for asking for the diaphragm is serious misinformation leading to an exaggerated fear of alternative methods.

10

Steroidal contraceptives

History

In 1775 Percival Pott operated to remove bilaterally herniated ovaries in a 23-year-old woman. He observed that she became thinner and 'her breasts, which were large, are gone; *nor has she ever menstruated since the operation*'.[274] However, the reproductive and endocrine function of the ovaries was discovered only slowly and not until 1897 did Beard suggest that the corpus luteum inhibits ovulation during pregnancy.[17] By the early twentieth century, the role of the ovaries in the sexual cycle was more fully understood, and in 1912 Fellner studied the effect of injections of ovarian extracts and showed that they promoted uterine and mammary growth. As early as 1921, the Austrian physiologist Ludwig Haberlandt explored the possibility of what he called 'hormonal sterilization'. Ovaries from pregnant does were transplanted into non-pregnant rabbits, rendering them infertile for several months, and in 1931 he wrote: 'It needs no amplification, of all methods available, hormonal sterilization based on biological principles, if it can be applied unobjectionably in the human, is an ideal method for practical medicine and its future task of birth control.'[115, 116]

For this vision to be fulfilled, several scientific and commercial steps had to be taken. The isolation of ovarian hormones and the role of the pituitary in controlling their output was fully elucidated in the 1920s and 1930s. Hartman (1932) suggested to a colleague that 'amniotin', a preparation of oestrogens from bovine amniotic fluid, might be used as a contraceptive. In 1936 MacCorquodale, Thayer and Doisy extracted 25 mg of pure crystalline 17β-oestradiol from four tons of sows' ovaries[171] and in 1940 Sturgis and Albright reported on the use of oestrogen to inhibit ovulation in order to relieve dysmenorrhoea.[293]

In the 1930s Japanese scientists isolated a compound called diosgenin from the sweet potato, or yam, and the next important step in developing cheap sources of hormones occurred in 1941, when Marker used diosgenin as a starting-point in the synthesis of steroids. Two years later he offered his skills to a commercial organization in Mexico which was to become the Syntex Corporation. The impact of his invention can be gauged by the fact that Marker presented, as his credentials, two jars filled with four and a half pounds of progesterone, which were worth about US $160 000 at the then market price. By 1950 steroid hormones were available at one-hundredth the price a decade previously.[233] Djerassi and his colleagues at Syntex went on to synthesize norethisterone, known as norethindrone in the US, which proved to be a most potent oral progestogen.[9] By 1945 Albright, at Harvard, had foreseen a potential use for orally active steroids beyond the narrow confines of gynaecology. He wrote: 'Since preventing ovulation prevents pregnancy, one could employ the same principles in birth control as in preventing dysmenorrhoea.'[5]

It took the drive of Margaret Sanger, then over 70 years old, and the philanthropy of Mrs Page McCormick of the family that owned International Harvester, to develop the first oral contraceptive. With a grant of US $115 000, Gregory Pincus and M. C. Chang of the Worcester Foundation together with the Catholic Boston obstetrician John Rock, began systematic experiments in animals which led to the first human trial of 19 norsteroids, the results of which were published in 1956.[242] Early studies were conducted in Puerto Rico, Los Angeles and Haiti. A satisfactory contraceptive effect was obtained but menstruation was irregular and in order to control this 'breakthrough bleeding' an oestrogen was added. In June 1960 the Searle Company marketed the first oral contraceptive, Enavid, a combination of norethynodrel and mestranol. The first British clinics began using the Pill in January 1962. In 1963 the Wyeth company achieved the total synthesis of norgestrel.

With the luxury of historical hindsight, the original Food and Drug Administration (FDA) approval of Enavid, which was based on a study involving only 132 women, has been criticized. But it should be remembered that when the Pill was developed governments did not support contraceptive research and that national drug regulations had not evolved in any area, least of all that of steroids. Finally, a drug which could, and perhaps should, have been a triumph of biology and pharmacology in the 1940s, was coaxed from a somewhat reluctant scientific community in the 1950s and began its widespread use in the 1960s under the control of a medical profession that was still deeply ambivalent about contraception. As early as 1961 the study of nearly 10 000 Pill users and users of barrier methods was launched but the logistics of such a large trial were not fully understood and long-term funding proved irregular.[232] Without doubt, it was the strong desire of the consumer for something better and less frustrating than messy diaphragms and uncertain condoms which catapulted oral contraceptives into widespread use in the 1960s and made the very word 'pill' gain a new significance in the language as well as in the lives of women.[147]

Production of bulk steroids is concentrated in relatively few firms in Europe, the US and Mexico, but prices remain competitive. Most of the patents on synthetic steroids were taken out in the decade following the registration of the first progestogen in 1953 and many have now expired. When millions of cycles are purchased for international programmes, a price of less than 20 US cents a cycle (1981) is possible. China[81] and Mexico are the only developing countries with the full capability to manufacture steroidal contraceptives while many developed countries such as Russia and Japan are still unable to do so.

Although the manufacture of oral contraceptives is one of the most complex modern industrial processes to be found anywhere, the total amounts of steroid involved are small. One tonne will meet the needs of five million women for a year. In the mid-1970s Mexico nationalized diosgenin production and raised the price by a factor of two and a half, but, unlike that of OPEC, this was a price rise that technology could circumvent and production rapidly turned to total synthesis and the use of other biological starting materials; as a result the Mexican share of current world production is small.[82] The problem in the 1980s may be to find international funds to subsidize the price for millions of very poor women who will wish to use oral contraceptives in the next 20 years in economically backward countries.

Natural and artificial steroids

All steroids have a common nucleus or ring, which is shared with cholesterol. The usual textbook method of illustrating the carbon skeleton molecule obscures its true three-dimensional structure (Fig. 10.1). Different steroid compounds can be obtained by substitutions of hydrogen atoms and side chains projecting above or below the plane of the ring and these compounds have different biological actions.

The sex steroids control reproduction and sexual differentiation, influence behaviour and are produced by the gonads, adrenal cortex and placenta. They are bound to specific protein receptors in certain areas of the brain and transported to the cell nucleus of target organs. Here protein synthesis is initiated and these proteins, in turn, become transmitters and receptors and the sources of cell differentiation. In addition to the output of steroids from endocrine sources, steroid production takes place through the conversion of androstenedione to oestrone and oestriol in fatty tissues. Natural steroids, when transported in the blood stream, are bound strongly to the sex hormone-binding globulin, but artificial steroids, with the exception of norgestrel, are bound weakly or not at all. The same metabolic pathways for hormone production occur in both sexes, although the relative proportions of hormones vary greatly. It is therefore a misleading

Fig. 10.1. Steroidal molecules.

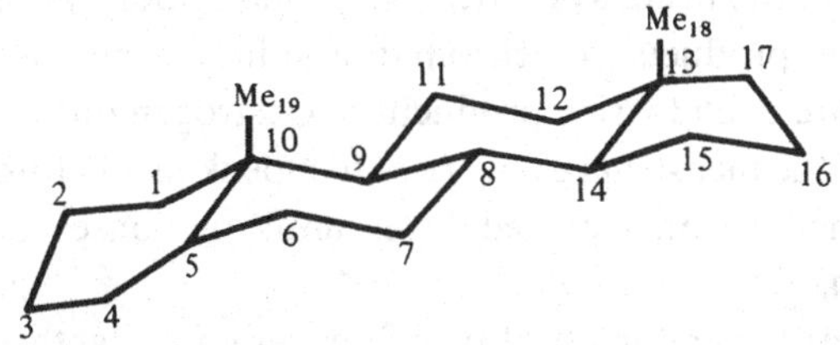

Three-dimensional representation
(Me is CH₃)

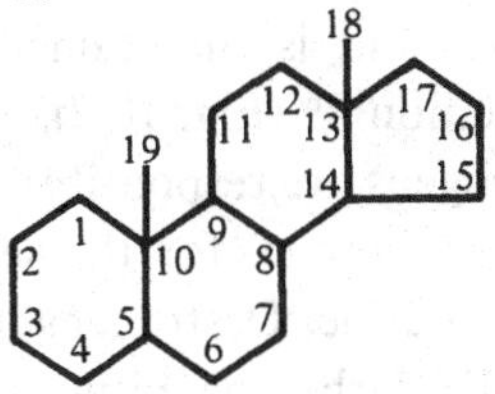

Conventional representation

Steroid nucleus

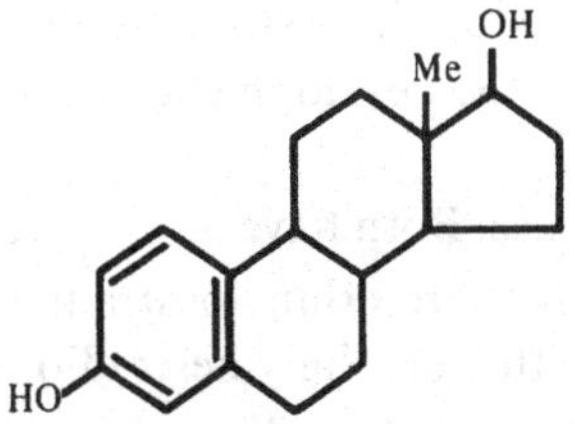

17β-oestradiol
(natural)

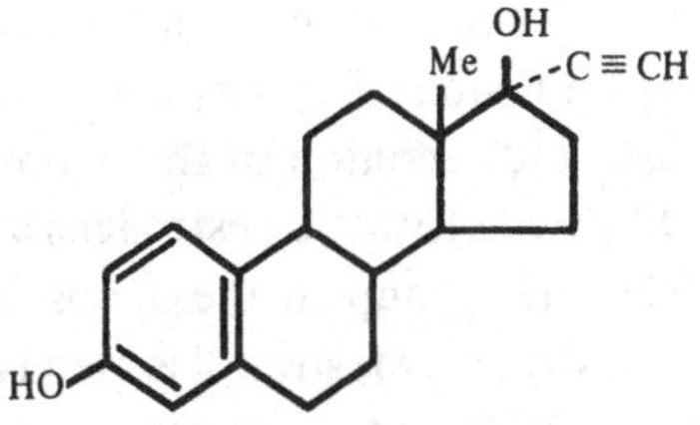

Ethinyl oestradiol
(synthetic)

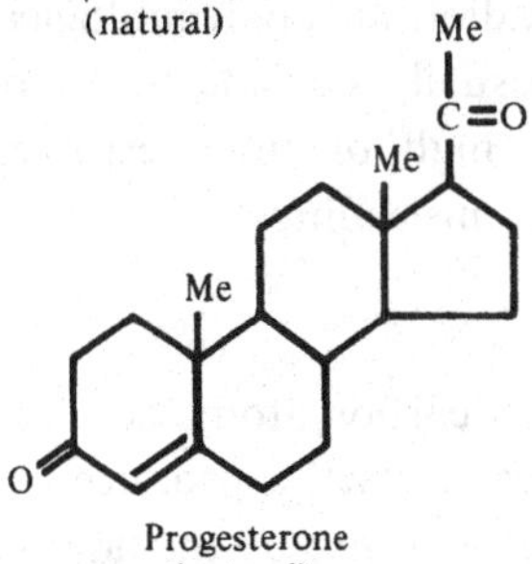

Progesterone
(natural)

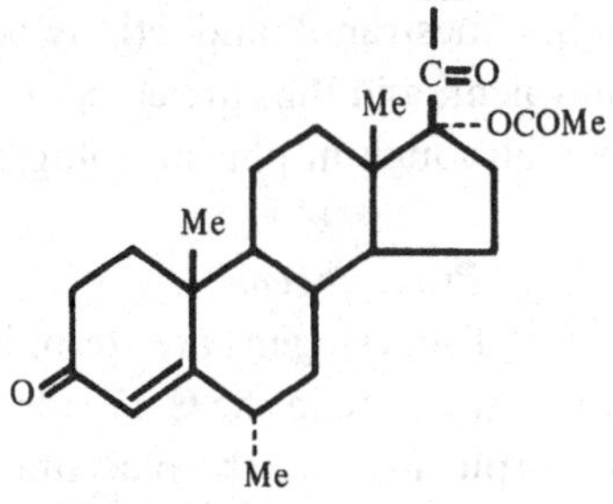

Medroxyprogesterone acetate
(synthetic)

simplification to think of oestrogen and progesterone as 'female hormones' and testosterone as the 'male hormone'.

Oestrogens

Oestrogens are steroids with 18 or 19 carbon atoms and 17β-oestradiol is the commonest oestrogen produced by the ovary. Oestrogens are conjugated by the liver to water-soluble sulphates and glucuronides which are excreted partly in free form and partly as sulphate esters in the urine. Some of the conjugates excreted by the liver in the bile are broken down by bacteria in the gut and reabsorbed again. About 20% of the total oestrogens secreted appear in the urine as oestriol, oestrone or oestradiol and measurement of these products by chromatographic techniques provides the simplest measure of endocrine production. Oestrogen output is lowest in the first week of the menstrual cycle, rises to a peak just before ovulation and is maintained at an elevated level until the onset of menstruation[286] (Fig. 10.2).

Oestrogens are responsible for endometrial proliferation and, together with progesterone, for the secretory changes in the second half of the menstrual cycle. Oestrogens inhibit secretion of follicle-stimulating hormone (FSH) by the pituitary but stimulate the release of luteinizing hormone (LH). These effects are mediated by the hypothalamus through the pituitary portal system. Oestrogens cause sodium, chloride and water retention but, unlike androgens, have little effect on nitrogen metabolism. The concentration of cholesterol in the α-lipoprotein fraction of plasma is increased and that in the β-lipoprotein fraction reduced. Oestrogens also promote fusion of epiphysial cartilage and cause the development of the breasts and secretion in the mammary ducts.

Only two synthetic oestrogens are in common use. Both have an ethinyl ($-C=CH$) group in the α position at C-17; they are ethinyloestradiol and mestranol. Mestranol is merely the 3-methyl ether of ethinyloestradiol; it is metabolized to the latter compound after absorption, and is only half as potent, weight for weight, as ethinyloestradiol. In epidemiological studies mestranol and ethinyloestradiol are usually considered to be equivalent, and Pills are categorized as being of 'high' or 'low' oestrogen dose, although in pharmacological terms this is misleading.

Progestogens

Progestogens are steroids with at least 21 carbon atoms of which two or more are in the C-17 side chain. Progesterone itself is produced by the corpus luteum, the placenta and, in minute quantity, by the adrenal cortex. It is the only naturally occurring progestogen found in the peripheral blood. It is produced in much larger quantities than the oestrogens and a total of up to 30 mg a day is manufactured in the corpus luteum in the second half of the normal cycle. During pregnancy plasma levels rise to several milligrams per 100 ml.

Progestational agents inhibit the pituitary secretion of gonadotrophins. As oestrogen-primed human endometrium will increase in thickness to maximum of 5–7 mm and its glands become tortuous and distended with a secretion rich in glycogen, the stroma becomes oedematous and the spiral arteries develop to their fullest extent. Menstruation normally occurs from an endometrium which has undergone such progestationally-induced

Fig. 10.2. Variation of hormone blood levels during the menstrual cycle. The hatched areas show the duration of the menses. (After Shearman, R. P. (Ed.) (1979). *Human Reproductive Physiology.* Oxford: Blackwell Scientific Publications.)

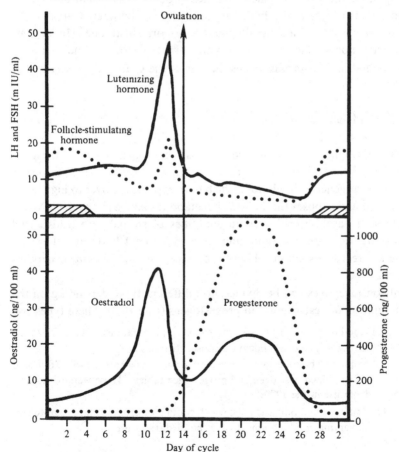

growth. Progesterone stimulates the formation of alveoli in the breast but outside the reproductive system it has fewer general effects than oestrogen.

Natural progesterone is a fragile molecule and its half-life in the blood is only 4 min. Its metabolite, pregnanediol, causes an increase in basal metabolic rate and is responsible for the rise in basal body temperature that occurs in the second half of the ovulatory cycle. Ten to twenty per cent of ovarian progesterone appears in the urine as pregnanediol.

Biological properties cannot always be predicted from the structural formula.[279] One group of artificial steroids is related to 17α- hydroxy-progesterone and methyl- and chloro- substitutions on C-6 in the steroid ring greatly increase the half-life in the serum and generate potent compounds which have a powerful proliferative effect on the endometrium. The second set of steroids is derived by substitution of the methyl group present in progesterone on C-19 by an ethinyl group. Most of these compounds show oestrogenic properties, probably as a result of metabolism to oestrogen in the body. A double bond between C-4 and C-5 makes them structurally analogous to 19-nortestosterone. (In organic chemistry nor stands for the German phrase Nitrogen ohne (without) radical and in the steroids means the loss of the C-19 methyl attached to C-10.)

Administration

Artificial steroids can be taken orally, given parenterally, absorbed through the vagina or even administered as an aerosol into the nasal cavity.[120] When given orally, they must pass through the liver before reaching the general circulation, which both exposes the liver to high levels of steroid and exposes the steroid to metabolic change in the liver. When given as a nasal aerosol, minute quantities of steroids are transported across the cribriform plate and enter the cerebrospinal fluid where they may have a direct but short-lived action on receptors in the central nervous system.

Oral contraceptives can be divided into different types depending on the combination of oestrogens and progestogens (Fig. 10.3). These types are:

(a) Combined oestrogen and progestogen preparations, where 21 or 22 identical tablets are taken on consecutive days.

(b) Sequential preparations, which used to contain oestrogen tablets followed by combined oestrogen and progestogen tablets. These were withdrawn from use in the 1970s.

(c) Triphasic and biphasic pills, which contain oestrogens and progestogens in varying combinations during the 21 days of use.

Fig. 10.3. The changing composition of contraceptive pills. Pill composition drawn to scale. (Open blocks, progestogen; filled blocks, oestrogen.)

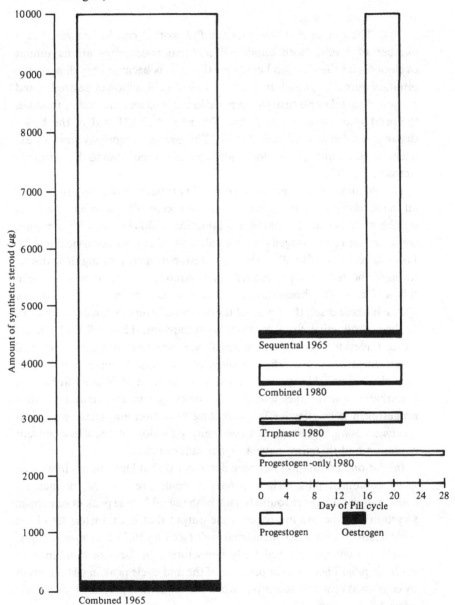

(d) Progestogen-only pills, which give the same daily dose of progestogen and are taken continuously.

Mode of action

The question 'How does the Pill work?' can be answered at a number of levels. Both combined and triphasic preparations inhibit ovulation and there is good evidence that this is because they depress the pituitary output of gonadotrophins. The feed-back action of oestrogen and progesterone takes place at the hypothalamic level and inhibits or modifies the production of releasing factors for FSH and LH and of the hypo-thalamic prolactin-inhibiting factor. The ovarian responsiveness to ex-ogenous gonadotrophins does not appear to be altered by artificial steroids.

The combined oral contraceptives modify tubal contractions and would affect the transport of an egg if ovulation did occur. They also have an effect on the endometrium, making implantation unlikely. In addition both combined and progestogen-only pills alter the character of cervical mucus. Progestogens may also affect the capacitation of sperm during their transit through the female reproductive tract. Among women who have been followed carefully, breakthrough ovulation occurs in about 2–10% of cycles. In these cases, the action of the combined preparation on other links in the reproductive chain is probably important. The ability of combi-nation tablets to make assurance doubly sure accounts for their exceptional effectiveness; very few pharmacological compounds have such a pre-dictable and reliable quality as the Pill. Modern Pills are effective at remarkably low dosages and 30μg of oestrogen in combination with a progestogen is as effective in preventing ovulation and altering cervical mucus as 50μg.[51] The progestogen-only pills do not regularly prevent ovulation and therefore have a higher failure rate.

Inhibition of ovulation has been demonstrated at laparotomy in women using combined pills. When urinary steroids are assayed, women on combination tablets are found to lack both the mid-cycle peak of oestrogen secretion and the rise in progesterone output that is characteristic of the second half of the normal menstrual cycle (see Fig. 10.2). Correspondingly, there is no change in basal body temperature in users of combined or triphasic pills. There is a suppression of the mid-cycle peak in LH secretion by combined oral contraceptives while the sequential preparations mainly affect FSH output.

One of the few studies that has been done to measure serum oestradiol in women using combined oral contraceptives observed levels corresponding to those found in the early follicular phase of the normal ovulatory cycle, which are somewhat higher than those found in the postmenopausal woman.[196] Exogenous oestrogens from the oral contraceptives themselves probably compensate for any deleterious effects which might arise from the relatively low level of ovarian output.

Variations in the absorption of exogenous steroids, the variety of metabolic pathways to which they are exposed, differences in patterns of transport and secretion, the interrelations of the feed-back between the ovary and the hypothalamus and pituitary, the reduction but not the elimination of endogenous secretion in the presence of exogenous contraceptive steroids, the fact that the actions of progestogens are modified by preceding exposure to oestrogens and the added complexity that, in appropriate doses, oestrogens and progestogens act synergistically, all make the pharmokinetics of contraceptive steroids a subject of great complexity. Some important questions remain unanswered, particularly in relation to metabolism.

Assessment

Pills are used by at least 50 million women, who range from those living in Chinese communes, through those living in the worst slums of Calcutta to those who constitute the elite of San Paulo or Stockholm. The information on which those who use the Pill and those who provide it make their decisions comes from a variety of sources, including highly sophisticated biochemical measurements, complex epidemiological studies and the crudest empiricism. Some occurrences of great rarity, such as an increased incidence of liver hepatocellular adenomas among users, are known with some accuracy, while facts as basic as why women do not fall pregnant during the week in which they stop steroids in order to have uterine bleeding remain difficult to explain.

Animal studies must be extrapolated with great caution to the human situation because of marked species differences in the physiology of reproduction. Does medroxyprogesterone acetate masculinize the human fetus if it has this effect in the rat? Does depomedroxyprogesterone acetate cause tumours of the breast in women because it does in beagle dogs? We have no evidence to suggest that either fear is justified but students of logic will appreciate the difficulty in proving a negative.

The literature on clinical studies is abundant but not always informative. Most short-term clinical trials of steroidal contraceptives have been on individual brands and it is difficult, if not impossible, to compare studies conducted at one centre with a specific Pill and on a particular population with another study on the same or a different Pill at another centre.[123] The side-effects reported by different authors for the same preparation vary widely (Table 10.1). In contrast to clinical trials, epidemiological studies are usually forced to lump all Pills together, often without taking dose or content into account. To compound these problems, it has been demonstrated that doctors prescribing oral contraceptives commonly make decisions based on the promotional material they have received rather than on the careful evaluation of clinical trials.[105]

Double-blind crossover trials, in which women switch from three or six months' use of one brand of the Pill to another, according to a random system of allocation, are difficult to conduct but are the most objective way of uncovering pharmacological differences between brands. It appears that whenever a woman changes from one brand to another there is an upsurge in side-effects, probably reflecting the time that it takes for liver enzymes to adapt to the new exogenous steroids, but studies have shown little demonstrable difference in clinical performance between different brands of Pill.[205, 239, 298]

While competition between manufacturers has led to important innovations, such as lower-dose Pills, the lack of difference between brands found in the few crossover trials which have been completed, inevitably casts doubt on some of the claims made by manufacturers on the basis of the large number of trials of individual brands.

When it comes to the study of certain short-term common side-effects, such as weight gain, then the use of placebos is likely to provide the most objective data, but for the obvious reason that the woman may get pregnant, this can only be done if volunteers are sterilized or prepared to

Table 10.1. *Side-effects reported by different authors for the same combined pill (4 mg norethisterone acetate and 0.05 mg ethyinyl oestradiol)*

Side-effect	Percentage of users experiencing side-effect	
	Lowest	Highest
First-cycle nausea	1.2	25.0
Breast discomfort	1.8	13.0
Weight gain (3 lbs (1.36 kg) or more)	1.5	54.0
Menstrual spotting	3.0	17.0
Breakthrough bleeding	2.1	5.2
Amenorrhoea	0.8	3.6

Source: Jeffery, J. d'A. & Klopper, A. I. (1968). *Journal of Reproduction and Fertility*, Supplement **4**.

use a barrier method. When such a trial was conducted, no difference was detected between various combination pills and a placebo in relation to weight gain.[106] In 1959 Pincus and his co-workers carried out a small-scale trial with three groups of women who used mechanical contraceptives and an oral tablet concurrently; one group was given a placebo, one group was given oral contraceptives without warning of possible side-effects and the third group was given the Pill and an explanation of possible reactions.[221] Those who had received the Pill without prior explanation had least side-effects (6.3%), while those on the placebo or receiving the Pill knowing about possible complications had most complaints (17.1% and 23.5% respectively). Today, most women in the developing as well as the developed world are well briefed about possible side-effects and it is now difficult or impossible to obtain objective information about certain aspects of oral contraceptives.

In the study of long-term rare but serious side-effects, many case-control retrospective studies and several cohort studies have been carried out (see Chapter 4). It needs to be emphasized once again that case-control retrospective studies can be carried out on relatively small numbers to help to confirm or refute clinical suspicions that relate certain diseases to the use of steroidal contraceptives. The validity of a study depends on the accuracy with which cases and controls are matched. For example, women who use the Pill often also smoke, and this itself can predispose to cardiovascular disease.

A number of important prospective studies of Pill users and non-users have been set up. Again, appropriate matching of cases and controls is important. In 1968 the Royal College of General Practitioners (RCGP) in Britain initiated a prospective study of more than 23 000 Pill users compared with approximately the same number of non-users. One thousand four hundred general practitioners notified the study co-ordinators every time that a woman attended her own physician or was referred to a hospital for in- or out-patient care. Well over 60 000 woman-years of oral contraceptive use have been followed, and all types of medical events, from excessive earache to cerebrovascular stroke were recorded and analyzed.[248–56] In the same year, Vessey at Oxford University launched a collaborative study with the Family Planning Association (FPA) to follow over 17 000 women using oral contraceptives (56%), IUDs and diaphragms. More than 50 000 woman-years of experience of Pill usage have now been accumulated.[310, 313, 314] The British tradition of the family practitioner, the existence of the National Health Service which provides free and comprehensive medical care and the compact nature of the country have made it easier to overcome the numerous logistic difficulties of large-scale prospective studies in Britain than in the United States. However, the Kaiser Permanente Health Insurance Scheme in California has provided a suitable base for such a study. In this insurance network, members have an examination on entering and all the records are cross-linked and computerized. Beginning in 1968, a prospective study on a total of 16 579 women was carried out and experience of approximately 65 000 woman-years of Pill use was accumulated.[236-8] The Walnut Creek area chosen for the study is a white middle-class area of California and the oral contraceptive users turned out on average to be taller, more physically active, more likely to smoke or drink moderately (although not more likely to be heavy smokers or heavy drinkers), to sunbathe more frequently, to have initiated sex earlier and to have had more partners than non-users. The study cost US $8.5 million over the 12 years of observation. Two studies were also carried out in the Boston area, partly using telephone interviews and hospital records. The larger involved nearly 20 000 Pill users and 46 000 non-users.[33] In Australia, 1370 Pill users were compared with 1253 non-users.[113]

The problems of assessing steroid use are legion. It is more difficult to study beneficial than adverse relations: the death that does *not* take place as a result of some protective effect is not as easily recognized as the one that is clearly correlated with Pill use. Most epidemiological studies include disproportionally fewer young women than are normally found amongst users, because the unmarried are difficult to follow in long-term prospective studies. It takes several years to design, finance, execute and publish an epidemiological study and the information which we have today invariably refers to yesterday's contraceptives. It should also be noted that the available epidemiological evidence relates almost exclusively to combined pills, with little or no data on progestogen-only pills. It will be many years, if ever, before triphasic pills are evaluated in anything except short-term clinical trials. It must also be emphasized that practically all the epidemiological data on oral contraceptives come from Europe and the United States. The World Health Organization (WHO) is conducting case-control studies on steroidal contraceptives and possible malignancy in a number of developing countries. The International Fertility Research Program has launched two studies of Reproductive Age Mortality Surveillance (RAMOS) with the intention of detecting some of the overall risks and benefits of using modern contraceptives in societies which have poor access to modern medical care.[134] When extrapolating western data to the developing world, it is imperative to remember the very much higher risk of maternal mortality (in the RAMOS studies about a quarter of all deaths of women aged 15–50 are pregnancy related) and the different patterns of disease (e.g. the high incidence of liver disease) in many developing countries. Ethnic differences may be important and Goldzieher has demonstrated that the metabolism of steroids differs between Nigerian slum dwellers and average American women.[107]

Scientific publications relating to the risk of steroidal contraception have been given wide publicity, largely according to the journalistic rule that good news is no news but bad news sells. There have been panic flights from the Pill on a number of occasions with many resultant unwanted pregnancies and otherwise avoidable misery.

In the western world, and especially in the United States, both the public and the medical profession have read the flow of publicity related to oral contraceptives in an increasingly pessimistic way.[141] Between 1976 and 1979 the number of American women using Pills fell from 9.1 million to 6.7 million.[259] Among women aged 20–24 there was a 12% decline in use and among those aged 35–39, a 52% fall. In Britain Pill use peaked at 3.4 million in 1976 and fell to 2.8 million in 1979; it then rose marginally, possibly because of the marketing of triphasic pills.

Has this overall flight from oral contraceptive use been justified and how does the Pill stand after 20 years of use and strong public medical scrutiny?

ORAL CONTRACEPTIVES

Preparations

Combined pills remain overwhelmingly the most commonly used. Many comprehensive reviews of combined pills have been published, [84, 102, 163, 225–30, 296] and *Population Reports* monitors the relevant literature regularly. Twenty-one identical tablets containing an oestrogen and progestogen are taken for three weeks followed by a break of seven days during which the withdrawal of exogenous hormones usually results in uterine bleeding. In China, 22 days of active Pills with six days off is the more common regime.

Pills are packaged in blister packs, which often also include seven vitamin, iron or placebo tablets, and are conveniently marked with the days of the week, something which allows the woman to check at once whether she did or did not take yesterday's Pill.

Most women find no difficulty in taking the Pill. It is easiest to remember the tablets if some regular time of day is chosen to take them. This is particularly important for progestogen-only pills.

Use of combined tablets can be started either on the first day of bleeding or day 5 of the cycle (see below). One tablet is taken daily until the packet is finished. If a woman forgets a tablet she must take it as soon as she remembers the omission and the next day's tablet should be taken at the normal time: this usually means she will have missed one day and taken two tablets in the course of the next day. Ideally, additional contraceptive precautions should be taken until the end of the cycle, but the very woman who forgets her Pills is often the one least likely to follow this advice. At the end of the course of combined tablets the woman must wait SEVEN days and begin the next packet regardless of the time of onset of menstruation.

If breakthrough bleeding occurs the woman should continue the medication. If a full period occurs she should stop taking the tablets and begin the next packet five days after the bleeding began.

Care should be taken when changing from one type of preparation to another because when changing to a preparation with lower oestrogen dosage, additional contraceptive precautions are advisable.

The effect of oral contraceptives on vitamins has been studied more than it deserves in developed countries and less than is truly needed in developing countries. A depletion of B_6 (pyridoxine) and B_2 (riboflavin) and folic acid has been described in Pill users as well as a rise in the mean serum vitamin A level.[336] The link between biochemical findings and clinical consequences is uncertain and the case for adding vitamins to the Pill pack is weak. Studies in Sri Lanka have demonstrated that vitamins do not influence continuation rates in the Third World.[193]

Conventionally, women taking oral contraceptives are instructed to begin on the fifth day after menstrual bleeding commences. In order to eliminate the risk of early ovulation and possible pregnancy in the first cycle, the user is sometimes advised to take additional contraceptive precautions when taking the first packet of pills. In practice it is easier to remember to begin oral contraceptive usage on the first day of bleeding and such instructions have the additional advantage of making sure that the ovulation due in the initial cycle is suppressed. The fact that the first cycle is a few days shorter than subsequent ones does not cause any problems and this regime has now become the standard instruction given by the British FPA. The manufacturers, largely because of the inertia of the drug regulatory authorities, still print package inserts instructing the first tablet to be taken on the fifth day of the cycle. In developing countries, it is easier to tell the woman to start on the first day of menstrual bleeding, but if there is already widespread use in a country, it can be confusing to have two apparently competing sets of instructions.

On the whole, the use of oral contraceptives has been dominated by a desire to imitate what is perceived to be 'normal' physiology rather than by consideration of social factors and user convenience. When a woman uses oral contraceptives she protects herself against pregnancy and gives herself extensive control over her pattern of uterine bleeding. The bleeding which occurs when a woman is on the Pill is a response to oestrogen withdrawal and physiologically quite unlike a normal menstruation and there is no 'ghost' pituitary cycle that continues while combined pills are in use. Therefore a user can choose, if she so wishes, to alter her pattern of uterine bleeding. Loudon *et al.* conducted trials with so-called 'tricycle pills' and found that there was no increase in breakthrough bleeding, nor was there delay in the return of uterine bleeding after 63 days of continuous Pill taking.[170] Therefore when there are personal reasons for delaying a period by taking tablets for more than 21 days, this is a safe and responsible procedure. Women who choose to have four rather than 13 episodes of bleeding a year will, however, ingest in aggregate more exogenous hormones.

In traditional societies, menstruation is often regarded in a negative way. For example, Moslem women cannot pray in the mosque, keep the fast of Ramadan, or, if on a pilgrimage to Mecca, visit the Holy places during menstruation and some Hindus are not supposed to cook their husbands' food at this time. Thus many unexploited ways of presenting oral contraceptives in a socially positive manner still exist. In the Indian subcontinent the astrologer commonly fixes the date of a wedding, and the young bride may find the use of the Pill helpful in altering the timing of menstruation.

The biggest difference in continuation rates for oral contraceptives does not lie between Pills of differing pharmacology, but in the way in which the same Pill is distributed. Siassi found in Iran that women given the Pill only had a 12% continuation rate six months after starting but when, in this male-dominated society, men in the same group were given oral contraceptives to pass on to their wives, more than 90% were still using them six months later (Figure 10.4).[276]

The dose of combined pills has fallen dramatically from a high of 10 mg of progestogen per tablet (OrthoNovum, 1962) to 1 mg in many contemporary preparations and from 1 mg of oestrogen (Enavid, 1964) to as little as 0.02 mg. Combined preparations with 0.03 mg (30 μg) of oestrogen first began to be widely used in Europe in 1970–74.

With two exceptions, the changes and possible improvements in oral contraception since the late 1960s have all been in the direction of lowering the dose. However, the introduction of triphasic pills in Europe (and of biphasic pills in the US) is an effort to mimic the hormonal changes of the menstrual cycle more closely and to achieve adequate fertility control with the minimum cumulative dose of steroids.[159] Triphasic pills are more complex to make than simple combined pills and are more expensive. In the 1980s, in Europe, the Organon company introduced desogestrel (0.15 mg) as a combination pill with ethinyloestradiol (0.03 mg) (Marvelon). Desogestrel is associated with a rise in high-density lipoproteins and long-term use could be associated with a reduced risk of cardiovascular disease, both in relation to other contraceptive steroids and perhaps even in absolute terms.[78, 318, 321] Desogestrel is also thought to reduce androgenic side-effects, such as weight gain and hirsutism. Neither triphasic pills nor desogestrel have been in use long enough provide any epidemiological data to confirm or refute the biological and clinical claims that may be reasonably made about them.

Most of a contraceptive pill consists of a filler designed to make it big enough to handle and not get lost if dropped in the fluff under the bed. The equal dispersion of the small quantities of hormone in each tablet requires careful quality control. The FDA allows an 8% variation in the content of a pharmaceutical tablet. While this may be tolerable in the case of antibiotics, most manufacturers set their limits at a 2% variation. It

Fig. 10.4. Continuation rate for oral contraceptives distributed to Iranian women (♀) and to men (♂) to pass on to their wives. (Redrawn from Siassi, I. (1972). The psychiatrist's role in family planning. *American Journal of Psychiatry*, **129**, 48.)

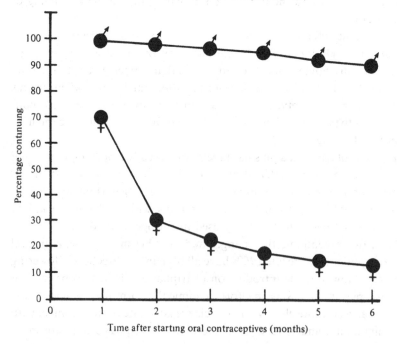

requires high levels of quality control to achieve such accuracy and this is one reason, in addition to low cost, why it is a wise policy to concentrate the manufacture of oral contraceptives in a few places around the world. The Chinese have tried to circumvent some of the technical problems associated with oral contraceptive manufacture by dipping carboxymethylcellulose paper in hormone solution and then drying the stamps as a 'paper pill'.[75]

Effectiveness

Steroidal contraceptives provide the only method of contraception which to all intents and purposes is completely effective and fully reversible. Indeed it is so effective that it is difficult to measure accurately the few failures that do occur. Few if any trials contain sufficient number of women to arrive at statistically significant conclusions. Supposing a contraceptive had a biological failure rate of 0.08 per hundred woman-years (HWY) of use (and the Pill seems to approach this level) and supposing, *ex hypothesis*, another preparation had twice the biological failure rate and if, as seems reasonable, it is assumed that 90% of pregnancies are due to mistakes in Pill taking, then a minimum of 2.4 million cycles of treatment would be required to detect the difference.[123] Clearly, no study can handle this many cases.

In the 1960s, Drill found a failure rate of 0.028 per HWY in over 116 000 cycles of use of the high-dose, original combined pill Enavid. Preparations containing 30–35 μg of ethinyloestradiol appear to have approximately the same failure rate as those containing 50 μg, but WHO studies suggest that when the dose is lowered to 20 μg, the failure rate rises.

Most failures are due to incorrect use, but fortunately the method is relatively tolerant of occasional mistakes. Some errors in tablet taking probably arise in at least 1 in 10 cycles. In about half of these cases a forgotten tablet is made good later, but in the remainder tablets are omitted altogether for more than one day. If 1–5 Pills are omitted, a pregnancy rate of about 2 to 3 per HWY occurs, and if 6 or more Pills are omitted, the rate jumps to as high as 40.

In some developing countries, pregnancy rates are considerably higher than in the West. However, certain traditional societies have found ingenious ways to reinforce regular Pill taking; in some Indonesian villages the temple gong is sounded daily to remind villagers to take their Pill and among the *Inglesea ni Cristo* Protestant group in the Philippines Pill packets are actually distributed after the Sunday service and at the Thursday prayer meeting.

The progestogen-only pill and some combined pills with low oestrogen doses are probably less tolerant of errors in tablet taking than the conventional combined pill. It seems likely that this may also be the case with the triphasic pill.

Oral contraceptives and physiology

Natural steroid hormones bring about widespread sustained and cyclical changes in adult women. Not surprisingly, the giving of exogenous hormones for prolonged intervals to regulate fertility also brings about extensive changes in the user's physiology.

In the small hunting and food-gathering communities in which the final stages of human evolution took place, there is some evidence that pregnancy intervals were extended for up to 3–4 years and were associated with long periods of lactation-induced amenorrhoea. Menstruation that is repeated perhaps several hundred times without interruption is an artefact of modern living. There is much that is artificial about the use of steroidal contraceptives, but failure to appreciate the above fact, by both the medical profession and educated users, has generated more fear of, and controversy over, oral contraceptives than there need have been.

The rapid return of normal pituitary function after prolonged use of oral contraceptives suggests that the integrity of the pituitary is not threatened by prolonged suppression of ovulation. No alteration in pituitary weight has been reported in monkeys on oral contraceptives. Secondary amenorrhoea following oral contraception is discussed later (see under Subsequent fertility). There is no evidence that oral contraceptives alter the pituitary at puberty or the menopause, although more data about the effects of artificial steroids in the early years immediately after the menarche would be useful. As oestrogen promotes closure of the epiphyses, the Pill could prevent a young girl reaching her full stature: oestrogens are sometimes used therapeutically for this purpose.

The ovaries of women using combined pills (or injectables) appear macroscopically to be like those of postmenopausal women, and, with rare exceptions, lack corpora lutea. Histologically there are no mature follicles and the tunica may be thickened; however, the ovarian response to gonadotrophin stimulation appears to be unchanged. The number of atretic follicles appears to be normal and there is no suggestion on the grounds of ovarian morphology or clinical observation that Pill use alters the time of the menopause.[289]

Oral contraceptives affect tubal motility. With combined tablets the endometrial glands are rapidly transformed through the proliferative phase so that the secretory phase, normally fully developed by days 19–20, occurs within a few days of commencing the tablets. The endometrium is hypoplastic and pseudo-decidual changes occur in the stromal tissue. With triphasic therapy the endometrial changes approximate more closely to those of a regular cycle. There is a rapid return to normal cyclical histological changes after the cessation of oral contraceptives.

Prolonged administration of norsteroids has no effect on adrenal histology but the oestrogens in oral contraceptives do cause an increase in the level of transcortin (corticosteroid-binding globulin), which leads to a raised level of total aldosterone. This appears to be unassociated with any increase in aldosterone output, although it may be responsible for changes in plasma pyruvate.

As in the case of the adrenal, oral contraceptives also cause alterations in the plasma carriage of thyroxine. The level of thyroxine-binding globulin rises during oral contraceptive use and as a consequence, protein-bound iodine increases from approximately 5 μg to 7–8 μg per 100 ml. This change is independent of dosage, is not progressive, returns to normal when the contraceptive is discontinued and has no demonstrable effect on overall physiology. Radiothyroid uptake is unaltered in oral contraceptive users, although changes in protein-bound iodine can lead to misinterpretation of clinical tests of thyroid function. Radio-iodine uptake and secretion give valid results in women on steroidal contraceptives but the resin uptake of labelled triiodothyronine and protein-bound iodine tests should not be done on anyone who has taken oral contraceptives within the previous six weeks. There is no evidence that long-term oral contraceptive use affects the pattern of thyroid disease.

Oral contraceptives, like pregnancy, and to a lesser extent the menopause, are associated with a wide range of metabolic changes. Not all of these changes are localized in the liver, but it is the organ predominantly involved.[4, 282] To date, up to 150 individual metabolic parameters have been measured and been shown to change when a woman takes the Pill, but the clinical significance, if any, of many of the alterations is difficult to interpret. The liver is the main source of serum proteins, with the exception of the α-globulins which are produced in the reticuloendothelial system. The cephalin flocculation and thymol turbidity tests (which reflect any imbalance in the serum proteins) and the serum bilirubin and alkaline phosphatase levels (which rise during biliary obstruction and hepatocellular damage) are all unaffected by oral contraceptives. Abnormal serum transaminase readings (which are elevated when there is cell damage) have not been found in users in Britain or the United States, but have been recorded in some Scandinavian women. Raised bromsulphalein (BSP) retention rates have been found in a few Pill users. The test is a measure of the liver's ability to concentrate a dye and excrete it in the bile; this ability to concentrate the dye rises to abnormal levels during pregnancy and in response to exogenous oestrogen. The percentage of abnormals declines as the length of time since starting the tablets increases and low-dose preparations produce fewest abnormalities or no effect at all.

The Walnut Creek study[236] conducted protein electrophoresis on sera from 6410 women. Pill users had lower serum albumin and γ-globulin levels, but higher α- and β-globulin levels. The effects were of a similar nature to, but of a lower degree than, those associated with pregnancy. Women on oral contraceptives also show changes in the levels of serum triglyceride, cholesterol, low-density and very-low-density lipoproteins; in general, levels of all these tend to be raised.[282] A rise in the levels of triglycerides and cholesterol also occurs in pregnancy. Progesterone decreases high-density lipoproteins (HDL). The triphasic pill appears to have no effect on HDL-cholesterol, but does raise the levels of triglycerides and thereby lowers the HDL-cholesterol/total cholesterol ratio. Oestrogens increase the production and removal of triglycerides and the total plasma pool increases, but these lipid aberrations return to normal shortly after discontinuing Pill use. (Interestingly, alcohol aggravates oral contraceptive induced hypertriglyceridaemia.) Studies show that there is a considerable variation in both low- and high-density lipoproteins during the menstrual cycle in normal women and in future base-line observations will have to take this into account. Women on the Pill show only minimal variations.[79] Norgestrel–oestrogen combinations cause the least rise in the levels of serum triglycerides.[337]

Unfortunately, it is impossible to make generalizations and to predict the effect of one Pill from what is known about others. On the whole, oral contraceptives alter the fats and proteins in the blood to make those of a fertile woman rather more those of a man, or a woman in an older age-group.

In some women, the response to a glucose tolerance test varies with the stage of the menstrual cycle, being greatest when circulating oestrogens are lowest. Abnormal glucose tolerance tests have been reported in nearly half the women taking high-dose oral contraceptives, although different observers have often used different criteria and many studies lack adequate controls. In the Walnut Creek study, the mean difference in serum glucose between users and non-users of older Pills in the 1-h glucose-tolerance screening test was 11 mg.[236] Pills containing 50 μg or less of oestrogen produce the least effect upon glucose tolerance, increased insulin secretion, changes in triglyceride levels and no change in the level of serum cholesterol. Since oestrogens by themselves do not alter glucose tolerance, it may be that their effect is an indirect one of potentiating the effect of the progestogen. Triphasic pills appear to have no effect on the plasma insulin response.[43]

The changes observed in women taking combined pills resemble those taking place in pregnancy. Pregnancy diabetes can be a precursor of frank diabetes but unfortunately the physiological basis of the condition is unknown. It may be significant that the incidence of abnormal tests in oral contraceptive users is greatest in women with a family history of diabetes.

User perspectives

Alterations which the Pill brings about in a woman's physiology are of immediate significance to her and she will require information about short-term side-effects, good or bad and long-term serious risks and benefits.

Useful side-effects

Those steroidal contraceptives that inhibit ovulation usually relieve the tiresome, and sometimes extremely painful, symptoms that are often associated with normal menstruation. A protection effect against the threat of ovarian cancer, endometrial cancer and pelvic inflammatory disease is discussed later.

Dysmenorrhoea is a colicky pain felt over the lower abdomen, often radiating down the inner aspect of the thighs, with or without backache.

and may include varying degrees of nausea or faintness. It can begin before, or coincide with, the onset of bleeding. Nearly half of western women experience some pain with their periods and in 10% the pain is severe and occasionally disabling. Raised intrauterine pressures have been associated with dysmenorrhoea and excessive prostaglandin synthesis is a possible cause. There is a negative correlation with both parity and age, and primary spasmodic dysmenorrhoea rarely accompanies anovulatory cycles. Between 60 and 90% of women using the Pill can expect dysmenorrhoea to be abolished and some relief of symptoms is almost invariable.[222]

Pain at ovulation, or 'Mittelschmerz', lasting for anything from a few hours up to a day, is less common than pain at menstruation, but is, of course, eliminated when ovulation is suppressed.

Premenstrual tension usually lasts for three or four days prior to the period, but sometimes goes on for up to 10 days and may end 24 h before the onset of the menses. There is depression and an inability to concentrate together with irritability characterized by variation in mood, emotional outbursts and perhaps episodes of crying. The woman may feel bloated, especially over the lower abdomen and breasts. About a third of normal women in western cultures complain of premenstrual irritability, and a quarter experience depression, anxiety or reduced physical activity. For some, life is appreciably disturbed. Dalton has shown a relation between phases of the menstrual cycle and numerous activities, such as examination performance, and has stated that over half the fatal accidents to fertile women occur during menstruation or the four days preceding it.[74] Most women taking the pill can expect relief of such symptoms[329] (Table 10.2).

When combined oral contraceptives are used, the periods can be

Table 10.2. *Effect of oral contraception on premenstrual tension and dysmenorrhoea*

	Rate per 1000 woman-years of exposure		
	Pill users	Non-users	Relative risk
Dysmenorrhoea	38.7	104.3	0.37
Premenstrual tension	64.3	90.0	0.71

Source. Berger, G. S., Edelman, D. A. & Talwar, P. P. (1979). The probability of side effects with Orval, Norinyl 450 and Norlestrin. *Contraception*, **20**, 447.

expected to come with clockwork regularity and to be lighter than normal. The reduction in menstrual flow should be socially and economically welcome. There is a reduction in the prevalence of iron-deficiency anaemia, and raised haemoglobin levels may be expected in women using oral contraceptives,[249, 338] which is useful in any society and can be critically significant among malnourished women from poor circumstances in the developing world.

As noted, menstruation is largely a product of civilized living: it tells a woman that she is not pregnant and at the same time reassures her about her future fertility. Certain groups of women have mythologized menstruation, believing it to be beneficial in ridding the body of dangerous poisons. A bright red loss is sometimes associated with health and may be described as 'pretty', for example by Caribbean islanders, whereas a light loss may be considered 'bad' and reassurance and explanation is necessary. Such beliefs, in modified form, are common among less educated women in westernized society.

A small group of women fail to have a period within seven days of stopping a course of tablets. Missed-menstruation occurs in only 1% of cycles, but up to one-fifth of women may experience this symptom at some time and all should be warned of the possibility. As noted, the continuous use of oral contraceptives for longer than 28 days is not associated with any increased incidence of breakthrough bleeding, or any delay in the return of menstruation when the tablets are finally stopped, and may be readily undertaken by any informed user for reasons of personal convenience.

Oral contraceptives produce a number of positive additional benefits to the user. Acne is an inflammation of the sebaceous glands, probably in response to the escape of sebum into the follicular wall. The rise in ovarian and adrenal androgens which occurs at puberty is responsible for female acne, and the condition improves in 80–90% of women on combined preparations, although it may take two or three cycles for the improvement to be noticeable.[235] Acne-prone women should be given a predominantly oestrogenic preparation. In less than 1% of women, acne is aggravated by Pill use. Some types of hirsutism are associated with raised serum testosterone and androstenedione levels and are also partially or wholly relieved by oral contraceptive use. For more than a decade antiandrogens, particularly cyproterone acetate, have been used in the treatment of hirsutism and alopecia in post-pubertal women. Tablets containing 2 mg cyproterone acetate combined with 0.05 mg ethinyloestradiol were first tried in Asia and later in Europe[124] to control severe acne and simultaneously to provide contraceptive security. Clinical results have been encouraging and the combination would seem to be contraceptively as effective as the ordinary 50 μg combined pill. Surprisingly, serum levels of cortisol, testosterone, dihydrotestosterone, androstenedione and dehydroepiandrosterone are not altered in women taking this preparation and it is possible that the skin target organs for androgens are selectively blocked. Clinical trials began in the UK in 1980.

A good deal has been written about possible changes in libido among Pill users. It is self-evident that human sexual behaviour is influenced by many factors and objective data are difficult or impossible to come by. In the first report on Enavid, Pincus found that coital frequency rose for 50% of oral contraceptive users and fell for 40%.[221] A placebo/Pill crossover trial in women using some other method of contraception found similar coital rates in the presence or absence of contraceptive steroids.[199]

In non-human primates a distinction has been made between female attractiveness to the male, female receptivity to male advances and female initiation of coitus. Female attraction appears to be influenced by ovarian hormones and the cyclicity observed in coital activity among monkeys is oestrogen dependent, but can be inhibited by progesterone and depends, in part, on the male responding to the odour of vaginal secretions.[13, 191] In women, use of oral contraceptives has an effect on the distribution of coitus in the cycle, abolishing premenstrual depression found in untreated women.[3, 305] Udry suggests that the Pill may abolish a progesterone-mediated suppression of desire in man, presumably through a pheromone. The addition of androstenedione to oral contraceptives did not improve sexual interest in Pill users.[14] However, for the vast majority of human beings, the wide range of cerebrate factors operating on human sexual activities, the role of fantasy, freedom from worry about unwanted conception and, above all, that complex of forces which we call love, all outweigh any pharmacological influence of oral contraceptives on sexual behaviour.

The majority of couples feel that their overall 'life situation' improves with the use of oral contraceptives and some benefits are far reaching. One family doctor in Britain found that the average number of surgery attendances dropped from 4.8 per year for average women to 1.8 per year for those taking oral contraceptives. He compared the 'alert, jolly, and bright-eyed woman calling for her repeat prescription' with the 'anxious, sullen-faced drab who, perhaps as little as six months previously, had . . . asked in hopeless tones, as an aside from her myriad complaints, for information on the pill'.[202] Today, such words, which were written by a doctor shortly after the Pill was first introduced, might be considered subjective and romantic but they may be worth recalling as a measure of the joy and relief brought by the introduction of oral contraceptives 20 years ago.

Annoying side-effects

Short-term symptoms noticed by a woman when taking the Pill can be sufficiently trying to cause her to abandon the method although they are likely to be less important than certain long-term changes, which may be less visible to her.

Breast tissue responds to circulating oestrogens and progesterone and each normal cycle is associated with some change in breast volume. Discomfort preceding menstruation is reported in about 1 in 6 European women. Engorgement and fullness appear to be a response to progesterone; pain, soreness and tenderness to oestrogens. Oral contraceptives expose the breasts to a somewhat different hormonal environment, and whereas some women who have previously had breast discomfort are relieved, in others the symptoms appear for the first time. The Pill can be associated with some breast enlargement. The relation between Pill use and lactation is discussed later in this chapter and in Chapter 6.

Probably, oral contraceptives are held responsible for weight gain more often than they cause it. Nevertheless, some women put on weight and the tendency is greatest in the first six months of use.[222] Part of any weight gain is usually fluid retention.

Headaches, and more specifically migraine, are a good example of symptoms which are difficult or impossible to measure and easily dismissed as subjective by the onlooker but may be of central importance to a user. Little is known about the incidence of headaches in normal populations and complaints amongst Pill users are difficult to evaluate. In a small group of women, steroid contraception appears to induce headaches, especially during the interval when tablets are not being taken, and if this symptom persists over several cycles and proves resistant to changes in preparation, then the method may need to be discontinued. Migraine may be reactivated or precipitated for the first time by oral contraceptives; on the other hand many migraine sufferers find great relief when they take the Pill. Some types of epilepsy are linked to the menstrual cycle but the condition is not a contraindication to use of the Pill.

Mucorrhoea, that is excessive secretion from the uterine cervix, is associated with high plasma oestrogen levels and may occur in some women on oral contraceptives. In some cases, the Pill may aggravate moniliasis by increasing the glycogen content in the vaginal cells; active treatment may be necessary for what can be a very trying condition, and a change in preparation may help.

Hypertrophic gingivitis is a rare complication of oral contraceptive use. It involves hypertrophy of the tissue around the necks of the teeth and is also a recognized complication of pregnancy. In extreme cases, an epulis may form, although more commonly the gums may be sore or the hypertrophied tissue may become a site of infection.[166] The condition is usually remedied by good oral hygiene.

Some women are less tolerant of contact lenses premenstrually and oral contraceptives have been reported to make contact lenses more difficult to use in a small number of users. Very rarely, the corneal oedema associated with Pill use can be severe and then the woman may either choose to return to spectacles or discontinue the tablet. The method is not contraindicated in glaucoma.

Chloasma, or pregnancy mask, the increased facial pigmentation that sometimes occurs in pregnancy, is a possible complication of oral contraceptive use. Both oestrogens and progestogens appear to be involved. It occurs in about 1% of Caucasian women but was reported in a quarter of early Pill users in Puerto Rico. It may be a complication of under-nutrition as well as of a more sunny climate.

As up to one-third of the fertile women in a population may be taking oral contraceptives, a large number of fortuitous relations occur between this form of contraception and various diseases. Possible relations have been reported with eczema and urticaria but remission, as well as a worsening, has been reported where the condition existed before the Pill. Alopecia has been reported in oral contraceptive users, but so has the arrest of hair loss.[46,222]

It is a consistent finding that the probability of a side-effect recurring after the initial cycle of use falls rapidly (Table 10.3).[28] The profile of side-effects reported in countries such as Bangladesh has been little studied but appears to be qualitatively different from that in the West with, for example, more reports of dizziness and 'eye problems'.[129]

Table 10.3. *Oral contraceptive side-effects (0.5 mg norgestrel and 0.05 mg ethynyloestradiol)*

Symptom	Probability of symptom recurring if present in first cycle	
	Second cycle	Third cycle
Breast discomfort	0.60	0.29
Nausea	0.47	0.23
Headache	0.33	0.20
Irritability	0.52	0.29
Breakthrough bleeding	0.20	0.13

Provider perspectives

The complex and widespread changes brought about by steroidal
contraceptives result in a series of effects which a potential user should be
warned may occur, and they may also be associated with risks, a small
number of which a provider can identify in advance. The woman user must
receive sufficient information to enable her to make an informed decision to
accept or reject the method. Those providing information may be well
advised to ask the woman to share what she already knows and then to
adjust and edit her knowledge in the light of known facts.

Prescription

If, as was technically possible, the Pill had been developed 10 or 15
years earlier, it might never have been made a prescription item, even in the
West. In parts of Europe, and in nearly all of the developing world, oral
contraceptives are available, *de facto*, without prescription. In 1973, the
International Planned Parenthood Federation (IPPF) issued a landmark
statement:

> When oral contraceptives were first introduced it was reasonable to
> restrict the use of these unknown, and relatively powerful drugs to
> medical prescription. However, as experience has extended over a decade
> and a half and grown to tens of millions of users, the IPPF Central
> Medical Committee is increasingly confident that this method of family
> planning is highly effective, relatively simple to use, and that the health
> benefits outweigh the risks of use in nearly all cases. It has been found that
> the complications that do occur are difficult to predict by examination
> prior to use . . . The limitation of oral contraceptive distribution to
> doctors' prescription makes the method geographically, economically
> and sometimes culturally inaccessible to many women. As a consequence,
> deaths and sickness of women and children, which might otherwise be
> avoided by voluntary limitation of fertility continue.[155]

In 1974 it was suggested that suitably trained 'state registered nurses,
midwives and health visitors' in Britain might prescribe Pills[240] and this
idea was upheld by a Working Party set up by the Department of Health
and Social Security. This recommendation, while medically well founded,
has not been implemented, possibly because no satisfactory way was
suggested for distributing the item-of-service payments for contraceptive
advice made by the British National Health Service.

In some developing countries, Pills are distributed by appropriately
trained and supervised personnel, but without the direct intervention of a
physician. Unhappily, however, in other countries, such as India, oral
contraceptives are only available to the rich (who buy them illicitly over the

counter) or on medical prescription to the poor, and are thus systematically denied to millions of potential users. In prescribing the Pill, the two most important facts in the case history are the woman's age and whether or not she smokes, and the most important physical signs are the blood pressure and whether or not she is obese. Most other aspects of clinical examination relate to preventive medicine or (at least in the US) are determined by medico-legal considerations.

Oral contraception and pre-existing disease

Hypertension. Among the 13 000 women using the Pill in the Walnut Creek Study the average rise in systolic blood pressure was 4.5 mm and in diastolic pressure was 1.3 mm of mercury.[236] These modest changes were unaffected by duration of use and involved a slight alteration in a large number of people rather than large changes in a small number, but they did push a small number of women over the arbitrary level of 140/90 mm usually chosen as a measure of hypertension. Blood pressure returned to normal after discontinuation of oral contraceptives. One double-blind crossover study found a reduction in *mean* blood pressure.[239]

The duration of Pill use appears to be important in relation to the risk of hypertension. The RCGP study found no demonstrable risk in one year of use, but that after five years the condition was 2.5 to 3 fold as likely among women using the Pill as among control cases.[249] American work rated the risk of Pill users developing hypertension to be about 1.76 times higher than for non-users and demonstrated that when the Pill was discontinued the blood pressure of those affected rapidly returned to normal.[94] In both surveys blood pressure changes were found to be related to age and weight. However, not all studies have found the same effect and the rate of new diagnosis of hypertension in the Oxford study was approximately the same among Pill users (1.6 per 1000 per year) as among diaphragm users (1.7 per 1000 per year).[310] Both studies mainly related to high-dose contraceptives that are no longer in use.

Increased aldosterone secretion and increased renin substrate have been detected in women taking the Pill, whether or not they developed hypertension.[160] Pill users who develop hypertension have a failure in the feed-back or shut-off of release.[40]

While blood pressure screening is desirable before a woman begins the Pill and at regular follow-ups, it is worth noting that only one-fifth of family doctors in Britain and slightly more than half of those working in family planning clinics actually carry out this task.[54] Certainly in developing countries, the possibility of giving oral contraceptives to hypertensive women, or of causing undiagnosed hypertension is an acceptable risk in relation to the hazards of unintended pregnancy.

Neither a history of pregnancy-induced hypertension,[234] nor pre-existing hypertension in younger women need be contraindications to oral contraceptive use. Spellacy found that when oral contraceptives were given to women with frank hypertension there was a fall of blood pressure in those using combined pills and an even greater decline in those using progestogen-only preparations.[283] Curiously though, the RCGP study suggested that the dose of progestogen might be related to the risk of hypertension arising.[250] Hypertension is a risk factor in the development of myocardial infarction and blood pressure should be monitored in known cases of hypertension and an alternative contraceptive, such as the progestogen-only pills or injectables, should be advised if the blood pressure rises. Certainly further rises of blood pressure make it unwise for older hypertensive women to use oral contraceptives.

Diabetes. Diabetes mellitus is associated with a raised risk of morbidity and mortality in pregnancy and childbirth. Intensive obstetric care is needed for the diabetic woman who chooses to become pregnant and highly effective reversible contraception must be available for the diabetic woman who wants to postpone pregnancy. Oral contraceptives, with their unique effectiveness can be tried in younger women, although the diabetes will require careful monitoring. The progestogen-only pill has proved useful in cases of insulin-dependent diabetes.[290] For the older diabetic, where the risk of cardiovascular disease will be greater, the dangers of pregnancy will also be high. The Pill is contraindicated and voluntary sterilization of her or her partner is likely to be a suitable choice. As a generalization, in a developed country where such women receive specialist care, the specialist would be wise to regard contraceptive advice as one of his obligations. In a developing country where diabetes often goes untreated, the risks of an unwanted pregnancy far outweigh any risk of giving the Pill to undiagnosed cases.

In women with a family history of diabetes or gross obesity, a test of the post-prandial blood sugar level may be taken and, if raised, and oral contraceptives are still chosen, then a full glucose tolerance test is indicated in order to establish the diagnosis of diabetes and decide upon treatment before oral contraception is started.

Liver diseases. Oral contraceptives are contraindicated in cases of idiopathic jaundice (Dublin–Johnson and Rotor syndromes), in those with a past history of recurrent idiopathic jaundice of pregnancy (benign recurrent cholestatic jaundice of pregnancy) or for women who have had recurrent generalized pruritis of pregnancy. These conditions are all rare (idiopathic jaundice of pregnancy occurs in 1 in 3500 pregnancies). They are aggravated by contraceptive steroids.

A past history of infectious hepatitis is not a contraindication to oral contraceptives, unless the liver function tests are still abnormal, when some alternative form of contraception should be advised until they return to normal. Acute intermittent porphyria can very rarely be precipitated by oral contraceptive use.[48]

Sickle-cell anaemia. Thromboembolic disease is more common in women with sickle-cell disease (SS and SC genes) than among the normal population and pregnancy may precipitate a crisis. By analogy, the condition is often considered a relative contraindication to the use of combined oral contraceptives.[2, 95] However, progestogens extend the interval between crises (see Chapter 14).

Other diseases. Oral contraceptives can be a satisfactory choice for most women with chronic diseases. In the Third World, where tuberculosis and leprosy remain common, it is important to note that oral contraception is suitable. Oral contraceptives may alter the pattern of epilepsy, but can be safely used if the woman is carefully watched. (See also The interaction of oral contraceptives with other drugs below.) There is no evidence that the Pill alters the progress of neurological diseases such as multiple sclerosis and, again, it can be a satisfactory choice.[192]

The interaction of oral contraceptives with other drugs

Drugs which induce the synthesis of hepatic microsomal enzymes, such as the antibiotic rifampicin, which is used in the treatment of tuberculosis, and phenytoin and perhaps other anticonvulsants such as phenobarbitone used in the treatment of epilepsy, are occasionally associated with breakthrough bleeding and lead to a small risk of accidental pregnancy.[41, 143] A higher dose of oestrogen should be used to counter this effect. Broad-spectrum antibiotics may interfere with the enterohepatic recirculation of oestrogens but the risk of unwanted pregnancy is low.[11, 45] An American physician might be wise to warn a potentially litigious woman, but for most sensible people variations in user compliance will override such therapeutic subtleties.

Matching users with Pills

The Chinese family planning programme uses two Pills; one for women with heavy periods and one for women with light periods. There are many situations in the world where hundreds of thousands of women have been satisfied without any choice of preparation and a certain amount of solemn nonsense has been written in the past about tailoring the preparation to a woman's hormonal balance. Part of this effort probably arose from competing manufacturers trying to promote their own product.

Important details have been discovered about particular preparations. Spotting and breakthrough bleeding are more common with low-dose Pills. Norgestrel appears to counter some of the effects of oestrogens on glucose metabolism, norethisterone is associated with the greatest reduction in breast disease and there is speculation that liver tumours may have been more common in women who used mestranol rather than ethinyloestradiol preparations. But, in general, prescribers should not be too earnest in attempting to fit a Pill to a woman's hormone profile. They should be aware of the factual evidence associating a certain preparation with particular advantages and disadvantages and they should be prepared to assist the woman who is having problems in using oral contraceptives by discovering exactly what side-effects she has developed and how she may benefit by changing to another preparation.

The number of women who give up using the Pill because of adverse side-effects is probably less than those who abandon it for irrational reasons. Absolute contraindications to its use are rare although there are several instances where caution may be needed.

Those distributing the Pill must be alert to the problems which worry women concerning oral contraceptives and willing to answer the unspoken as well as the overt questions. In some groups questions are based on folklore which surrounds human reproduction or arise from dullness of comprehension. In educated women the questions are more likely to be of the sort that the woman is suspicious of upsetting her 'hormonal balance'. Objections to taking the Pill can be deep-seated and unexpected, as in a patient who refused the Pill because she was a vegetarian and thought it was made from animal hormones: she took it with alacrity when told it was manufactured from yams.

The partner is an important factor in a woman's attitude to contraception. The phrase 'my husband won't let me take the Pill' is sometimes heard. Unfortunately, labourers or mechanics are less likely to come and discuss their reservations with a doctor than are solicitors or bank clerks, but a great deal can be done to answer a husband's questions by face-to-face interview or through the embassy of the wife. From Manchester to Manila there is an awareness that dangerous side-effects have been reported in women taking the Pill; the risks can be fitted into the context of the dangers which everyone is forced to take in their daily life (see Table 16.1). The magnitude of lay misunderstanding of the Pill is brought out by the fact that some people think oral contraceptives are synonymous with thalidomide.

A small percentage of women need more than usual help. Such women may be particularly forgetful or unable to grasp even the simplest instruction. Some women will remove tablets from a packet so as to produce a pattern which pleases them, or will limit their tablet taking to the days when they have intercourse, or will share their prescription with friends, neighbours and unmarried sisters or take the Pill for only one week out of four. Women of this kind need repeated, calm instruction and, in the context of a domiciliary family planning service, numerous visits. The husband or boyfriend may provide a suitable path to regular Pill taking but there remains a tiny residual group of women who do not have a capacity to take oral contraceptives and for whom, other considerations apart, alternative methods appear preferable.

Failure to replenish supplies of Pills is more common than gross errors in Pill taking. Lack of foresight, a domestic life which makes it difficult to visit the doctor, clinic or chemist, or straightforward lack of housekeeping money may make a woman miss getting a fresh supply of Pills. Once a woman is established on oral contraceptives it can be helpful to prescribe for six- or twelve-month intervals.

Pills, like other contraceptives, are sometimes used in odd ways, such as 'feeding' them to drawing-room plants in the hope of better growth: doctors should, perhaps, be aware of the sydrome of a pregnant woman with a beautiful aspidistra! Women should keep Pills in a safe place. The well-known story of a daughter replacing her mother's Pills with aspirins has a basis in fact and one case of a husband replacing his wife's contraceptive pills with grandfather's digoxin occurred before the easily recognized packages were introduced. Such substitutions are very unlikely in the future. Young children and toddlers may swallow large numbers of Pills, taking them to be sweets, unless the mother keeps them beyond their reach. Fortunately, there are no toxic effects and reassurance, not gastric lavage, is indicated. In nearly 100 cases of accidental ingestion by children no ill effects were reported, except for three cases of vomiting.[103]

The tendency in recent years has been to prescribe the lowest dose of oral contraceptive possible. In the case of thrombotic disease and hypertension, and by implication for all side-effects, it is assumed that the lower the dose the less is the risk. On the other hand, in relation to some of the beneficial effects of the Pill it could be that higher doses may have advantages. Therefore, even today it is not possible to generalize that the lowest dose is always or unequivocally the best, although in the absence of other information, it is a reasonable guideline to follow. Some, but not all combined pills with less than 50 μg of oestrogen have poor cycle control and there may be less relief of dysmenorrhoea. The disadvantages of progestogen-only pills are irregular cycles, less reliability, less tolerance of errors in use and occasional episodes of breast discomfort for some women. It seems probable that information will continue to accumulate in this field and those prescribing the Pill should attempt to keep up to date, avoid panic reactions and fashions in relation to isolated pieces of information, but not lose sight of priorities, such as discouraging cigarette smoking in all users (see Chapter 14).

When oral contraceptives were first registered by the US FDA they received, like all new drugs, a two-year provisional licence. Somehow this bureaucratic fiat became translated into a clinical guideline and there are still doctors who teach that a woman should come off the Pill, 'to give her body a rest', after two years' use. This is incorrect. The physiological changes that do occur are more marked in the first few months of use and it is irrational to stop and start the therapy. Once a woman is on the Pill, she should continue taking it until she wants a child, runs into unacceptable side-effects, selects another method, enters an age that puts her at demonstrably higher risk of cardiovascular disease, is silly enough to begin to smoke, or no longer needs contraceptive protection.

Some major issues in Pill usage

Several key issues, such as the return of fertility, cardiovascular disease and neoplasia, need to be understood by both the provider *and* the user of the method, although the vocabulary and details of understanding may well vary greatly between the two groups and in different cultural circumstances. There is an exceedingly large literature on oral contraceptive use, but most of it can be reduced to relatively few principles.

Subsequent fertility

Large-scale studies on the return of fertility following the discontinuation of oral contraceptives usually show a slight but measurable delay in the mean time taken to conceive (Fig. 10.5), but in any large population the proportion of women conceiving is unaltered by prior use of the Pill.[109, 117, 316, 317] Care should be taken in calculating the expected date of delivery in a woman who has previously used the Pill as the first ovulation may have been delayed.

Spontaneous episodes of amenorrhoea lasting for six months or more occur in up to about 1% of women who are actually taking the Pill. Post-pill amenorrhoea has been reported in 0.3–2.7%[90] of women. Some cases of post-pill amenorrhoea are related to the suppression of pituitary function by oral contraceptives, although others no doubt would have occurred even without Pill use.[304] The probability of post-pill amenorrhoea does not appear to be correlated with the age when the women start the medication. In both spontaneous and post-pill amenorrhoea approximately half the women complaining of the condition have a history of menstrual irregularity from earlier in life.[186] Many others have undergone recent rapid weight loss and in one series from Scandinavia only 8% of women with post-pill amenorrhoea had no additional reasons to explain their clinical situation.[99]

Galactorrhoea occurs in both spontaneous and post-pill amenorrhoea and may be associated with high serum prolactin levels. Pituitary adenomas have been detected in some cases of amenorrhoea.[181] It is not known if the Pill was ever a causative factor, or if Pill use masked the development of an adenoma. Reports of cases primarily reflect the development of the technology to measure prolactin, conduct pituitary tomography and the type of case on which suspicion falls.[272] It is worth noting that pituitary microadenomas are found at postmortem in 10–20% of *men* and prospective[328] and case-control studies[65] have not confirmed any causal relation between pituitary adenomas and Pill use.

Whatever the relation between the use of contraceptive steroids and secondary amenorrhoea, spontaneous cure is common and the outlook excellent for any woman with the condition. As far as is known virtually all cases respond to the use

Fig. 10.5. The return of fertility following the discontinuation of steroidal contraceptives. (Sources: Vessey, M. P., Wright, N. M., McPherson, K. & Wiggins, P. (1978). Fertility after stopping different methods of contraception. *British Medical Journal. i*, 265; and *Second Asian Regional Workshop on Injectable Contraceptives* (1982). Oklahoma City, Oklahoma: World Neighbors.)

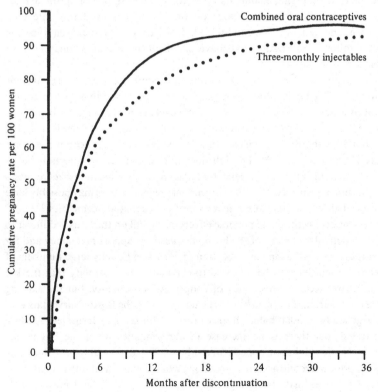

of clomiphene. Ninety-five per cent of women in one study of post-pill amenorrhoea gave birth by 30 months after starting treatment.[130]

There seems no reason to refuse the Pill to women with irregular cycles, episodes of amenorrhoea or oligomenorrhoea, although they, and all other Pill users, must understand that fertility can never be proved in advance of becoming pregnant. When secondary amenorrhoea occurs it is not related to the duration of Pill use and, as noted, there is no reason to discontinue the use of oral contraceptives after arbitrary intervals.

Effect on the offspring

One of the reasons Rock & Pincus chose to develop a female, as opposed to a male, Pill was that the primary oocytes in the female are all formed before the mother's birth, whereas sperm production is an active process throughout adult life. The first chromosomal reduction division takes place before birth but the second reduction occurs at the formation of the first polar body, shortly before ovulation and theoretically could be affected by changes in hormonal environment. Exogenous hormones could also alter critical stages of embryogenesis, perhaps particularly, but by no means exclusively, of the reproductive system. It is also known that in some, perhaps all, mammals circulating sex hormones imprint a male pattern of neuro-endocrine behaviour on the hypothalamus during late fetal development and under certain conditions individuals with a female genotype can be made to follow a male pattern of behaviour, which only becomes apparent when the animal reaches adulthood.

Rarely, pregnancy occurs during routine oral contraceptive use, use may be accidentally initiated in an already pregnant woman or a woman may deliberately take oral contraceptives (perhaps even a whole packet) in an attempt to bring on a 'late period'. Although all these events are unusual, the scale of Pill use is such that several hundred thousand embryos may be exposed to contraceptive steroids annually in the US alone.[206] The Pill does not actually cause abortion but is relatively commonly taken in the belief that it might do so in locations where access to safe abortion is restricted. So-called hormonal pregnancy tests may possibly have been associated with an increased incidence of congenital abnormalities.[111]

The evidence concerning the possible effects of the Pill on the fetus is difficult to assemble and involves review of the hormones used to support pregnancy and for other purposes, as well as in contraception.[24, 334] Exceptionally large numbers of pregnancies would have to be followed to eliminate any possibility that the Pill increases, or reduces, the frequency of congenital abnormality, but the existing evidence is reassuring. The British cohort studies,[255, 310] the Boston surveillance[246] and a large study of 3000 babies born to former Pill users in Jerusalem[117] have demonstrated that there is no increase in abnormalities when the Pill is discontinued. Neither did the Connecticut study of 1370 abnormal babies show any increase in prior oral contraceptive use among women with the abnormal babies.[37] Studies of national birth defect registers in Hungary and Finland make it 95% certain that Pill use has no effect on visible malformations.[71, 263] Perinatal mortality is lower in women who used the Pill, probably because the wanted pregnancies were better spaced than the control deliveries. An increase in multiple births after discontinuing Pill use was reported by Bracken[36] but was not seen in the Jerusalem study.[117]

Respiratory distress syndrome has been reported to be less common after Pill use and this merits further study.[69] There is no alteration in any complication of pregnancy or labour other than a slight excess of cervicitis among nulliparous former users.[118] It is possible that a different situation obtains if the fetus is exposed to exogenous hormones at a contraceptive dose. One syndrome of multiple defects involving the heart, limb reductions and abnormalities of the oesphagus and vertebrae (VACTERL = vertebral–anal–cardiac–tracheal–oesophageal–renal–limb) has been reported to be more common in Pill users although the numbers are not large enough to reach statistical significance.[121, 137] There is no evidence that contraceptive hormones at the doses used can masculinize a female fetus or that sexual behaviour is in any way modified in children born to Pill takers.

Human reproduction is an imperfect process, with up to half the fertilized eggs either failing to implant or else aborting (Chapter 13). Most serious chromosome anomalies appear to lead to spontaneous abortion. Some studies of Pill users have suggested a changing pattern of chromosome abnormalities among women who used the Pill before conception or during pregnancy,[53] but weaknesses in understanding the biology of the situation make it impossible to assess these observations quantitatively.[31, 156]

The rule that a pregnant woman should avoid all drugs is a sound one. Hormonal pregnancy tests have been withdrawn in many countries and should be abandoned where still available. There is no place for diethylstilboestrol in the treatment of threatened abortion and the use of progestogens should be restricted to cases where progesterone deficiency has been demonstrated as the cause of a previous abortion[56] even though progestogens have been used in the UK for 30 years with minimal complications and no long-term ill effects reported.

The instruction to discontinue Pill use and use a mechanical method for two or three cycles prior to a wanted conception is sometimes given, and may be reasonable for the most pessimistic but it should be understood that there is no objective evidence that it is worth the effort.

In the developing world, powerful drugs are sold over the counter and polypharmacy by physicians is all too common. In the United States 1 in 8 pregnant women still smoke. A recent study in the US found that 55.6% of pregnant women still received at least one drug prescription during the pregnancy[38] and although many drugs may be harmless, tranquillizers, narcotic analgesics and smoking over 20 cigarettes a day seem to present particular risks.[58]

In summary, in the case of oral contraceptives, 99 women out of 100 can expect minimal delay in conceiving a wanted pregnancy after use. For the remaining 1% some months of post-pill amenorrhoea may occur, which nearly always resolves spontaneously, but occasionally requires treatment which, in turn, always appears to be successful.

There is no statistically significant evidence of any greater probability of congenital abnormality in the offspring of women who stopped taking contraceptive pills to become pregnant, or who accidentally took Pills when pregnant, although additional information is required in the case of certain rare conditions.

The possible effects of oral contraceptives on lactation and the passage of steroids into the breast milk are discussed in Chapter 6.

Cardiovascular disease

After more than a decade of work a great deal is now known about patterns of cardiovascular disease among Pill users by age, duration of use and other risk factors. Sometimes oral contraceptive dose and distribution policies can be devised to reduce the hazards to users.

The first report in the British literature of a thrombotic episode in an oral contraceptive user was made in 1961.[142] Subsequently, both case-control and cohort epidemiological studies have measured an increased, but low risk of deep vein thrombosis and pulmonary embolism in Pill users. The risk of death from myocardial infarction, especially among older users, is actually higher than that from pulmonary embolism, but this was only established some years later. It is now known that oral contraceptives are also associated with a measurable rise in cerebrovascular disease. The magnitude of oral contraceptive use in developed countries and the scale of the risks involved encourages analysis of age-specific mortality rates among women of fertile age, by comparing data for years before and after the widespread use of the Pill. This approach suggests that, in reality, death rates may be *less* than were suggested as a result of case-control and cohort studies.

Apparently dramatic associations can be coincidental and the possibility of bias in clinical observation is well illustrated by a doctor in the 1960s who gave a prescription for Enavid to a woman who, six weeks later, had an episode of thrombophlebitis: on further investigation it was found that she had failed to have her prescription dispensed. Epidemiological observations require care and time to carry out.

The balance of hormones during pregnancy appears to protect against thromboembolic disease and in a review of the world literature Drill[84] found a rate of only 0.73 cases per 1000 pregnant women per year as opposed to 1.2 and 2.9 per 1000 non-pregnant women. However, use of oestrogens to 'suppress' lactation raises the incidence of puerperal thromboembolism.[138] It is also known that large doses of oestrogen used in the treatment of cancer of the prostate are associated with an increased incidence of thromboembolic disease in men. Together with the changes noted in clotting factors all this information helps to explain the relation between the Pill and cardiovascular disease.

A suspicion that the level of risk might be partially linked to the type of Pill first arose with the work of Sartwell on combined and sequential oral contraceptives in 1969.[261] The synergistic action of additional risk factors, in particular smoking, has been brought out by Ravenholt & Frederiksen[98] and Jain.[136]

Overall perspectives in relation to the Pill and cardiovascular disease have been reviewed by Vessey,[306,307] Ory, Rosenfield & Landman[215] and Stadel.[287]

Blood clotting is one of the most complex physiological processes known, involving as it does platelets, tissue damage, surface contact and a number of clotting factors which may be pre-enzymes that are activated by other enzymes. Obviously there are evolutionary reasons for an interlocking system of checks and balances to control the process of clot formation to meet the body's need to repair breaks in the vascular system without obstructing normal blood flow. Inhibiting factors rapidly destroy the activating factors in clot formation.

No single laboratory test satisfactorily predicts the clinical risk of thrombosis; this is also true in relation to long-term hazards such as myocardial infarction. The exact effects of steroid hormones on blood clotting, on the make-up of the serum and on the architecture of the vascular tree are still being unravelled. Oral contraceptives bring about a reduction in the clotting time but leave the bleeding times unaltered. The platelet count and prothrombin time decrease, while fibrinogen concentration, fibrinolytic activity, Factor VII and Factor VIII all increase. Antithrombin III, which is the main plasma inhibitor of thrombus formation, appears unchanged in level but less active in oral contraceptive users.[224] Activated Factor X (Xa) is also reduced.[325] Overall, high-dose combined pills appear to reduce the body's ability to stop the progression of intravenous coagulation and dissolve fibrin clots. The observed changes taking place in clotting factors are mainly oestrogen dependent and preparations with low oestrogen content should carry less risk.

Progestogens alone, either as injections or as Pills, have little or no effect on blood clotting. However, as noted earlier (see Oral contraceptives and physiology), steroidal contraceptives also have an action on serum lipoproteins and cholesterol and here the progestational component may be important. Norethindrone acetate and norgestrol-containing Pills appear to decrease HDL.[319] High levels of HDL bound to cholesterol in the bloodstream are believed to predispose to a reduced risk of heart disease. Men of 40 years and over have a higher rate of myocardial infarction and less HDL than women at the same age. Women who smoke and take the Pill have HDL levels that are somewhat closer to those of men.

A direct effect of oral contraceptive steroids on the architecture of the vascular epithelium has been postulated.[135]

The effect of smoking. It is logical to deal with risk by order of magnitude and there is no doubt that the single most important factor relating to Pill use and cardiovascular disease is cigarette smoking. Whether a woman smokes should be the first question, and in some cases the only question, to be asked when screening prior to oral contraception. Among men in Britain, the average number of cigarettes smoked rose consistently between 1920 and 1940 and then reached a plateau, but unhappily the prevalence of smoking in women is still increasing and they seem to be determined to catch up with men in the use of this dangerous and addictive drug.

Moreover, statistically, women who take the Pill smoke more than those who do not.[148] Discouragement of smoking, always an important medical responsibility, becomes mandatory when oral contraceptives are used.

There is a strong and spectacular relation between the use of combined contraceptives and smoking. Both smoking and the Pill alone raise the risk of heart attack, subarachnoid haemorrhage and haemorrhagic stroke. The two together have a synergistic effect which may result in a hundred-fold increase in the risk taken by a woman who both smokes and takes the Pill when compared with a woman who does neither (Table 10.4).[244]

Smoking has a number of effects on the cardiovascular system: the amount of carbon monoxide in the circulation rises, atherosclerotic changes are accelerated and nicotine causes contraction of blood vessels. However, there is no physiopathological explanation why the effects of Pills and cigarettes should have a multiplying rather than an additive effect. It is known that steroid levels do not differ in Pill users who smoke,[68] and that smoking does not appear to affect venous thromboembolic disease.[161] In the western world the probability of death from all causes for women aged 20–50 in the absence of smoking and oral contraceptive use is about 4%. If non-smokers take the Pill for the whole of this same interval, they have an additional chance of death of 0.3%. If women smoke and take the Pill then the additional risk is 1.9%.

Myocardial infarction. Myocardial infarction is rare in the fertile years, but rises in prevalance after the menopause or surgical oophorectomy. The possible relation between oral contraceptive usage and coronary thrombosis was first suspected in the 1960s but it was not until the 1970s that case-control and prospective studies began to measure it.[133, 176, 178, 179, 180, 244, 269, 280]These studies, most of which involved high-dose Pills no longer in use, demonstrated the following points.

(a) Oral contraceptives appear to multiply the risk of myocardial infarction by three to four times in women aged 24–49. It must be emphasized that the risk of myocardial infarction is low in young women but rises in the later fertile years: for example a twelve-fold increase in risk for a group

Table 10.4. *The relative risk of non-fatal myocardial infarction in contraceptive users*

Group	Relative risk
Controls	1
Oral contraceptive users	3
Smokers (non-oral contraceptive users)	5
Hypertensives (non-oral contraceptive users)	8
Women with hypertension who use oral contraceptives and smoke	170

aged 25–29 would not be as damaging as a five-fold increase in risk at age 40–44.

(b) The higher the oestrogen content of the Pill the higher the risk.

(c) The dose of progestogen appears also to influence the risk, 3–4 mg of norethindrone acetate or norgestrel increases the risk to about 1.5 to 2 times that experienced by those who take only 1–2 mg of these same progestogens.[187]

(d) As already pointed out, there is a remarkable synergism between cigarette smoking and oral contraceptive use.

(e) The risk of myocardial infarction does not appear to be related to the duration of Pill use, but among women who have used oral contraceptives for five years, there is a suspicion of a carry-over effect that leaves the previous user with approximately twice the risk of myocardial infarction compared with the woman who has never used oral contraceptives. The effects may persist for up to 10 years. Slone and colleagues compared 566 women aged 25–49 years with myocardial infarction with 2036 age-matched controls (Table 10.5).[280] The degree of persistent risk was related to the duration of use, suggesting a genuine biological effect.

Although the risk of morbidity and mortality due to myocardial infarction is serious, the majority of these risks can be avoided by applying simple rules when distributing oral contraceptives. The switch from Pills containing up to 100–150μg of oestrogen to Pills containing only 30μg may have reduced the incidence of myocardial infarction by up to 80%, so that the present generation of Pill users may well be relatively safe.

Venous thromboembolic disease. Deep vein thrombosis is a condition that is particularly difficult to diagnose. There may be unilateral swelling, especially of the calf, although venous anastomoses reduce the usefulness of this sign. Pain is often absent, even on pressure over the affected area or dorsiflexion of the foot, and the condition may be totally silent. Clinical findings and post-mortem observations agree only in a minority of cases and careful observers miss two-thirds of venous

Table 10.5. *The risk of myocardial infarction by duration of oral contraceptive use*

	Relative risk (95% confidence limits)
Controls	1.0
Current users	3.5 (2.2–5.5)
Past users who stopped the Pill: < 5 years ago	1.0 (0.8–1.4)
5–9 years ago	1.6 (1.1–2.8)
10 + years ago	2.5 (1.5–4.1)

thrombosis while, conversely, experienced surgeons diagnose deep vein thrombosis in twice as many cases as demonstrated by phlebography. Biases in diagnosis are important. In the US deep vein thrombosis is suspected twice as often among Pill users on clinical grounds as it can be demonstrated by more objective tests[16] and a Pill user is 20–40% more likely to be admitted to hospital for this reason. Such bias is less apparent in Britain and has been adequately handled in several epidemiological studies.

The FDA reviewed early reports of thromboembolic disease among Enavid users and found that the Pill had no demonstrable effect. However, in 1967 the British Committee on the Safety of Drugs concluded that 'there can be no reasonable doubt that some types of thromboembolic disorders are associated with the use of oral contraceptives'. Thrombosis of the central vein of the retina has been reported as an exceptionally rare complication of oral contraceptive use.

Since these pioneer studies in Britain, confirmatory material has come from the United States[261] and studies involving pooled samples from Britain and Scandinavia have also been published.[182, 262, 292]

As a result of this research the following facts appear to be established for western women.

(a) The use of oral contraceptives is associated with an increased risk of thromboembolic disease which commences within one month of starting the medication and ceases within one month of stopping.

(b) The relative risk for the user is approximately 2–4 times that of the non-user.

(c) The risk of death is rare, being less than 1 in 100 000 users per year.

(d) The degree of risk is correlated with oestrogen dose and following the changeover to low-oestrogen combined contraceptives there is epidemiological evidence that the hazard of thromboembolic disease has declined.

(e) The risk of thromboembolic disease in normal women who do not use oral contraceptives but belong to blood groups A, B, and AB is twice that of women with blood group type O. Among oral contraceptive users, the risk of thromboembolic disease is 3 times as high in women with A, B and AB groups than in women with group O.

(f) The risk is slightly greater in users whose mothers or sisters have had thromboembolic disease.

It is not known if the risk of thromboembolic disease applies to third-world women. One study on post-operative thrombosis, which compared patients in Oxford and Bangkok, Thailand, found the condition less common in Asians after comparable operations.[60]

Stroke. In the 1960s there were conflicting reports about women suffering cerebrovascular accidents when taking the Pill.[139] In 1973 the Collaborative Group for the Study of Stroke in Young Women established that the incidence of thrombotic stroke was 3–4 times higher in Pill takers than in other women.[62] The attributable risk is about 37 episodes per 100 000 users per year. Approximately 5–10% of cases are fatal and morbidity can be severe in those who survive.[70]

The risk of thrombotic stroke does not appear to be related to the duration of oral contraceptive use and reverts to normal after use, while that of haemorrhagic strokes is thought to increase with duration of use and to apply to past users.

Stroke is rare in women of fertile years, so much so that in the case of thrombotic stroke insufficient observations exist to determine if either cigarette smoking or the dose of hormones influences the risk, although it might be assumed that one or both factors are important. In the case of haemorrhagic stroke cigarettes appear to exacerbate the risk. Petitti found that haemorrhagic stroke was 6.5 times as common in Pill users as in non-users but 21.9 times as frequent in women who smoke and use oral contraceptives as in non-smoking non-users.[219] High-dose Pills appear to carry a greater risk than low-dose Pills.

Migraine may be a prodromal sign of stroke and its occurrence, particularly in new Pill takers and should always be regarded as serious. The Pill should be discontinued, particularly if there is a concomitant rise in blood pressure.

Subarachnoid haemorrhage. Three out of five epidemiological studies have shown a statistically significant increase in subarachnoid haemorrhage among oral contraceptive users. It is not clear if the effect is a direct one or secondary to the small rise in blood pressure that occurs in Pill users.[132, 253, 315]

Post-operative thrombosis. Deep vein thrombosis is a common but unpredictable complication of surgery. Women who are using oral contraceptives at the time of operation are at slightly greater risk of deep vein thrombosis than are non-users.[110] In a study of 30 women who developed post-operative thromboembolism and 60 matched controls the increased risk appeared to be three to four fold.[308]

Patients approaching scheduled surgery should therefore be advised to discontinue Pill use before the operation. It is thought that the most important inhibitor of coagulation is an α_2-globulin which inhibits Factor Xa, sometimes called anti-Xa or antithrombin III.[258] A reduction in anti-Xa is found in Pill users and also correlates with an increased risk of deep vein post-operative thrombosis in any type of patient.[288] The advice to discontinue the Pill must be accompanied by adequate alternative contraceptive counselling; apart from the social consequences of an unplanned pregnancy, this will also increase the operative risks.

Intestinal thrombosis. The symptoms of mesenteric thrombosis are often vague, slow in onset and include abdominal pain, vomiting, diarrhoea and haemorrhage into the bowel. The patient may be febrile and have abdominal tenderness.

Mesenteric vein and artery and hepatic vein thrombosis have been reported in Pill users.[47, 127, 150] Arterial thrombosis is less common than venous thrombosis but more dangerous. Small bowel ischaemia has a high mortality and those who survive require radical surgery. In one sequence of 21 cases of oral contraceptive users who developed mesenteric thrombosis, 12 died: most were taking high-dose Pills and smoked, and several were hypertensive.

Overall picture of cardiovascular disease and Pill use The oestrogen component of combined pills appears to act mostly on the blood-clotting mechanisms, while some progestogens, such as norethisterone acetate, may exert an effect on the vascular tree, removing part of the protective effect exerted by HDL on the atherogenic process.[39] Progesterone may also influence hypertension and glucose metabolism, exacerbating possible arterial disease. Therefore, while a very high ratio of progestogen to oestrogen lowers the thrombotic risk, such a combination could be related to a greater risk of hypertension. Some progestogens have an oestrogenic effect, for example norethinynodrel, while others, for example norgestrel; have no such effect.

Epidemiological studies express probabilities but rarely prove causal relations. In the case of oral contraceptives and cardiovascular disease, the findings of prospective and retrospective studies together with collateral biological and clinical evidence are convincing. However, the demonstrable cardiovascular hazards of using combined contraceptives can be greatly reduced by the following measures:

(a) Stopping smoking or recommending an alternative method to those women over 35 who are rash enough to continue to use cigarettes.
(b) Selecting low-dose Pills whenever possible.
(c) Recommending alternative methods to most women over the age of 40.

If any of the following symptoms appear in women using oral contraceptives, their continued use should be carefully assessed:

(a) Sudden onset of severe chest pain.
(b) Sudden, severe headache.
(c) Calf pain with swelling of the leg.

The shift from high- to low-dose Pills in Britain was followed by a 25% reduction in reports of venous thrombosis.[248] A large decline in venous thrombosis, but not in arterial disease, also occurred in Sweden as low-dose Pills replaced high-dose Pills.[34] However, Meade and his colleagues,[187] using data from nearly two thousand fatal and non-fatal reports to the British Committee on the Safety of Medicines between 1964 and 1977, both confirmed the increased safety of low-dosage oestrogen Pills and found a reduced risk of arterial disease with lower doses of progestogens. Only 1 in 9 of the few deaths of oral contraceptive users in the Oxford study involved a woman *without* a predisposing risk factor such as heart disease or smoking.[177]

In the developing world, safe legal abortion to back up less effective contraceptive methods is often unavailable and maternal mortality is also much higher than in the West, so the women in their late thirties who smoke and most women over 40 are safer continuing on the Pill than choosing an alternative method. Fortunately, the few older women who smoke in the developing world often also belong to the social group that has access to modern medical services.

Where medical services are available to supervise oral contraceptive use and distribution, and where alternative methods of contraception are available and acceptable, it is prudent to deny the use of oral contraceptives to a woman with any of the following conditions:

(a) Previous deep vein thrombosis.
(b) Severe heart disease.
(c) Previous severe toxaemia of pregnancy.
(d) A personal history of hypertension.
(e) Demonstrated Type 2 hyperlipoprotinaemia.
(f) Blood dyscrasias, such as polycythaemia.

It is also wise to substitute an alternative method of contraception six weeks before major elective surgery and during the immediate post-operative period.

Up to 20% of the population may have one or more relative contradictions to oral contraceptive use and it must be appreciated that the guidelines which have been established are not absolute rules. A woman over 40 has the right to insist on using oral contraceptives just as she has the right to continue smoking or skiing down a mountain slope. In diseases such as leukaemia or diabetes mellitus, individual clinical judgement is needed but the Pill is not necessarily contraindicated.

Routine biochemical tests for hyperlipoprotinaemia are not recommended. A family history of the loss of the first degree relative from heart disease at or under aged 50 is a more practical guide in deciding whether to use oral contraceptives in doubtful cases.

Mann and his colleagues have attempted to put the data gathered from retrospective case-control studies based on 52 deaths from myocardial infarction in British women aged 40–44 into perspective (Table 10.6).[178] They assume that women not using pills might adopt the diaphragm and while using it have a failure rate of 10 per HWY. In a second comparison they estimate that cardiovascular deaths attributable to oral contraceptive use in the 20–35 age-group are equivalent to half the road accident death rate for the group, but in the 35–44 age-group, a woman using the Pill has twice the risk of death from her contraceptive method than from road accidents. It should be noted that the data were collected predominantly from women using Pills with at least 50μg oestrogen.

It is particularly important to note that, while epidemiology says something about yesterday's Pills, intensive clinical studies can give clues about the performance of today's. For example, Notelovitz found in women on 0.4 mg norethindrone and 35μg ethinyloestradiol (Ovacon) that antithrombin III activity was maintained, and no change occured in activated partial thromboplastin time, throughout 13 months of study.[207] He concluded that with low-dose Pills there was no evidence of enhanced intravascular coagulation.

Only limited data are available about blood clotting in the presence of progestogen-only pills and injectables and no epidemiological observations whatsoever are yet available. It may be guessed that the absence of oestrogen will obviate the clotting changes observed with combined pills,[224] but some residual risk of adverse cardiovascular effects could still exist due to the progestogen component. Perhaps injectables or progestogen-only pills would be more suitable for older women than combined pills, but this possibility has not been investigated and in the US, the FDA has so far chosen to deny the choice of injectable contraceptives altogether.

Epidemiological studies on oral contraceptives always receive widespread public attention and sometimes misinterpretation. When the relation between the oestrogen content of the combined pill and thromboembolic disease first became available from Britain and Scandinavia in 1970, a recommendation was made by the then Committee on the Safety of Drugs in Britain that low-oestrogen Pills should be used whenever possible. In

Table 10.6. *Overall death rate (annual mortality per 100 000) due to cardiovascular disease or maternal mortality. (Oral contraceptive users and non-users England and Wales)*

	Age-group	
Cause of death	20–34	35–44
Oral contraceptive users		
Myocardial infarction	1.1	8.1
Pulmonary and cerebral thromboembolism	1.3	3.4
Total cardiovascular disease	2.4	11.5
Maternal mortality	0.1	0.5
Overall risk	2.5	12.0
Non-users		
Maternal mortality	1.1	2.5
Excess risk of taking the Pill	1.4	9.5

reality it was a statement that a small risk could be made even less, but the lay press, and some doctors, took it as a signal of some previously undiscovered danger and a significant number of women temporarily gave up using oral contraceptives with the consequence that many unwanted pregnancies occurred. In America the situation was worsened by the fact that the findings came at a time when the Committee of the US Senate under the chairmanship of Senator Nelson was pursuing an emotional and not always objective account of the side-effects of oral contraceptives.

Epidemiologists nearly always state their findings with caution because controls and cases can never be perfectly matched. Data on the same problem using different methodologies are always welcome. Tietze has reviewed deaths due to cardiovascular disease in American men and women from 1950 onwards spanning pre-Pill and post-Pill years. Pill use rose to a maximum in the mid 1970s when over one quarter of all women in the 20–25 age-group were using the method. Between 1950 and 1976, the age-specific mortality rate of deaths attributed to diseases of the circulatory system fell in men by approximately 50% and in women even more rapidly. The greatest decline was in younger women. In view of the widespread use of oral contraceptives it is surprising that the national data show a decline in cardiovascular disease. Tietze developed his analysis by assuming a rise in cardiovascular disease among Pill users as predicted by the RGGP studies and then calculated the rate at which deaths from non-users would have had to have fallen to create the *average* rates which are measured in the nationwide records. The results suggest that a decline of 76–79% in deaths to women not using the Pill would have had to occur over the 24 years studied. Such decline seems unlikely, especially as women were smoking more heavily during this interval and entering a more competitive work environment. It seems more reasonable to conclude, as Tietze did, that 'In the case of cardiovascular disease, the levels of risk attributed to the Pill (based on 24 deaths of users and former users and five deaths of controls) in the RCGP study appears to be exaggerated'.[301] A WHO group led by Belsey[20] conducted a similar analysis on 21 developed countries, including Japan (where oral contraceptives are used by less than 10% of fertile women), the United States (10–19%) and Sweden and Australia (over 20%). They conducted regression analyses on national cardiovascular disease mortality data for pre- and post-Pill years, and again found trends which were less than those which the prevalence of use of oral contraceptives and the mortality measured in case-control studies suggested. Shearman has shown that the death rate from myocardial infarction in Australia declined significantly during the 12 years of maximum oral contraceptive use during which up to 32% of Australian women between the ages of 15 and 44 were using the Pill at any one time. Yet deaths due to coronary heart disease fell by 25.5% between 1968 and 1980 and those from cerebral thrombosis fell by 55.3% between 1952 and 1980.[271] Similar studies have been conducted in England and Wales (Fig. 10.6).

In conclusion, it is reasonable to accept the trends which so consistently appear in the prospective and retrospective studies carried out in Britain, Europe and North America and which have been used to set policies to advise women who may be at particular risk from oral contraceptive use. At the same time, the degree of risk seems to have been overstated and such

Fig. 10.6. Deaths of all women aged 15–44 from cardiovascular disease in England and Wales. (CVD, cerebrovascular disease; IHD, ischaemic heart disease.) (Redrawn from Wiseman, R. A. & MacRae, K. D. (1981). Oral contraceptives and decline in mortality from circulatory disease. *Fertility and Sterility*, **35**, 277.)

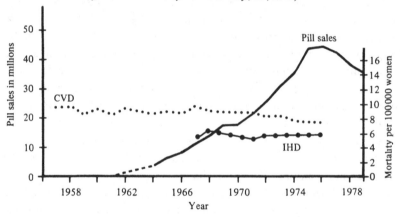

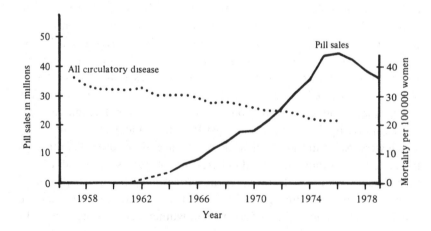

policies need to be applied wisely. As Shearman has pointed out, guidelines set up by regulatory authorities 'often acquire an apostolic aura, if not quite reaching the authority of an *ex cathedra* dictum'.

The many factors that must go into establishing an overall perspective on the risk and benefits of contraceptive use are also discussed in Chapters 4 and 16.

Neoplasia

Both users and providers of oral contraceptives are aware that their use might affect patterns of malignant disease. Several types of neoplasia, particularly of the reproductive tract, are influenced in their growth and development by endogenous and exogenous ovarian hormones. The importance of this potential problem is emphasized by the fact that in the US cancer of the breast and reproductive tract account for nearly half of all female malignancies.

The relationship between Pills and cancer is one that sometimes generates more heat than light. Between 1977 and 1980, 3735 papers on oral contraceptives and cancer were published in the world medical literature but only a handful presented any new data.[322]

The problems surrounding animal studies designed to predict the effect of hormones on the incidence of neoplasia and especially malignancy, have been emphasized earlier. The British Committee on the Safety of Medicines reported that contraceptive steroids given in up to 450 times the weight-equivalent dose throughout the life-span of rats and mice produced no evidence of carcinogenesis.[64, 333] Further, artificial steroids have been used therapeutically since 1938 and for more than 20 years in oral contraceptives, so that epidemiological studies on human use are now possible and are broadly reassuring. The latent interval for the growth of cancer can be long: if a malignant cell divides every 100 days, in 7 years it will form a clump of cells 1 mm in diameter, in 10 years a lump 1 cm across while in another 3 years it will form a tumour weighing a kilogram.

Cancer of the breast. One in 14 US women will develop cancer of the breast and 1 in 18 will die from the disease. Treatment is often disappointing and, overall, therapy has improved little, if at all, in the last 50 years. Breast cancer is the disease where an adverse effect of oral contraceptive use would be most catastrophic and where, by the same token, even a hint of a protective effective could have revolutionary implications for the health of women.

Breast cancer can arise in the nipple, ducts or alveoli and several types of alveolar cancer can be defined histologically. It is likely that these various forms of cancer respond in different ways to endogenous and exogenous hormones but in epidemiological studies data are usually pooled.

Many factors point to the significance of reproductive hormones in the aetiology of the disease. Less than 2% of mammary cancers occur in men and these men often have high oestrogen levels.[76] Cases of breast cancer have been reported in men receiving very high dosages of oestrogens for the treatment of prostatic cancer and also in transvestites taking oestrogen to enlarge their breasts. (In South-East Asia, transvestites sometimes consume a whole packet of contraceptive pills a day as a cheap and ready source of hormones, but no systematic study of this group has been performed.) In women, the disease is rarely found before puberty and in those women who have both ovaries removed between the ages of 20 and 40, a protective effect can be demonstrated. Established breast cancer responds in different ways to steroids, ovariectomy leading to remission in up to half premenopausal cases. Progestogens have also been used in treatment. Long-term use of postmenopausal oestrogen may possibly increase the risk of breast cancer.[125,162] High doses of contraceptive steroids in animals have been associated with breast tumours in beagle bitches on several occasions and in monkeys once, but controls also get the disease and the significance of 10 or 50 times the weight-equivalent human contraceptive dose is difficult to interpret.

The most important variable in the epidemiology of human breast cancer is the age when a woman bears her first child. Worldwide multicentre studies have demonstrated a linear relation between the age when a woman has her first child and the likelihood of her developing breast cancer later in life: the earlier the first pregnancy the less the risk. (Fig. 10.7).[173,174] Like those of many epidemiological studies these findings have been criticized on grounds of biases in matching controls, but increasingly careful studies appear to confirm the relation.[12] Where women marry and have children early (e.g. Ibadan, Nigeria) the incidence of breast cancer may be as low as 6 per 100 000 per year, while in societies where childbearing is postponed it is often ten times as high (e.g. 90 per 100 000 in Saskatchewan, Canada and 70 per 100 000 in Scotland).[229] Among Japanese women now in their forties and fifties, breast cancer is rare, but among those who migrate to the US it becomes more common and the incidence in their children reaches the high Caucasian levels.[50] Overall, the disease has many aspects of an environmentally induced cancer and it seems likely that varying incidences follow variations in the way in which women use their reproductive systems. It is not known how pregnancy early in life reduces the risk of mammary cancer. A pregnancy ending in abortion has no protective effect. It is the first pregnancy that exerts the effect and the effect is life long. Breast-feeding is more common in women who have their children early and may have a direct effect in addition to the age of pregnancy variable.[131]

The human breast seems more sensitive to oestrogens than that of even closely related primates and we are unique among animals in that the female breast develops at puberty rather than during the first pregnancy. In animals such as cats, breast cancer is most common in intact females that have never mated. In women the breast undergoes changes in volume during each menstrual cycle and Short and Drife have suggested that the greater the number of menstrual cycles that elapse between puberty and the first pregnancy, the greater is the risk of breast cancer.[275] The declining age of the menarche in western women (Japanese women now in their fifties had a later menarche than their contemporaries in the West[201]) might also be a factor in the dramatic differential in breast cancer rates in different parts of the world.

It is also true that women with a female relative who developed breast cancer have a two to three fold higher risk of the disease. Women who develop benign breast disease are more likely to develop breast cancer later in life.[32, 173] Variations in the pattern of metabolism of oestrogens in early

Fig. 10.7. Relative risk of developing cancer of the breast with age when first child born. (After MacMahon, B., Cole, P., Lin, T. M., Lowe, C. R., Mirra, A. P., Ravuihar, B., Salber, E. J., Valaoras, V. G. & Yuasa, S. (1970). Age at first birth and risk of breast cancer. *Bulletin of the World Health Organisation*, **43**, 209.)

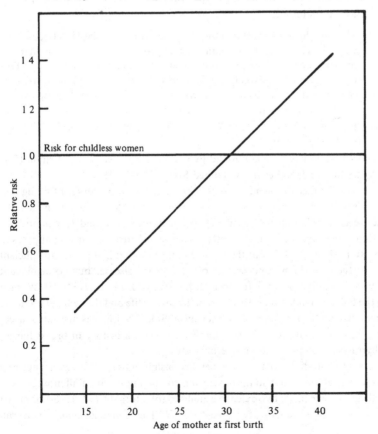

life have been suggested to be important in the aetiology of breast cancer, and it is possible that oestriol is less carcinogenic than oestrone or oestradiol, so that details of the balance of oestrogens in a young woman might be important in relation to cancer 20 or 30 years later. It is the level of oestriol which rises most markedly in pregnancy itself and which is relatively higher in Oriental than in Caucasian women.[172] An alternative explanation is that the fetus in the mother's womb immunizes her against the later development of breast cancer.[188] Such an effect can be simulated in animal experiments, although it would be reasonable to expect it to apply to all cancers, not just that of the breast.

It is against this background that the limited data on Pill users must be reviewed. Biopsy studies on women using the Pill are few. Pinotti *et al.* found dysplasia of glandular tissue and some fibrosis among users.[223]

The first important study on oral contraceptives and benign breast disease was published by Vessey, Doll and Sutton in 1972.[309] In a case-control retrospective study, 345 women with breast disease were interviewed in hospital to determine whether they had used oral contraceptives. The authors concluded:

> The data do not suggest that the use of oral contraceptives is related in any way to the risk of breast cancer, but provide some evidence that the preparations may actually protect against benign breast disease. This protective effect is largely confined to women who continue to use oral contraceptives and have used them altogether for more than two years. Such women appear to have only 25% as great a risk of being admitted to hospital for a breast biopsy as women who have never used oral contraceptives at all.

This initial finding has been confirmed by more extensive studies in Britain (Fig. 10.8) and additional studies in the United States.[91, 149, 216, 311]

In view of the fact that benign breast disease can be a precursor of malignant disease, is it possible that when more data are available on long-term use the protective effect of oral contraceptives might be demonstrated to extend to a reduction in the incidence of malignant breast disease? So far the answer appears to be no. By 1981 the RCGP and the Oxford cohort studies had gathered sufficient cases to study cancer as opposed to benign breast disease, but no significant alteration in relative risk was found in either study (Table 10.7).[252, 313] Women using the Pill may tend to have their first child later in life and this will have a direct adverse effect on the incidence of breast cancer. Since the Pill was first introduced, doctors have avoided giving it to young women with a history of breast lumps, thereby further complicating long-term study.

Case-control studies promise more detailed insight into specific age-groups and certain other relations, but so far have given conflicting results. Paffenbarger and his colleagues have made two extensive analyses (of a total of 1423 cases) of breast cancer from the San Francisco Bay area.[91, 217, 218] They found no change in overall risk among Pill users, but a relative risk of 1.38 in women using the Pill for two years or longer. The initial Paffenbarger studies suggested that women who used the Pill before the birth of their first child had a three-fold increase in the relative risk of developing breast cancer, but later, more extended analysis failed to substantiate this finding. More recently, Pike and his colleagues reviewed 163 cases of women who developed breast cancer at age 32 or less and found a relative risk of 2.2 among

Fig. 10.8. The incidence of benign breast lumps in Pill users. (After Royal College of General Practitioners (1974). *Oral Contraception and Health.* London: Pitman.)

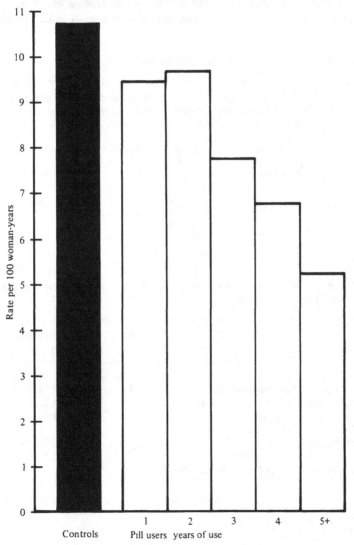

women who had used the Pill for four years or more to postpone the birth of their first child.[220] The Centre for Disease Control (CDC) Atlanta, Georgia, is conducting studies which have so far shown no difference in the incidence of breast cancer amongst those who started the Pill before or after a diagnosis of benign breast disease, before or after their first delivery or who had, or did not have, a relative with breast cancer (Table 10.8). Finally, Vessey's group analyzed 1176 pairs of breast cancer and case-controls (210 under the age 35), but found no association between Pill users and breast cancer even after up to four years' prior to the first pregnancy.[311] In view of the apparent effect of the first pregnancy on the pattern of breast cancer later in life, these results, while in need of confirmation with larger numbers, are important. At the other end of fertile life, Jick, using data from the Group Health Cooperative of Puget Sound, Washington State, found a positive

Table 10.7. *Breast cancer rates per 1000 woman-years*

	Woman-years of observation	Rate	Risk ratio: users vs controls (95% confidence limits)
RCGP cases (133)			
Current users	98 551	0.50	1.2 (0.7–2.2)
Former users	78 142	0.45	1.14 (0.7–1.9)
Controls	129 593	0.39	–
Oxford cases (72)			
Current users	47 206	0.52 ⎫	0.96 (0.59–1.63)
Former users	41 402	0.45 ⎬	
Controls	53 353	0.54 ⎭	–

Table 10.8. *Relative risk of breast cancer among oral contraceptive users[a] (n=687) and controls (n=1072)*

	Relative risk	(95% confidence limits)
All cases of breast cancer	0.96	(0.8–1.1)
First degree relative had breast cancer	1.1	(0.6–2.3)
Second degree relative had breast cancer	0.9	(0.4–1.2)
No relative with breast cancer	0.8	(0.6–1.1)
Used oral contraceptives prior to 1st birth:		
Unstandardized	1.8	(1.3–2.7)
Standardized for age at first birth	1.2	(0.8–1.8)
Cases with preceding diagnosis of benign breast		
disease	0.8	(0.5–1.3)

[a] Combined and sequential pills.
Source: Ory, H. (1982). Personal communication.

association between oral contraceptive use and breast cancer in women over 45.[140] The relative risk was four fold (95% confidence limits 1.8–9.0) for women aged 46–50 and 15.5 fold (5.2–46) for women aged 51–55. However, as in other studies the number of cases was small, being only 11 in the older group. Again, additional studies with specific age-groups are necessary.

A rather strong protective effect of the Pill on breast cancer was suggested in a study of 242 women with breast cancer carried out by Gambrell, using US Air Force medical records.[101] The incidence of breast cancer among current users was 17.7 per 100 000 women per year and among past users was 22–44 per 100 000. The weakness of the study lies in a lack of controls and a comparison was made with an incidence of 53.3 per 100 000 women in the Third National Cancer Survey. Current users appeared to have a better prognosis than non-users and Vessey (in the Oxford Study)[313] and others have made similar observations[183, 285] (Fig. 10.9).

In summary, the incidence of breast cancer has risen in western women

Fig. 10.9. Survival of women with breast cancer (treated by radical mastectomy): Pill users and others. (Redrawn from Matthews, P. M., Millis, R. R. & Hayward, J. L. (1981). Breast cancer in women who have taken oral contraceptive steroids. *British Medical Journal*, **282**, 774.)

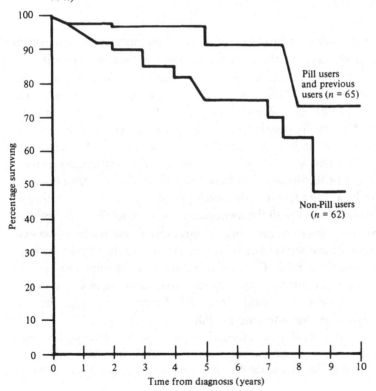

largely in response to changing patterns of childbearing. This change occurs regardless of the means used to postpone the first pregnancy and is more significant than any proven or possible alteration in mortality due to oral contraceptive use.

Animal studies remind us to be wary and avoid false assurance, but a number of epidemiological studies on Pill use and breast cancer give reassuring results and occasionally even suggest a protective effect. More than one type of response to oral contraceptives may occur. For example, women who have never been pregnant, particularly young women, could react in one way while older women who have had children might react quite differently. It is important that data are now becoming available on some of these subgroups, for example on women who used Pills prior to the birth of their first child. There can be no doubt that possible relationships between breast cancer and the oral Pill need continued monitoring. In establishing an overall perspective, newly established facts about the Pill and breast cancer allow open speculation about possible preventive measures rather than treatment and, even though the present oral contraceptives do not seem to meet this exciting goal, their use has certainly helped to define it.

Cancer of the Cervix. In the United States, cervical cancer is the second most common malignancy of the reproductive tract in women. But, although neoplastic changes in the cervix are readily accessible and widely observed in routine diagnostic Papanicolaou smears, the aetiology and even the natural history of cervical malignancy are still disputed. There is some evidence of a sexually transmitted carcinogen affecting the cervix and the herpes virus seems to be one factor. Age at first intercourse, frequency and number of partners and low socio-economic status all statistically increase the incidence of the disease. The hormonal status of the woman does not appear to be a major factor in the development or outcome of the disease, but its incidence rises until the menopause and then levels off or declines.

In the nulliparous woman oral contraceptive use leads to cervical growth and the endocervical cells become exposed to the vaginal environment for the first time. Cervical adenosis and adenomatous polyps sometimes develop during pregnancy and have also been observed in oral contraceptive users.[52] A histologically florid picture may arise, but the lesions regress on discontinuing the Pill.

The cellular changes of intra-epithelial cervical neoplasia (CIN) vary from mild dysplasia to carcinoma-in-situ and are in fact progressive in step-like form from one to another, but the timing and the degree to which each step may be reversible are disputed. Currently the generally held opinion is that lesions more advanced than severe dysplasia (CIN2) are unlikely to regress spontaneously. The more crucial step to early invasive cancer is also a part of the continuum of change but is irreversible.

Routine cervical screening, case-control studies and cohort studies have all been used to look for possible relation between cervical intra-epithelial neoplasia and oral contraceptive use. Such screening has shown no difference in the prevalence of cervical malignancy in users and non-users.[63] Case-control studies in Canada (308 cases of carcinoma in-situ)[335] and the US (378 cases of class III to class V smears[300] and 689 cases of carcinoma-in-situ and invasive cancer)[35] all found no relation between the disease under investigation and the use of oral contraceptives. A second series of studies that was built around comparisons between oral contraceptive users and diaphragm or IUD users found small changes in prevalence. In a study by Melamed *et al.*,[190] published in 1969, which is possibly invalidated by the fact that the oral contraceptive users were predominantly black and Puerto Rican women from New York and were compared with mainly white diaphragm users, an observed variation in the prevalence of carcinoma-in-situ (6.6 per 1000 for pill users and 3.8 per 1000 for diaphragm users) possibly reflected no more than their different lifestyles,[85] though there may have been a protective effect of diaphragm use. A follow-up study by Ory and colleagues in Atlanta[210] compared IUD and Pill users and found a higher rate of dysplasia in the latter (2.3 versus 1.3 per 1000) and the risk of carcinoma-in-situ rose from 1.3 per 1000 in the first year of use to 4.7 per 1000 after 36 months or more.[214] The Oxford study, the RCGP study and the Walnut Creek cohort study all showed no significant difference in cervical neoplasia among users and non-users.

One of the most interesting studies is that of Stem[291] who matched 300 women with cervical dysplasia and 300 with normal smears and followed the group for seven years, taking a cervical smear every six months. Women who were found to have normal smears when they entered the study had no increased incidence of abnormalities if they took the Pill, but women with dysplasia developed carcinoma-in-situ more rapidly, although the relationship only involved long-term users, the numbers involved were small and a high-dose (0.1 mg mestranol) Pill was used. In the original randomized trial of the Pill in Puerto Rico[222] there was no overall difference in cervical abnormalities among users and non-users, but women who entered with class III smears (approximately equivalent to CIN2) deteriorated more rapidly if they were taking the Pill.[100]

The uncertain biology of cervical neoplasia, and the lack of consistent epidemiological evidence, suggest that there is no strong, direct relation between the disease and oral contraceptive use, although the rate at which the dysplastic disease progresses may possibly be accelerated by prolonged use. It is likely that study will always be difficult because of a possible connection between particular sexual lifestyles and oral contraceptive use, either of which might predispose to cervical disease. In the US, at a time of explosive oral contraceptive use, annual mortality from cancer of the cervix fell dramatically from over 10 per 100 000 women in all age-groups in 1955 to just over 5 per 100 000 in 1975.

Cancer of the endometrium. While carcinoma of the cervix is more common in women of high parity the opposite applies to cancer of the endometrium, often known as cancer of the body of the uterus. Obviously for this reason cancer of the endometrium is more common in developed than developing countries, and in the US accounts for approximately 7% of all female cancer. Progestogens are used in the therapy of established endometrial cancer[93,324] and frequently cause premalignant changes to revert to normal.[153] The disease is more common in the obese, in diabetics, in women with Stein-Leventhal syndrome and apparently also after long exposure to unopposed oestrogens. It is rare in women under 40.

The study of the use of oestrogens for menopausal symptoms overlaps with the study of oral contraceptives, but unfortunately the area is an epidemiological minefield. Studies of women taking menopausal oestrogens have proved difficult because of possible biases due to unequal rates of follow-up among takers[126] and non-takers, inadequate history of dosage and duration of exposure and problems of classification. It is not surprising that some reports show increased risks while others do not.[6] Among endogenous oestrogens, oestrone seems to be the causal factor. At this stage it would be wrong to group all exogenous oestrogens together.[8]

Sequential contraceptives gave unopposed oestrogen for 14–16 days of each cycle, followed by oestrogen and progesterone. In one series of 30 cases of invasive endometrial cancer in women under 40 years of age in the US, 20 had used sequential preparations and 9 had used combined preparations[277] but the population base from which the cases came was unknown, and although an increased risk due to sequential use seems likely, the effect could have been overestimated due to the protective effect of combined pills. Whatever the final explanation, sequential pills have been withdrawn from use.

None of the cohort studies of oral contraceptive use have shown any evidence of increased risk of endometrial cancer and more recent case-control studies have shown evidence that the Pill exerts a protective effect against the development of endometrial cancer.[146,323] CDC studies show that the protective effect takes at least a year to demonstrate itself but persists for up to 10 years after Pill use. Among 187 cases of endometrial cancer and 1320 controls the relative risk of cancer among ever users of oral contraceptives was 0.6 (0.4–1.0). For nulliparous women it was 0.6 (0.4–1.0) but for those with three or more deliveries it was 1.0 (0.6–1.6). The annual incidence of cancer of the endometrium has risen slightly in the past 20 years in several countries, but the rise began before the Pill was introduced and appears to stem from entirely unrelated causes.

Cancer of the ovary. Ovarian cancer is responsible for 1 in 20 cancers of the female reproductive tract in western women, is often diagnosed late and carries a high mortality. It is a complex of pathological conditions some of which are not likely to be related to the woman's reproductive history.[167] It is less common in developing countries and, like breast cancer, often appears to be associated with voluntary or biological infertility.[55]

The RCGP study found a reduction in ovarian tumours in Pill users but numbers were insufficient to separate true primary ovarian cancers. In the Boston study Pill users were one-fourteenth as likely to develop functional ovarian cysts as non-users.[211] Although benign, such cysts often lead to surgery.

One case-control study involving 162 cases of epithelial ovarian cancer found a reduction among Pill users and it has been suggested that cancer is more likely if the ovary is 'wounded' repeatedly by ovulation, a hypothesis that would explain the protective effect of the Pill and observed effects of repeated pregnancy and prolonged long intervals of breast-feeding on reducing ovarian cancer (Table 10.9).[55] Rosenberg and colleagues found a 40% reduction in ovarian cancer and could detect a protective effect up to 10 years after the use of oral contraceptives was discontinued.[245] CDC studies have confirmed this finding and also show that the relative degree of protection falls with parity, being 0.3 (0.1–0.8) for nulliparous women and 0.7 (0.4–1.2) for women with three or more children. The protective effect was also demonstrated to continue for 10 years or more after the discontinuation of Pill use.

Table 10.9. *Relative risk of ovarian cancer with duration of supression of ovulation.*
(n = *162 cases of epithelial ovarian cancers and 150 controls*)

Cause of supression of ovulation	Duration of suppression	Relative risk
Number of live births	0	1.0
	1–2	0.75
	3+	0.59
Oral contraceptive use (months)	<6	1.0
	7–83	0.73
	84+	0.62

Other tumours. Uterine fibroids were widely believed, a decade ago, but without statistical evidence, to be encouraged by taking the Pill, and some physicians still avoid giving oral contraceptives to women with clinical evidence of fibroids. In fact, the development and rate of growth of fibroids is extremely capricious and it may be that the early belief that fibroids grew rapidly in some women on the Pill arose for the simple reason that Pill users received regular pelvic examinations and the irregular and sometimes sudden growth of fibroids came to be more widely appreciated. The RCGP study showed that fibroids were less common among Pill users than among controls and there was some evidence that the higher the progestogen content the greater the protection afforded.[249] There is no evidence to suggest that giving the Pill increases the size of pre-existing fibroids, although it is wise to advise the woman who has fibroids and chooses the Pill that they may still grow and cause symptoms in the future. It is good practice to keep any woman of reproductive age known to have fibroids under regular monitoring, regardless of whether she uses the Pill or not.

Hepatocellular adenoma is an exceptionally rare disease in women of the fertile years, occurring spontaneously in one or two women in a million. The tumour is benign but highly vascular and can cause death by haemorrhage. Oral contraceptives cause a marked rise in the disease and, although it is of great rarity, the association is a strong one. Biologically, the liver is exposed to circulating steroids in much high concentration when they are taken orally than when they are secreted by the ovaries or given by injection. The disease has become more common in the US since the Pill was introduced and in case-control studies there is a correlation with the duration of use, the relative risk rising rapidly from 9 times after 1–4 years of use to over 100 times in women who have taken Pills for 4 years or more.[10,86,151] High-dose Pills may carry more risk than low-dose Pills and, in at least some cases, withdrawal of the drug is associated with regression.[87]

Sometimes the tumour is discovered at routine laparotomy but it can present with pain or shock due to rupture. While the relation is a strong one the risk to the woman remains small (perhaps three to four deaths per million users a year).[243] To get the risk in perspective it is worth noting that, for example, the Scottish National Diagnostic Index, covering 5 million women between 1968 and 1974, when Pill usage was at its maximum, does not record a single case and Vessey found no cases in over 83 000 woman-years of exposure.[312]

Malignant melanoma occurred in more cases (24.1 per 100 000) of oral contraceptive users in the Walnut Creek study than non-users (17.6 per 100 000).[27] However, the explanation possibly lies with the fact that Pill users also sunbathe more often than non-users,[238] and it is an interesting illustration of how a single set of epidemiological findings needs to be interpreted cautiously.

Pituitary adenoma has been associated with Pill use in isolated case reports but there has been no published evidence of causal relation.[44]

Trophoblast disease varies greatly in its incidence around the world and is common in some developing countries. There is no evidence that either molar or other pathological pregnancies are in any way linked to prior Pill usage and recent data suggest that there is no increased risk of postmolar tumours if oral contraceptives are used following a molar pregnancy.[30]

Overall picture of neoplasia and Pill use. There is no doubt that the age at first pregnancy, the pattern of childbearing and such factors as lactation affect the development and outcome of some female cancers. The volitional control of fertility with mechanical methods of contraception or the use of periodic abstinence has already exerted a powerful documented and predominantly adverse effect on the pattern of reproductive neoplasia in the modern woman. The rise in the incidence of breast cancer with the postponement of the first pregnancy is the single most adverse change.

The use of oral contraceptives could affect the incidence and prevalence of benign and malignant disease in a particularly complex way, both by changing the pattern of childbearing and by having a direct effect mediated through alterations in the levels of circulating hormones. Some of these effects are beneficial, as in the reduction of ovarian cancer, while others are harmful, as in the increased risk of benign but potentially lethal hepatic tumours. However, the significance of a relative risk lies more in the intrinsic frequency with which the disease occurs than in the magnitude of the change. In the case of breast disease, which accounts for nearly one quarter of *all* cancers in women, there is good evidence of a reduction in benign tumours but increasingly convincing evidence about no change in malignant disease.

The story of high doses of diethylstilboestrol (DES), given to women as a supposed therapy for threatened abortion, and the increased incidence of clear cell adenocarcinoma of the vagina and cervix in their daughters is well known.[122] As the risk occurs in another individual many years after exposure, it has a particular poignancy. It also seems as if the mothers themselves have a higher risk of several diseases later in life.[26] In the lay mind the DES story has become a paradigm for contraceptive risks. In fact there was no real similarity because of differences in the way the hormone was given, the dosage and the hormone used. Nevertheless, the episode is a sober warning of the complexity of hormone interactions with cancer and a sad reflection on the medical profession's tendency to be swayed by fashion: the original treatment had no biological reason behind it and, indeed, was shown to have no therapeutic effect.

The use of contraceptive steroids, as their effectiveness demonstrates so strongly, is based on sound biological principles. This does not mean to say that they are free from the risk of altering the pattern of human malignant disease, they obviously do just that, but it seems likely that in the past 20 years most neoplasms that could be altered by the use of combined oral contraceptives have been reviewed. It is of course possible that additional adverse or beneficial effects could still be discovered, but as our experience grows year by year this seems less and less likely. Overall, Pill users have not been shown to have any greater risk of cancer than non-users and indeed there may in certain cases be a protective effect. In the contemporary US up to 5000 less cancers may develop each year as a result of present or past Pill use.

Other diseases
In addition to effects on the cardiovascular system and alterations in the profile of neoplastic disease, the use of combined oral contraceptives also has good and bad effects on several other diseases.

Gall bladder disease. The mean level of cholesterol saturation in bile is higher in women using Pills. In addition the proportions of the different bile acids alter. The exact mechanism behind these changes is not understood, but they are probably the basis of the observed rise in gall bladder disease (cholecystitis and gallstone formation) found in both the RCGP study[249] and the Boston Surveillance Program.[33] Surgically proven gall bladder disease occurred in 79 cases per 100 000 non-users and 158 cases per 100 000 users.

The risk of gallstones appears to rise with the dose of progestogen.[248] After four to five years of Pill use, a woman has approximately twice the risk of gall bladder disease as would a non-user. In the US Pills may contribute up to 10 000 of the 800 000 new cases of gall bladder disease that occur annually.[25] More recent studies suggest an even lower risk.[7]

Rheumatoid arthritis. In contrast to causing gall bladder disease, combined oral contraceptives protect against rheumatoid arthritis, and a woman who uses the Pill has approximately half the risk of developing the disease. The effect has been demonstrated in the RCGP study[256] and appears to be confirmed by community statistics in which cases of rheumatoid arthritis in men have plateaued since 1960, while among women they have fallen.[168]

The protective effect of the Pill does not appear to be dose dependent nor is there evidence that it changes with time. It is not known whether contraceptive hormones suppress the autoimmune responses or if some other action is involved.

Infectious diseases (including pelvic inflammatory disease). Hormones influence host resistance to infection: for example, diabetics are at greater risk of infection than healthy individuals and adrenalectomy in experimental animals increases susceptibility to infection. Pregnant women get more urinary tract infections than non-pregnant women.[145] It is not surprising that the Pill affects a number of infectious diseases.

Infectious hepatitis is reported in Pill users more often than in non-users, but it is uncertain whether this is a causal relation or a coincidental one related to lifestyle[200] and to the fact that Pill takers are in closer contact with doctors so that the disease, which is notoriously easy to miss, is therefore more likely to be diagnosed. The fact that the effect is more pronounced in women under 25 suggests that sexual transmission of the disease may be important.

The RCGP study found urinary tract infections to be 25–50% more common in Pill users,[249] although most cases are asymptomatic.[89,297] The study also suggested that the trend was more marked with higher doses and longer usage.

Oral contraceptives exert a significant protective effect against pelvic inflammatory disease.[268] Possibly this effect is mediated by changes in the cervical mucus. The protective effect is large (a 50% or more reduction in risk (Table 10.10)) and involves a disease that is common in many societies and which is Of particular long-term significance for young women who are also those most likely to use the Pill. In many parts of the world reduction in

Table 10.10. *Incidence of pelvic inflammatory disease in contraceptive users and non-users (Swedish women aged 20–29 years)*

	Rate per 1000 woman-years of exposure
Sexually active non-contraceptive users	34.2
IUD users	52.1
Oral contraceptive users ($n = 16311$)	9.1
Barrier users	13.9

Source Weström, L., Bengstsson, L. P. & Mardh, P. A. (1976). The risk of pelvic inflammatory disease in women using intrauterine contraceptive devices as compared to non-users. *Lancet*, ii, 221.

pelvic inflammatory disease may be the single most important benefit of the Pill.

Endometriosis. There is a clinical impression that endometriosis is less common among users of combined oral contraceptives and either the Pills themselves, or similar oestrogen–progestogen combinations are used therapeutically for this purpose, but there is no systematic epidemiological confirmation or refutation of this possibility.

Ectopic pregnancy. All oral contraceptives, by reducing the chances of conception, reduce the incidence of ectopic pregnancy, but the reduction is less in the case of progestogen-only pills than in combined pills and therefore the *ratio* of ectopic to intrauterine pregnancy is *higher* when progestogen-only pills are used.[29,281] Possibly progesterone induces changes in tubal motility, further changing the pattern of ectopic gestation.

The diagnosis of ectopic pregnancy should not be overlooked in oral contraceptive users. In the case of progestogen-only pills menstrual irregularities brought about by the method may confuse the diagnosis.

Evaluation
Combined pills

Combined oral contraceptives are remarkably effective, relatively cheap, simple to use and unrelated to intercourse. They greatly reduce the blood loss and pain associated with menstruation and most side-effects that a user notices are mild and get less after a few cycles of use. Pills have been tested more meticulously than any other medication and found to have widespread systemic actions, from a possible reduction in the incidence of acne to a virtually certain rise in the incidence of cardiovascular disease.

The hazards and benefits of oral contraceptive use are curiously well balanced: how does the user or provider balance an increase in the acute pain of cholecystitis against a reduction in the chronic discomfort of rheumatism; a reduction in benign breast disease versus a rise in a rare benign but potentially lethal liver tumour and a reduction in ovarian and endometrial cancer against a rise in cardiovascular disease? Clearly the Pill has changed the profile of diseases among users, but has it changed it for the worse? In the contemporary US, with an estimated 9 million current Pill users there may be 500–1000 episodes of cardiovascular disease each year, half of which may be fatal, that can be attributed to the use of combined oral contraceptives, while among current and past users the Pill may prevent up to 5000 cases of ovarian and endometrial cancer. It may yet be proved that, all considerations of contraception apart, the Pill may prevent more deaths than it causes.

Neither the risks nor the advantages of oral contraceptives were discovered chronologically in the same order as their clinical or numerical significance. Media reporting and the reactions of the medical profession and the lay public have often been irrational. The discovery of deep vein thrombosis sparked more controversy than some later more important findings about coronary thrombosis. Conversely, important advantages, such as protection against pelvic inflammatory disease and some pelvic cancers are not yet widely known. Only recently has the impact of the Pill on general surgery been assessed and it is estimated that each year there are 270 *fewer* operations per 100 000 Pill users due to the reduction in breast disease and ovarian tumours as well as a massive reduction in pelvic inflammatory disease (Table 10.11).[212, 213]

'Everytime there is a new pill scare', remarks Christopher, 'pills are thrown away, women become pregnant and then may want an abortion. This phenomenon has been seen several times, particularly among domiciliary family planning patients who are least able to evaluate the risks associated with the pill.'[59]

The medical profession as a whole, like users, has sometimes been bewildered by the onslaught of information about oral contraceptives, occasionally building up clinical guidelines to deal with one piece of information but then failing to dismantle such defences when additional facts become available.

Table 10.11. *Rate and total number of hospital admissions prevented annually by oral contraceptive use*

Causes of hospital admission	Rate per 100 000 users	Total hospital admissions	
		UK[a]	USA[b]
Benign breast disease	235	7 000	20 000
Pelvic inflammatory disease	156	4 600	13 300
Ectopic pregnancy	117	3 500	9 900
Ovarian retention cysts	35	1 000	3 000
Endometrial cancer[c]	5	150	2 000
Ovarian cancer[c]	4	120	1 700

[a] Estimated 3.0 million current users.
[b] Estimated 8.5 million current users.
[c] Estimate includes protection offered to past users.
Source: Modified from Ory, H. W. (1982). The noncontraceptive health benefits from oral contraceptive use. *Family Planning Perspectives*, **14**, 182.

In the case of combined oral contraceptives caution is sometimes recommended in their use by teenagers. There is very little objective information to guide the clinician, partly because the age-groups involved tend to be socially mobile and are therefore excluded from many of the epidemiological studies, but the very low incidence of serious side-effects found among women in their twenties can probably be extrapolated to the youngest age-groups. Certainly the Pill meets the social needs of the young unmarried for a highly effective, easy-to-use method. The protection against pelvic inflammatory disease can be particularly significant. The Pill is not necessarily contraindicated in women with irregular and scanty periods and could even be the method of choice as it will, at a minimum, ensure monthly exposure to progestogens in women who are otherwise at a somewhat greater risk of developing endometrial carcinoma later in life. Therapeutic pessimists will argue that young women with oligomenorrhoea may later prove to be infertile, even if the data on the return of fertility after oral contraceptive use appear to be reassuring. There would seem to be good reasons for making the Pill widely available to young people who need it, but to ensure that every woman who has not borne a child (and particularly those with menstrual problems suggesting irregular ovulation) understand that fertility cannot be proved in advance of pregnancy.

The Pill, like pregnancy, presents greater risks to the older woman, but there is no need to routinely deny its use to all women over 35. Some couples will choose an alternative method (e.g. voluntary sterilization or an IUD) of their own volition but others may benefit from being offered new choices and additional counselling on the relative risks and benefits of oral contraceptive use as they get older.

Experience has shown that oral contraceptives can be taken by women with many chronic diseases (e.g. tuberculosis) including, in selected circumstances, diabetes. Epidemiological studies suggest that there is no need to deny the Pill to women with breast or pelvic disease, as was once thought necessary. In the case of follicular ovarian cysts, the combined pill is the treatment of choice.

When all the current data on combined oral contraception are reviewed, it seems reasonable to use low-dose Pills when possible.[152] In certain instances long-term use may lead to cumulative problems such as the possible long-term risk of myocardial infarction, hepatocellular adenoma and gall bladder disease. It must also be noted that some beneficial effects for example the reduction in ovarian cancer, also increase with duration of use. In practice most women discontinue use after a few years and there is no indication for setting a strict limit on how long a woman may use the Pill.

The lifestyle of women who choose the Pill in rich countries may exacerbate some risks (e.g. the association between smoking and cardiovascular disease[320]) and present certain hazards unassociated with Pill use, but which will nevertheless appear more frequently among users (e.g multiple sex partners with cervical cancer, and sunbathing with malignant melanoma).

As far as can be ascertained, the risks of oral contraceptive use in the developing world are no greater and may be less than in the West. Smoking and obesity are less common among third world women and physical exercise more common. The dangers of childbearing are much greater, and often abortion is illegal and sometimes voluntary sterilization hard to come by.

Deaths from ectopic pregnancy that would otherwise occur will be prevented by widespread use of oral contraceptives. It is in the health interests of women in the developing world to make the Pill freely available, and clinically and ethically necessary to modify guidelines about relative and absolute contraindications so that local needs are met with full understanding of local risks and benefits (see Chapter 4). A possible deleterious effect on breast-feeding must be considered (see Chapter 6) in designing a distribution system.

The practice of distributing Pills through community outlets in developing countries is a responsible one.

Progestogen-only pills

Combined pills have given rise to most controversy, but progestogen-only pills[227] have perhaps been the most under-utilized.

Progestogen-only pills bring about less extensive physiological changes than combined pills. They have a higher failure rate and are less tolerant of irregularities in use than combined pills and this might prove of particular importance in the developing world. They have been less extensively studied, so at the same time they appear to be both more bland medications and lack evidence of specific advantages: for example, might they also reduce the incidence of pelvic inflammatory disease? Although epidemiological evidence is lacking, progestogen-only pills are likely to be associated with less risk of cardiovascular disease and of metabolic changes. Therefore the method may have a valid place for some older women who reject permanent methods of contraception, as well as for some diabetic and hypertensive women. From a developing world perspective, progestogen-only pills are associated with a less beneficial pattern of ectopic pregnancy, but also carry less of a question mark against their use by lactating women and, once again, advantages and disadvantages appear to be evenly balanced.

PERI-COITAL STEROIDS

Oestrogens and progestogens are both capable of preventing pregnancy when given shortly before or after coitus.[231] Such methods have obvious attractions for those who have had unpremeditated or unprotected intercourse, where a mechanical method is thought to have failed or in the tragedy of rape. The hormones may act on the endometrium and/or tubal motility. The altered hormonal environment probably upsets the sequence of events necessary for implantation.

Post-coital pills are marketed in Hungary and China (the visiting Pill) and the practice of giving steroids after unprotected intercourse is spreading in Europe. Being discontinuous in use, the method is difficult to evaluate. Possible teratological effects must be recognized. It would be biologically rational to limit post-coital preparations to places where legal abortion is available, but the social pressure for use is likely to be greatest because abortion is illegal. (The post-coital use of IUDs is discussed in Chapter 11).

Ethinyloestradiol (2–5 mg) and diethylstilboestrol (25–50 mg) have both been used as post-coital agents, taken on five consecutive days after unprotected intercourse and beginning within 36 h. In 3016 cases, 17 pregnancies were reported (0.05%) and only five pregnancies occurred in those cases where total doses of at least 3 mg of ethinyloestradiol or at least 30 mg of diethylstilboestrol were given.[119] The schedule is associated with nausea in many women and vomiting in some. Subsequent menstrual irregularities can occur.

Another compound that has been used post-coitally is D-norgestrel and the combined oral contraceptive tablet (0.25 mg D-norgestrel and 50μg ethinyloestradiol) taken two at a time and repeated 12 h later appears to act as a post-coital preparation and is recommended as an emergency treatment within 72 h of unprotected intercourse by the IPPF and is used by clinics and family doctors in Britain.

LONG-ACTING STEROIDS

Injectables
Long-acting progestogens were first synthesized in the 1950s and

occasionally used in the treatment of gynaecological disease. A variety of progestogens and combinations of progestogens and oestrogens have now been used as injectable preparations or as subdermal implants, and promising work is now being conducted on the microencapsulation of steroids. The Chinese have developed a once-a-month Pill. However, these products, and in particular the injectable preparations, while popular among users, have been perceived as highly controversial by certain public groups and use has not grown as rapidly as demand would otherwise have allowed.

Medroxyprogesterone acetate was synthesized in 1954 and the depo preparation (DMPA or Depo-Provera) was first tested as a contraceptive by Tyler, Coutinho and others in the early 1960s.[67] In the 1960s and 1970s DMPA was used by many thousands of women within the US and by the 1980s was approved as a contraceptive in 80 developed and developing countries, including Sweden, Belgium and New Zealand. In 1967 the Upjohn Company asked the US FDA to extend the registration of DMPA as a therapeutic agent to include contraceptive purposes. In 1974 the FDA published a letter of approval, but it was immediately withdrawn following pressure from both the public and Congress. In 1978 the Obstetrics and Gynecology Subcommittee of the FDA recommended registration a second time, but the FDA rejected this expert advice, partly on the grounds that there was no significant demand for this type of contraceptive in the United States. The FDA Commissioner pointed out that non-approval of DMPA in the United States does not mean that the drug could not be acceptable in other countries with a different pattern of health problems. The Upjohn Company is appealing the decision about US use. In 1982 the British Committee on the Safety of Medicines approved DMPA as a contraceptive; however, implementation was vetoed by the Minister of Health. This unprecedented action was claimed to be because the medical profession might misuse the drug, giving it, for example, to mentally retarded patients in inappropriate circumstances. But, of course, an IUD, abortion or a tranquillizer could be similarly misused and the Minister's action merely reflects the lack of a coherent philosophy towards the control of human reproduction and really represented an immediate reaction to political pressure rather than any comment on injectable contraceptives.

In the world as a whole, approximately one and a quarter million women are using Depo-Provera as a contraceptive and over 10 million women have used it at some time or other, approximately one half of them being in developed countries. Eight hundred scientific references exist to DMPA and the drug has been extensively reviewed.[21, 23, 97, 228]

The patent on DMPA has now expired and it is distributed by a number of manufacturers in the developing world. Depo preparations consist of a crystalline form of the hormone which is slowly absorbed at a rate determined by particle size and other physical chemical properties. It is normally given as a three-monthly intramuscular injection of 150 mg, although regimens extending to six months or more have been used. Within 24 h of injection, serum levels reach 2.6–7.8 nmol/L and plateau at 2.6–3.9 nmol/L over the next two to three months.[209] Once released from the depo site, DMPA is cleared from the blood stream within about 24 h. Unlike other contraceptives, DMPA has been used in large doses in the therapy of endometrial cancer and blood levels of 100–200 times as high as those found using the contraceptive regimen have been recorded; there do not seem to be obvious ill effects.[154, 257, 260] DMPA has also been used in the treatment of endometriosis, precocious puberty and even sleep apnoea. It has also been used in attempts to control male fertility (see Chapter 16, Future developments in fertility regulation).

Other long-acting injectables include chlormadinone acetate, 17-hydroxyprogesterone acetate, lynesternol phenyl-propionate and norethisterone enanthate (NET-EN).[330, 331] Only the latter has achieved widespread use, but still on a more limited scale than DMPA. A number of monthly injectables (e.g. the combination of DMPA and oestradiol valerate and other progestogens plus an oestrogen) have been developed.[67, 88, 303] Monthly injectables are widely marketed in Mexico, where more than 100 000 women use the method.

Croxatto and Segal first described the sustained release of steroids from silastic capsules in 1966. The Population Council undertook multicentre, double-blind trials of a number of steroids and found L-norgestrel to be the most suitable candidate for acceptability trials. Each silastic capsule is 2.4 mm in diameter and 36.0 mm long and releases around 4 μg of drug per 10 mm of capsule per day. Six more capsules are usually implanted giving a blood level of around 1 ng/ml, although there is considerable variation between individual women.[204]

Capsules are usually placed under the skin of the forearm and remain easily visible. Infection and irritation are a rare complication of use. Unlike a depo preparation, implants can be removed by operation. Insertion requires a local anaesthetic, skin incision and use of a large trocar. Selected women have accepted the method well and net 12 month continuation rates of 75 per 100 women and higher have been reported. It is not known if medical workers will feel any reluctance to insert these novel devices.

A new concept in injectable contraceptives has been developed by Beck and associates who have microencapsulated steroids with polylactic acid to produce microspheres that range in diameter from 10 to 250 μm and which are slowly degraded biologically.[18, 19] They have the advantage of relatively constant steroid release associated with implants, but the convenience of an injectable which can be administered by anyone with a clean syringe and needle. They may represent an important step forward and could displace depo preparations and overtake implants.

Physiology

Depomedroxyprogesterone acetate, like oral contraceptives, abolishes the cyclical release of LH and FSH, probably by an action at the hypothalmic level. Implants and once-a-month pills appear to have the same effect. Injectable contraceptives seem to have less effect on overall bodily physiology, for example on liver or thyroid function, than do oral contraceptives but they may have a more profound effect upon the genital tract. DMPA is a particularly potent progestogen, binding to progesterone receptors with approximately 30 times the affinity of the natural hormone.[299]

The 17-acetoxy progestogens do not produce any oestrogenic products on metabolism and, unlike oral contraceptives, injectables and implants do not have to be absorbed from the gut and pass through the liver.

Effectiveness

Injectable contraceptives are the most effective reversible contraceptives known. The reported pregnancy rates for DMPA vary between zero and 0.35 per HWY.[97, 267] In the WHO comparative trials, the cumulative gross pregnancy rate per HWY was 3.6 ± 0.7 for NET-EN and 0.7 ± 0.4 for DMPA, and the continuation rate for NET-EN was 83.1 and for DMPA 76.6 per 100 users at 12 months, the difference being due to the larger number of women who had discontinued DMPA because of amenorrhoea.[22, 247] L-norgestrel implanted in silastic capsules had a 12-month net pregnancy rate of 0.6 per 100 women.[66]

Side-effects

In the well-documented Chiang Mai programme in the north of Thailand, one million injections of DMPA have been given without serious adverse reaction at the time of injection and without a single death attributable to the drug in the group of users at any time. In the world literature, only one case of anaphylactic shock at injection is recorded.[49]

The major side-effect of long-acting steroids is on patterns of menstruation. These are least disrupted in the case of monthly preparations but severely altered in the case of three- and six-month injectables. The discontinuation rate for L-norgestrel implants due to menstrual disturbances was 12.3 per HWY. In the case of DMPA, not only is the menstrual cycle grossly irregular, but there is a high incidence of amenorrhoea, particularly after three or four injections. In a double-blind comparative trial of NET-EN and DMPA in Bangladesh, less than 15% of users of either drug were having regular menstrual bleeding after four or more injections.[295] The overall blood loss is usually reduced, but occasionally there are episodes of heavy bleeding.[158] If necessary, these can be halted by oral steroids (four Norinyl-80 or comparable Pills will usually prove effective) or an oestrogen injection.

Depomedroxyprogesterone acetate reduces the incidence of vaginal moniliasis and may, like oral contraceptives, reduce pelvic inflammatory disease, but this remains to be fully documented. DMPA causes an important reduction in the symptoms of sickle-cell disease in women homozygous for the disease.[77]

Many women gain weight on DMPA or NET-EN, often as much as 0.5–2 kg (about 1–4 lb) in the first year.[330] Interestingly, weight gain appears to be *less* among obese women.[164] Weight gain has also been reported in women with L-norgestrel implants. Some women complain of headaches, abdominal discomfort and mood changes. Although all these alterations may be genuine side-effects in some cases, they are difficult to measure and are only rarely reported by users as reasons for discontinuation.

Apart from serious disruption of the menstrual cycle and weight gain, long-acting steroids seem to have less side-effects than oral contraceptives. There is no evidence of significant changes in blood coagulation or fibrinolytic systems.[241, 326] It would seem reasonable to conclude that most of the cardiovascular risks associated with oral contraceptive use do not apply to the two injectable contraceptives DMPA and NET-EN or to implants, although some of the long-term risks that may depend on progestogens rather than oestrogen might still occur. It seems unlikely that any study which can totally confirm or refute such a possibility will be carried out in the near future, but the limited evidence that does exist suggests that thromboembolic disease occurs no more frequently in DMPA users, and may perhaps be less than among non-users.[203]

In contrast to women using oral contraceptives, no consistent rise in blood pressure has been demonstrated among women on injectables. Women with high blood pressure at the time of commencing the drug were more likely to experience a fall than a rise.[164]

There appears to be a small increase in fasting glucose and insulin levels in the case of DMPA users.[284] Most studies on DMPA have shown no change in fasting triglycerides or in cholesterol levels, although one study found a small reduction in HDL.[42] The data on NET-EN are more limited but no changes have been detected in blood glucose, insulin, growth hormone, total lipids or cholesterol levels. A WHO study in Thailand found that Depo-Provera could be safely used by women with liver fluke (*Opisthorchis viverrini*) infection.

Return of fertility

Numerous studies have shown that the use of injectable steroids is associated with a slow return of fertility (Fig. 10.5).

The first analyses of the return of fertility after DMPA use were limited to only one year after discontinuation and it was suggested that some women might be permanently infertile after using the drug. However, further analysis has shown that the median time to conception is about 10 months after the last injection with fertility returning to 75% of women within 15 months and to 95% in 24 months.[184, 266, 302] NET-EN appears to be associated with a more rapid return of fertility, although study has not been as extensive as in the case of DMPA. There are no substantiated cases of failure of fertility to return after the use of injectables, although a potential user should be warned of a delay in conception of several months discontinuation. Ectopic pregnancies have occurred during the use of implants and after DMPA use, but are exceptionally rare in the latter case.[294]

Teratology and effect on the infant

Neither DMPA nor NET-EN has any adverse effect on the amount or duration of lactation and infants of DMPA and NET-EN treated mothers gained weight more rapidly than controls.[144]

It is possible that DMPA increases milk volume[157] and a direct effect by raising serum prolactin has been reported.[57] In the case of DMPA, there is a 1:1 ratio of the drug in plasma to milk, while in the case of NET-EN there is a 10:1 ratio.[264] The appearance of artificial steroids in the milk has raised concern for possible effects on the infant, which overlap in part with discussion on possible effects on the fetus. However, the absolute level of DMPA in the milk is low and an infant would have to be breast-fed for 500 years to receive the amount of DMPA contained in a single adult dose. Follow-up babies where the mother received DMPA postpartum has not revealed any differences with controls.[73, 128]

While the effect of long-acting steroids on the suckling infant has probably been exaggerated, possible effects on the fetus require more discussion. In this regard, injectable contraceptives differ from oral contraceptives in two ways. First, if a depo steroid is given inadvertently to a pregnant woman or if accidental pregnancy takes place, there is no way of discontinuing the dose once it has been injected. Second, steroids remain present in the body for many months after the last injection and could still be present at low levels when conception occurs. However, during use for contraceptive purposes, injectable preparations are even more effective than oral contraceptives and accidental exposure of a fetus is exceptionally rare. For this reason, it is unlikely that a definitive epidemiological study on the human teratology of injectable steriods will ever be conducted. The small number of studies on DMPA provide neither total reassurance nor cause for alarm.[265, 339] No relevant information is available for NET-EN. Providing the woman returns early in pregnancy, implants can be surgically removed in cases of unintended pregnancy.

In high doses, medroxyprogesterone acetate has a masculinizing effect on the female rat, rabbit and dog and a single case of a masculinized human baby has been reported in a woman who received DMPA during pregnancy for non-contraceptive purposes.[327] Overall, DMPA has an *anti*androgenic effect in human use[1] and normal babies have been delivered to women who received as much as 400 mg of medroxyprogesterone acetate during pregnancy.[104]

Neoplasia

The greatest debate concerning the use of long-acting steroids has revolved around possible carcinogenicity. The issues are similar to those surrounding oral contraceptives. In theory, exogenous hormones could raise, lower or leave unchanged the incidence of a number of cancers and could have different effects on different tumours and on the same tumour at different stages in its evolution. In practice, the use of injectables has remained relatively limited and most series still fall short of the number of cases necessary to provide a definitive answer to the questions that can be asked. In the case of subdermal implants, it might be decades before appropriate studies could be mounted.

In some studies, a higher prevalence of abnormal cervical smears has been recorded in DMPA users[169] but not in others.[72] The rate falls with duration of use and the change would appear to be a reflection of the lifestyle of those selecting the drug rather than any biological effect. There is no evidence of any change in the risk of invasive cervical cancer.

Oral contraceptives reduce the incidence of ovarian cancer and, if this benefit is the result of reduced ovulation, it could extend to users of long-acting steroids, although the only data available are limited in value. Liang *et al.* found a relative risk of 0.8 (95% confidence limits 0.1–4.0) for ovarian cancer in American users of DMPA.[165] Benign liver tumours have been reported in users of oral steroids and it could be argued that this risk will either be less, or eliminated, when steroids are given parenterally.

The main problem with long-acting steroids revolves around the interpretation of toxicology experiments using DMPA in animals. Two out of 12 rhesus monkeys given DMPA at 50 times the human dose for 10 years developed neoplastic changes in the endometrium.[332] As DMPA given in high doses is an effective therapy for human endometrial cancer,[61] and in contraceptive doses produces endometrial atrophy, these unexpected results have been doubly difficult to interpret: do they reflect a species difference in response to steroids (the rhesus endometrium is unlike that of the human in having a midline thickening[15]); do steroids at a high dose have an effect they do not show at lower doses; is it a statistical accident; or could it be indicative of a similar but lower risk when the drug is used in contraceptive doses in women? No cases of endometrial cancer among DMPA users have been found in northern Thailand, where use has been especially extensive, although the numbers available for study are small and do not yet provide statistically significant results.[185] Among 60 000 woman-years of observation in Atlanta, Georgia, US, a relative risk of 1.2 (95% confidence limits 0.1–6.7) was found when the number of cases of endometrial cancer among DMPA users was compared with National Cancer Institute data.

The major area of concern, however, as with oral contraceptives, is perhaps a possible relationship between continuous low levels of progestogens and the incidence of breast cancer. Benign and malignant breast tumours have been found in beagle dogs given 125 times the human dose of DMPA and benign tumours have been found in rats given NET-EN.[97, 332] However, the tumours occur spontaneously in many bitches, dogs lack the sex hormone-binding globulin so that blood levels are correspondingly higher, the bitch breast responds to progestogens in a way that the breast does not in women[80] and, finally, unlike humans, dogs release massive amounts of growth hormone in response to progestogens.[96, 108] The UK Committee on the Safety of Medicines and WHO have both concluded that the beagle results are not of value in predicting possible human risks.

Direct observation on the human use of DMPA and breast disease is now becoming possible and to date has been broadly reassuring. Two cases of breast cancer among DMPA users have been reported,[340] but this is not unlikely in the case of a common disease. The best data, and even these have their limitations, come from a study of a population of more than 10 000 predominantly black women who used DMPA as a contraceptive in Atlanta, Georgia. In a case-control study, 16.7% of women with breast cancer had received DMPA at some time, as against 17.9% of control cases.[112] Liang *et al.* followed up 5000 women for 4–17 years after their initial DMPA injection and found that relative risk of breast cancer for DMPA users was 0.7 (95% confidence limits 0.3–1.4).[165]

Vaginal rings

Drug absorption through the vaginal walls is good and pharmacologically active compounds pass directly into veins draining into the inferior vena cava, and, as with injectables and implants, bypass the liver on their first pass. A number of progestogens have been made into sustained-release systems that can be left in place for three weeks and removed for one, during which menstruation occurs.[92, 197, 278]

The technology is similar to that of a cat or dog flea collar and a polysiloxane ring is impregnated with medroxyprogesterone acetate, norgestrel or some other steroid. Cycle control is usually good. The ring sometimes gives rise to a discharge and the acceptability of inserting such a device, leaving it in place for three weeks and then removing it, cleaning it and storing it for one week has not been extensively investigated.

The rings are 50 mm or more in diameter and release 250–290μg L-norgestrel and 150–180μg oestradiol daily. A study of over 1000 users found a gross pregnancy rate of 3 per HWY. Subjective symptoms such as headache and nausea may be less than for oral contraceptives, perhaps because oestradiol is used and systemic absorption avoids immediate passage through the liver. The use of L-norgestrel/oestradiol rings reduces HDL levels and raises the cholesterol/HDL–C ratio. There is no way of knowing, pending widespread use, if these changes cancel one another out or if use might raise the risk of cardiovascular disease.

Once-a-month pills

Quinestrol is an oestrogen which is absorbed into the body fat and then slowly released over the next three to four weeks. Combined with an oral progestogen it can be used as a once-a-month pill which acts by suppressing ovulation.[208] Use was pioneered in the late 1960s by the Warner-Lambert Company in America and an effective and acceptable product developed.[114] However, when clinically tested in the US a higher pregnancy rate was discovered and when further clinical studies showed that a small change in the dose of quinestrol was necessary, the potential expense of meeting the mechanical requirement of the regulatory authority to repeat the whole of the investment already made in animal toxicology studies proved a deterrent to further research. Quinestrol is marketed for the treatment of menopausal symptoms. However, the Chinese continued to work on a once-a-month pill and eventually developed a formulation containing 12 mg norgestrel and 2 mg quinestrol. (Both hormones are FDA-approved and have undergone extensive toxicology studies, but as noted have not been approved in this particular combination in the West.) The Chinese recommend a routine of one Pill on the fifth day of each cycle and a second Pill on the twelfth day of the first cycle only. The pregnancy rate appears to be 2 or 3 per HWY of exposure and is probably better than the observed use-effectiveness of the combined pill in many developing countries.[194] Women sometimes complain of nausea on the day the Pill is taken, but the method has proved popular in China and deserves active study elsewhere.

As with vaginal rings, use causes changes in blood lipids[83] which require further investigation in an effort to forecast any possible effect on the cardiovascular system.

Conclusions

In comparison with oral contraceptives at a similar stage in clinical use, long-acting contraceptive steroids have performed slightly better than daily oral contraceptive steroids, while toxicology experiments in animals have raised a somewhat greater number of issues. However, long-acting steroids have been introduced in a different political environment than was the Pill and have become the focus of a passionate public debate.[175, 189, 195] Long-acting steroids are certainly popular among many users (Fig. 10.10) and often have better continuation rates than Pills or IUDs. DMPA, in particular, has been the subject of more emotion than common sense and it seems that preparations such as NET-EN and subdermal implants may come to be more widely accepted than DMPA for the very reason that *less* is known about them.

EVALUATION

Steroidal contraceptives are the only geniunely twentieth-century method of contraception. They have been simultaneously oversold and over-criticized. Slow in development, often abused in the media and sometimes misunderstood by physicians, nevertheless they have wrought a social and medical revolution.

Fig. 10.10. Contraceptive choice made when DMPA was freely available (Matlab area of Bangladesh 1977–81).

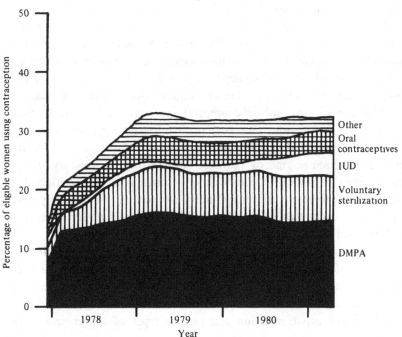

In all developed countries, oral contraceptive use grew rapidly soon after the method became available. By 1972, sales in non-communist countries had reached about 20 million women and users in China were estimated to be 13–20 million. In Britain and America the Pill became the single most popular method of contraception, overtaking older methods such as condoms and eclipsing IUDs. In Australia, one-quarter of all women (aged 15–44) were users as early as 1969 and by 1974 the proportion had risen to one-third. In the United Kingdom, acceptance was slower, reaching 20% by 1977 (Fig. 10.11).

The prevalence of oral contraceptive use began to decline in several developed countries in the late 1970s[270] but continued to grow in the developing world. In a very real way, women in the rich world had been the guinea-pigs for women in the developing world. The United States Agency for International Development (AID), under the leadership of R. T. Ravenholt, became the major supplier to overseas aid programmes, providing 100 million cycles of so-called blue lady Pills annually.

If family planning is to continue to succeed, it must be expected that the total worldwide use of steroidal contraceptives will continue to increase and that the greatest use is yet to come. However, a decade's publicity of adverse effects and frequent misreporting has taken its toll in the developed world and, in addition, voluntary sterilization has become more available than previously, taking away some of the need for the Pill. At the same time, a whole generation of potential users and physicians has grown to adulthood in the new world of the Pill. Ignorant of the bitter experiences their parents often had in the pre-Pill era, they began returning with naive enthusiasm to the barrier methods their parents had abandoned so happily. Perhaps the pendulum will swing back in the 1980s to some reasonable position where methods are neither oversold nor over-criticized but used in complementary ways to solve the important problem of fertility regulation.

A much larger investment has been made into studying the effects of the Pill than was put into developing it in the first place. Over the last 20 years, the Pill has become one of the best studied drugs in history. If the controversies surrounding the use of long-acting steroids can be lifted, they may also come to be used by tens of millions of women in a relatively short time. If this occurs, then a great deal of additional information is likely to be discovered about this important class of contraceptives.

The mechanism of steroid action is known in considerable anatomical and even molecular detail. Side-effects of exceeding rareness have been measured with considerable accuracy. Steroidal contraceptives have proved uniquely effective as contraceptives and the Pill has been shown to protect against pelvic infection and certain types of cancer and to be acceptable to nearly all younger women. Rare deaths have been associated with Pill use in older women, especially if they smoke, but to date (1983) no deaths have ever been reported with the use of long-acting steroids. Even with the Pill, if the estimated 10% of all users over 30 who smoke were to stop smoking it would reduce the number of heart attacks among users by 75%.

Perhaps it was predictable that the first agents in history to provide totally reliable, fully reversible, simple and acceptable ways by which

Fig. 10.11. Estimated minimum number of women aged 15–44 supplied with oral contraceptives in selected countries. (Modified from *Population Reports* (1974). Oral Contraceptives – 50 million users. Series A, 136.)

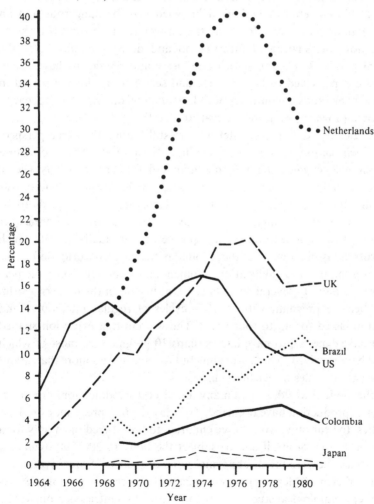

human beings could gain control over the wonder and joy of bearing a wanted child, should have proved too great a challenge to some individuals with insufficient understanding to handle such a freedom. It is this human fact, as much as anything unique about the pharmacology of the agents themselves which has made the interpretation of their side-effects such a persistently controversial issue. There are, of course, a great many reasonable questions to be asked about the biology, physiology and epidemiology of steroidal contraceptives. As in all scientific fields, every question answered tends to raise two more that can be asked. As with most creative human endeavours, it is easier to destroy than to build. Painstaking, responsible and expensive efforts to improve contraception by a whole team of professionals can be set back by one amateur with access to a medical library, enough biological knowledge to be dangerous and an unscrupulous publisher. However, the answer to this problem must be more, not less, sharing of information and decision-making with the general public. The manufacturing industry and physicians have sometimes been perceived to be defensive and secretive by those involved in using new methods of contraception. Fortunately, opinion does appear to be moving towards more positive attitudes.[147, 189, 198, 213]

Biologically, contraceptive steroids are still finding their true perspective. Their action is seen as something 'unnatural'. Some of those professionally engaged in family planning look forward to the day when a non-hormonal alternative will be discovered which is as simple and safe as the Pill. But in a way, this might be a retrograde step. It needs to be appreciated that the human reproductive system has been tailored over millions of years of evolution to a sequence of reproductive events which are profoundly different from those found in the modern world. Before the pressures of modern civilization, women underwent the physiological changes of puberty several years later than they do in the modern world. Most became pregnant within a few cycles of regular intercourse and lactation lasted for up to four years. The woman that evolution shaped could have expected to have had perhaps 10 pregnancies, most of which would have survived to breast-feeding but to have had no more than about 50 menstrual cycles in her lifetime.

In the modern world, a great many 'unnatural' modifications of normal human reproduction have occurred. To delay the first pregnancy until the twenties, to bear only two or three children, to breast-feed them only for a few months or not at all and to subject the body to 200–300 ovulatory menstrual cycles, is a highly abnormal series of events.[273] Moreover, it is a pattern of changes demonstrably associated with certain pathologies. As noted, epidemiological studies from a number of countries demonstrate a correlation between the age of the first pregnancy and the probability of developing malignant disease of the breast later in life: the earlier the women has her first term pregnancy, the less the chance of developing cancer of the breast later on.[173] In the US, 1 in 14 women can expect to develop breast cancer and 1 in 18 to die of the malignancy. Modifications in the 'natural' patterns of childbearing may also be associated with an increase in endometriosis, ovarian cancer and other forms of pelvic pathology. Evolution has left women with a reproductive system geared to early and continuous childbearing but no-one would suggest that young girls should have babies in order to avoid breast cancer and other reproductive pathologies in later life. The world needs effective contraception and preferably in a form which mimics the life-long pattern of reproduction associated with protection against such diseases. Up to the present time, steroidal contraception, possibly in particular when it involves suppression of ovulation, is the nearest we have come to this ideal. Those who condemn the Pill as unnatural have forgotten their biological history and pre-history.

The answer to the question posed earlier in this chapter: has the flight from oral contraceptives in developed countries been justified? seems to be that users and providers have been going through a period of unjustified apprehension. Steroidal contraceptives, after more than 20 years of use, have been found to have several defects, but they remain the only fundamental contraceptive innovation of the twentieth century and it is hoped that appropriately monitored evolution of the method will continue and that its use will increase.

11

The intrauterine device

History

More or less any foreign body placed in the uterus prevents pregnancy in the majority of cases and intrauterine contraceptive devices (IUDs) have a lengthy history. Guttmacher called attention to anthropological evidence showing that such appliances were used by preliterate people.[33] Casanova recommended a gold ball[13] and as recently as 1950 one women was reported to have used her wedding ring as a do-it-yourself intrauterine device.[25]

The medical forerunner of the modern intrauterine device was a stem pessary first described and illustrated in the *Lancet* in 1868. Originally intended to treat retroversion of the uterus, its contraceptive function was soon noticed and 10 years later Dr C.H.F. Routh complained to the British Medical Association that his colleagues were inserting stem pessaries and 'teaching a way to sin without detection'. As might be expected such condemnation popularized the method and by the end of the nineteenth century intrauterine devices were prominently featured in surgical catalogues. A wide range of models had by then been elaborated, including gold or gold-plated 'wishbone' pessaries. The structure of these pessaries was such that, when fitted, a V-shaped intrauterine device held a device like an enlarged drawing pin in the cervix. It was claimed that 'they regulated the menses'. It was through the accidental fracture of such pessaries, which resulted in the retention of a portion within the uterus when the cervical part was lost, that the contraceptive efficacy of the completely intrauterine body was discovered. At the turn of the century Dr Richard Richter, a practitioner near Braslaw in present-day Poland, fashioned an IUD with two threads which hung through the cervix thus facilitating removal of the device. In 1909 he published an article, entitled 'A means of preventing conception', which capably summarized much of what we know about

IUD use.[73] Richter described how women 'sacrificed their health and happiness every year for the sake of child-bearing' and concluded 'it becomes a matter of obligation and conscience under these circumstances that the physician attempt to restrain the excess of children. After many years of testing and improving I am able to offer my colleagues a simple and safe contraceptive. This is a silk-worm gut suture which is inserted into the uterus. Irritation of the endometrium by the thread is so slight that the majority of women do not feel it at all, yet it is sufficient to prevent pregnancy.' Despite the need, the medical profession turned its back on the opportunity.

In the 1920s Grafenberg (1881–1957) in Germany and Norman Haire in Britain began a second effort to use the IUD, this time a coil of silk-worm thread secured by silver wire and later an 18-mm diameter pliable ring of coiled silver wire.[27] The devices were inserted by dilatation of the cervix and the women was examined annually. Ota independently devised a ring-shaped device in Japan in 1925.[64] At the 1929 Zurich Birth Control Conference, Grafenberg reported 3% failures amongst 1100 women fitted with his devices. 'The method is not suitable for every doctor, nor is it suitable for every patient . . . We must differentiate very carefully between individual cases, . . . the important point is that it must not be regarded as the only method: *every physician must select the method that in his opinion* is the right one for the individual patient.'[28]

Grafenberg was arrested by the Nazis in 1937, partly because of his IUD work, and his freedom was purchased with money raised by Margaret Sanger. Subsequently, he practised in New York[54] but his advice on IUDs was not followed and IUDs fell into disrepute as cases of pelvic inflammatory disease and peritonitis and at least one death was reported. A standard textbook of contraception, first published in 1938, classified the Grafenberg ring among 'harmful' methods and even the 1960 edition states 'the use of intrauterine devices for birth control is advisable only when other methods have failed repeatedly or are unacceptable'.[82] Only a handful of doctors, notably Jackson in Britain, Ota in Japan and Knock in Indonesia, had the insight and courage to use IUDs during the next generation.

During the Second World War and into the late 1950s, a sophisticated clinic serving London's Mayfair fitted modified Grafenberg rings by dilatation and curettage (D and C) under general anaesthetic with the provision that any women whose menses became delayed should return at once for D and C and change of device. Naturally the zero pregnancy rate was much appreciated by a clientele who could afford the expense.

In the 1950s several doctors re-examined the intrauterine device and two in Japan, Kondo[51] and Ishihama,[43] achieved considerable success using rings constructed from nylon and polythene. Their results attracted the attention of the Population Council in America which between 1959 and 1962 spent US $1.5 million on work designed to improve and re-habilitate the IUD. In 1962 Margulies devised the first flexible plastic IUD which did not require dilatation of the cervix.[60] In the same year Dr Jack Lippes of Buffalo published a report on the first six months' experience of 264 women fitted with similar open, pre-stressed plastic devices of superior design which bear his name and are still used throughout the world.[57] Closed devices of various forms were devised by Zipper in Chile, Ragab in Egypt, Szontagh in Hungary and a number of Chinese scientists,[59] and continue to be widely used in the Far East, though in the West they are no longer used for fear uterine perforation may cause intestinal obstruction.

Today it is thought that 60 million IUDs are in use worldwide, of which over 40 million are in China, a country where it is the single most commonly used contraceptive method. In Britain and the US about 1 in 14 married fertile women use the method but in some Scandinavian countries more that 1 in 4 women are using an IUD. In most developing countries IUDs are used by only a small percentage of sexually active women. Copper devices have captured a large proportion of the European market but are unknown in China. IUDs, it would seem, like shoes, are influenced by fashion.

Mode of action

It is surprising, after so many years of use, that it is still not known for certain how IUDs work in human beings. Almost certainly they produce no systemic hormonal effect. One early explanation was that they cause increased tubal motility, this being shown in monkeys but never confirmed in women.[49] It has been suggested that a foreign body in the uterus increases prostaglandin secretion, but again animal experiments have not been confirmed in women. The insertion of an IUD post-coitally appears to prevent pregnancy and this is strong empirical evidence that at least one of the actions of the IUD must occur after fertilization.[6] Further, if an IUD is removed mid-cycle and careful mechanical precautions are used for every intercourse thereafter, pregnancy can occur, suggesting that fertilization must have taken place before removal of the device.

The most straightforward, and perhaps the most likely explanation of IUD action, is that a foreign body in the uterus causes a migration of white cells into the cavity. Leucocytes do not normally penetrate above the basement membrane of the endometrium. However, in the presence of any IUD migration of leucocytes has been demonstrated in both women and experimental animals. Electron microscopic observations in the mid 1960s demonstrated that devices removed from users were covered in a thin layer of leucocytes,[68] but it was the elegantly simple experiment by Nuri Sagiroglu from Turkey of smearing removed loops on a microscope slide which enabled the role of leucocytes to be followed in particular detail.[75] Within a few hours of insertion massed cells migrate to the region of the device and within a few days numerous monocytes can be found. After about a week more than 100 000 macrophages will be present on any one device.

Sagiroglu removed devices between 2 and 16 h after coitus and found macrophages containing phagocytosed sperm. It is clear that this capture of ascending sperm has, of itself, a contraceptive action but its importance in the total process is not known. Fertilization certainly occurs in women using an IUD more often than pregnancy is diagnosed.[9] Exactly what happens in women is speculative but when mice or rhesus monkeys are fitted with IUDs, blastocysts are altered and destroyed by leucocytic infiltration (Fig. 11.1).[40-2]

The fact that the clinical effectiveness of IUDs appears to be propor-

Fig. 11.1 Drawing from electron micrograph showing an intact leucocyte *inside* a degenerating blastocyst (Rhesus monkey fitted with an IUD). (Redrawn from Hurst, P. R., Jefferies, K., Eckstein, P. & Wheeler, A. G. (1977). Intrauterine degeneration of embryos in IUD-bearing mice. *Journal of Reproduction and Fertility*, **50**, 184.)

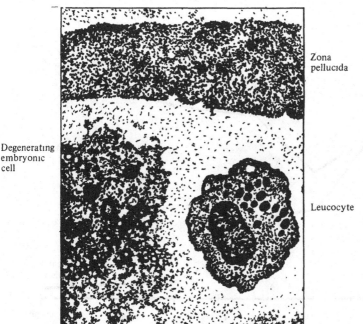

Zona pellucida

Degenerating embryonic cell

Leucocyte

tional to the surface area (Fig. 11.2)[50] fits well with the hypothesis that white cell invasion is one essential factor in their effectiveness. It is not a response to infection, because the same leucocytic outpouring occurs in germ-free animals. Women receiving immunosuppressive therapy after renal transplant have conceived using an IUD.[97]

The early stages of mammalian development are somewhat similar in man and laboratory rodents: the blastocyst is small, invasive and the timing of development comparable. A foreign body can be placed in one horn of a bicornuate rodent or rabbit uterus, where it inhibits pregnancy, while the other horn can sustain normal development. If a thread is placed at the time of mating but removed before implantation then development proceeds normally. A short thread placed at the tubal end of the uterus will inhibit implantation throughout the experimental horn but a similar thread placed near the cervix prevents implantation in that area only. The experimental transfer of blastocysts has shown that the IUD-treated horn is lethal to the early embryo, and if a culture of leucocytes is injected into one horn of a rabbit uterus, pregnancy will not occur in that horn.

Fig. 11.2. The effect of IUD surface area on rates of removal and accidental pregnancy. (After Kessel, E., Bernard, R. & Thomas, M. I. (1976). *Performance and Hypothesis Testing in International Clinical Trials*. Research Triangle Park, North Carolina: International Fertility Research Program (IFRP).)

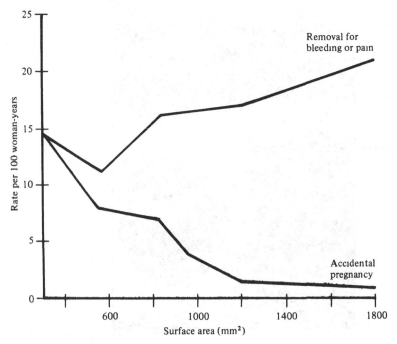

From present evidence it seems likely that the contraceptive mode of action, or at least the main action of inert IUDs is achieved by inducing phagocytosis and absorption of the very early embryo.

Devices
Design

A satisfactory intrauterine device must be easy to insert and remove, remain in place for as long as desired and be associated with a low rate of side-effects and even lower pregnancy rates. No such ideal device exists as the very plethora (Fig. 11.3) of different models produced, some of which look as if they come from packets of breakfast cereals, demonstrates.

It is difficult to determine the normal shape and dimensions of the human uterus as most methods of investigation have the potential of distorting the lumen. In addition, the living uterus is a muscular organ undergoing contraction and relaxation. In practice, therefore, the geometry of IUDs often reflects little more than an intelligent guess about uterine shape or a commercial need to avoid infringing someone else's patent rights. After many years of effort it is humbling to recall that the Grafenberg ring remains one of the most widely used devices (most IUDs are in China and the Chinese use the device widely) and few inert devices perform

Fig. 11.3. A selection of IUDs.

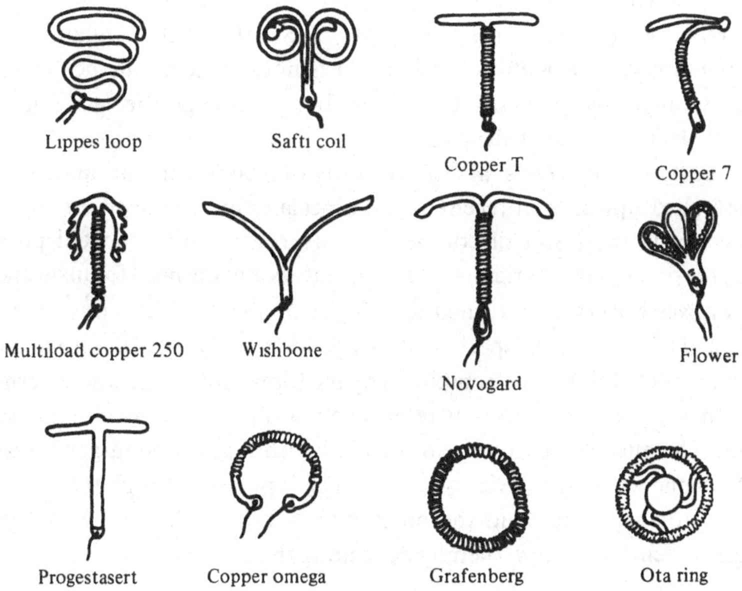

Lippes loop Safti coil Copper T Copper 7

Multiload copper 250 Wishbone Novogard Flower

Progestasert Copper omega Grafenberg Ota ring

significantly better than the aesthetically, economically and mechanically satisfactory Lippes loop.

While large devices have low pregnancy rates they do have more side-effects. In an effort to escape from this dilemma a second generation of IUDs was developed in the 1970s. Zipper wrapped copper wire around a small device.[98] A low concentration of copper ions is released into the uterine cavity and there is a direct relation between the area of copper exposed and contraceptive efficiency. Copper ions have no inhibitory effect on ovulation or fertilization but may be spermicidal, and certainly stimulate the migration of white cells into the uterine cavity.[34, 46]

A second type of biologically active device employs the slow release of a progestogen.[36] In theory, the intrauterine release of the progestogen could render the endometrium unsuitable for implantation, or the cervical mucus hostile to sperm or alter tubal transport in addition to the leucocyte migration caused by the presence of the device. The Progestasert device releases daily 65 μg of natural progesterone which is probably all metabolized in the uterus itself. The synthetic hormone D-norgestrel is used in other devices.

In 1970 Davis described a plate-shaped IUD, the Dalkon shield, which covered most of the uterine cavity and had a low expulsion and pregnancy rate. This device was widely promoted and became widely used.[19, 37] Within five years, however, use was associated with serious infection and, in a few cases, death, where women wearing the devices became pregnant and developed a septic abortion, often in the second trimester of pregnancy. The device was withdrawn and over 4000 women and their lawyers have claimed a total of nearly US $100 million against the manufacturers A. H. Robins, although it is not yet clear whether or not there was anything qualitatively different between the performance of the Dalkon shield and other devices.

The cost of many IUDs, and particularly of second-generation devices, has spiralled upwards in recent years, especially in developed countries. This is partly the result of competitive advertizing, sophisticated packaging, the occasional avariciousness of inventors and the need for insurance as dissatisfied users have turned to suing manufacturers and physicians.

Most IUDs come with specially designed inserters which fall into one of two categories. The first is exemplified by the Lippes loop where an external tube remains stationary while an internal plunger pushes the device into the uterus. The alternative arrangement, used with many second-generation IUDs, is one where the device within its tube is passed through the uterine cavity[80] to the fundus and the outer tube is then withdrawn while the plunger is held stationary, thereby depositing the device high in the uterine cavity. The later design is less likely to be associated with perforation because the device and the tube, moving as one unit, can be smoothly passed through the cervical canal and can then be used to 'sound' the uterus. With the old type of introducer any sticking between the device and introducer had to be overcome by force directed inwards towards the uterine fundus and a sudden overcoming of such friction disposed to perforation.

In the West it is usual to incorporate a string, or tail, to an IUD. This string passes through the cervical canal and into the vagina. The primary purpose of the string is to assist in removal, but it also acts as a marker to health professionals and to the woman herself to demonstrate that the device remains in situ. A sudden shortening or disappearance of the string may indicate pregnancy, uterine perforation or the unwanted expulsion of the IUD, whereas a sudden lengthening invariably indicates that it has moved downwards into the cervical canal and that expulsion may be imminent or the device no longer effective. In China few devices have tails and removal is performed with a small hook.

Biologically active devices have to be removed and reinserted regularly, although devices with sleeves of copper will remain effective for a decade or more.

Performance

The Population Councils' Co-operative Statistical Program multi-centre trials of the International Fertility Research Program (IFRP) and numerous individual investigators have produced a great deal of information on IUD performance[38, 67, 88] (Table 11.1). Fortunately, this large literature can be distilled to a relatively small number of useful generalizations. Firstly, the experience with the same device in different centres can be as great or greater than differences between different devices in different centres (Fig. 11.4). Secondly, as noted, the larger the area of an IUD the higher the number of side-effects but the lower the pregnancy rate. The addition of copper lowers the risk of pregnancy, even for small devices, and the addition of a progestogen reduces menstrual loss and lowers the pregnancy rate. However, progestogen-releasing devices have virtually disappeared from the UK following reports that they appeared to be associated with an increased incidence of ectopic pregnancies relative to other IUDs.[78] No unequivocal epidemiological study on this problem has been published and they continue to be used elsewhere. Thirdly, pregnancy rates, the possibility of expulsion and the incidence of infection are much more closely related to the age of the user than to the type of device used. The older the woman, the lower the pregnancy rate with any IUD (Table

Table 11.1. *One-year net cumulative life-table rates per 100 women for selected IUDs*

Device	Pregnancy	Expulsion	Removal for medical reasons
Lippes Loop A	5.3	23.9	12.2
Lippes Loop B	3.4	18.9	15.1
Lippes Loop C	3.0	19.1	14.3
Lippes Loop D	2.7	12.7	15.2
Copper 7[a]	1.9	5.7	10.7
Copper T 380[a]	0.8	9.2	27.5
Progestasert[a]	1.8	3.1	11.2
Chinese Flower[b]	2.9	5.9	7.5

[a] Parous women only.
[b] Chinese data, unlike western data, have not been prepared by the life-table technique.
Sources: Population Council, Family Health International and Lu Zilan (1980). Flower intrauterine contraceptive. *Chinese Medical Journal,* **93**, 528.

Fig. 11.4 Rates of pregnancy, expulsion and removal for users of Lippes loop D. (Data from Cole, L. P. & Edelman, D. A. (1980). A comparison of the Lippes Loop and two copper-bearing intrauterine devices. *International Journal of Gynecology and Obstetrics,* **18**, 35.)

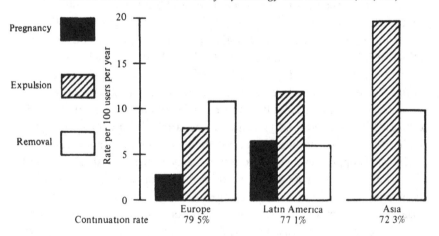

11.2) and the less the possibility of developing local or pelvic infection.

Menstrual loss has two components: volume (or heaviness) and duration of bleeding. Each component is affected differently by different IUDs. Surface area is related to volume of loss and copper-bearing IUDs, which have small areas, cause less menstrual loss than larger, inert devices. Most IUDs increase the duration of bleeding above the average found before IUD insertion. Only progesterone-loaded devices reduce menstrual loss to a level below the average prior to insertion.

IUD use has been well reviewed by Edelman, Berger & Keith.[21] Some of the longest follow-up of IUD users has been conducted in Japan and extends over 12 years.[35, 43, 62]

Storage and sterilization

An IUD must be placed in the uterus in a sterile condition. Metal devices can be autoclaved or boiled. Polythene devices soften at 98°C (200°F) and cannot, therefore, be sterilized by heat; if acquired loose they must be stored in antiseptic solutions. Benzalkonium chloride (Roccal or Zephiram 1:750) is a suitable solution and devices can be stored indefinitely in such a solution in screw-topped jars. Alkaline glutaraldehyde sterilizes copper devices effectively. Unfortunately the action of most antiseptics is slow and devices and introducers must be soaked for a minimum of 24 h prior to use. Iodine is an effective bactericidal and viricidal agent in concentrations of 1:100 to 1:1500 (12 ml tincture of iodine to 100 ml of water). It is cheap, readily available and quick acting, although some women are allergic to iodine and in concentrations above 1:1500 it is

Table 11.2. *Age and IUD use (12 month net rates per 100 users)*

	Age of women	
Complication	Less than 30 yrs (95% confidence limits)	30 yrs and more (95% confidence limits)
Pregnancy		
Lippes Loop C	1.6 (1.3–1.9)	0.7 (0.5–0.9)
Copper 7	2.7 (2.5–2.9)	0.6 (0.4–0.8)
Expulsion		
Lippes Loop C	9.7 (9.0–10.4)	3.9 (3.3–4.5)
Copper 7	13.7 (13.2–14.2)	6.3 (5.7–6.9)

Source: Snowden, R., Williams, M. & Hawkins, D. (1977). *The IUD: A Practical Guide*. London: Croom Helm Ltd.

irritant and in theory could cause tubal inflammatory response. Many commercial devices, particularly copper devices and all hormone-containing devices, are sold in sealed sterile packs.

Counselling on IUD use

The family planning worker must be prepared to devote far more time to explaining the method to the woman and answering her questions than is necessary to insert the device itself. It may be wise to ask why she has chosen the method; an unwillingness to use other methods of contraception can be a good reason for having a device, but belief that it is less trouble than alternatives is not always valid. A brief history should be taken and if current or recent uterine infection or salpingitis is uncovered, then in most cases the woman should be counselled against IUD use. Particular attention should be paid to the woman's future desire for children, especially if she is young and has more than one sexual partner, when an IUD may be contraindicated. A history of menorrhagia is not necessarily a contraindication although its cause should be sought before insertion. It is argued below (see Ectopic pregnancy) that there is no evidence which establishes the IUD as a cause of ectopic pregnancy. Logically, therefore, a history of previous ectopic pregnancy is not a contraindication to fitting a device. Any woman who has had an ectopic pregnancy has, however, a more than average risk of having another. If her first ectopic pregnancy occurred when using an intrauterine device she is liable to feel convinced that the method was responsible and if she is unfortunate enough to suffer again she will then blame both her ectopic pregnancies and her subsequent infertility upon the devices and upon her contraceptive adviser. For this reason, following a previous ectopic pregnancy, both adviser and woman herself may well feel happier to avoid the method.

Uterine malformation may make use of an IUD impossible or more liable to failure. Where two uteri are present an IUD can sometimes be fitted to *each* with success. Submucosal fibroids are not a contraindication, but the presence of fibroids which distort and/or enlarge the uterine cavity can be associated with failure. Endocervicitis is relatively common and if severe is best treated before IUD insertion. A woman who has had an abnormal cervical smear and who is under investigation can be fitted with an IUD while follow-up continues. Colposcopic examination with biopsy, and even when followed by laser destruction of a pre-cancerous lesion, can be carried out with the IUD in situ.

The woman should be shown the device and its position in the uterus explained, preferably with the aid of a model or diagram. For some women it is reassuring to know that the Fallopian tubes are tiny and there is no possibility of the device 'getting lost inside'. In developing countries, for example in Mexico, some women may make no distinction between the uterus and the 'stomach'. Sometimes a woman's knowledge of her own body literally stops at the labia and it may not be out of place to emphasize that the device goes into the uterus and not in 'the front passage'. The husband may be interested in the technique and it can be helpful to counsel the couple together.

The likelihood of heavy periods following insertion must be pointed out. An honest warning is the first step of dealing with the menorrhagia which complicates IUD use for most women. (Vaginal tampons can be used when an IUD is in place.) It is especially important to warn the user about hypogastric pain, backache, fever, increased menstrual loss and dysparunia, all signs of pelvic infection, especially if she plans future pregnancies. It is essential to tell the couple that IUDs have a failure rate. For most women exact figures, or the personal experience of the doctor inserting the device, may be useful.

Sometimes IUDs are used by women who cannot manage any other type of contraception, but for such a woman it is more than usually necessary to point out the possible drawbacks of the method. The real test of a contraceptive method is often what is said over the garden fence, in the supermarket or, in developing countries, at the village well. A pregnancy failure that is known to be possible is more acceptable than one which is entirely unexpected. The risk of spontaneous expulsion must also be explained.

If appropriate, the woman should be taught to feel the thread and it is usually sufficient to check this after each period. It is important to remember that sexual customs vary among different social, religious and ethnic groups. For example, menstruation is a time of uncleanliness for Moslem women and they are forbidden to pray, have intercourse or observe the feast of Ramadan while menstruating. Thus slight intermenstrual spotting may be seen by them as menstruation and what might be a minor nuisance to a western woman is perceived as a major objection in another culture. Hindus, who believe in reincarnation, have been known to ask whether the device will still be there when they are reborn.

Clinical use

The factors which almost certainly cause most variation in IUD performance relate to differences in the skill and experience of the individual inserting the devices and in the anatomy of the uterine cavity. Kamal has conducted patient and prolonged studies in Egypt using hysterography and has convincingly demonstrated that the most troublesome side-effects occur when a given device is so large that it distorts the uterine cavity, while pregnancy is most likely when a device is so small that it does not completely cover the uterine cavity.[30, 48] A skilled operator will avoid both errors. Just as variations between women provides a reasonable well-documented explanation of differences in clinical outcome, so variations between those who insert the devices account for most of the remaining variations in performance. Snowden and others have shown that the same device may have a wide range of outcomes in different clinics[18, 79] (see Fig. 11.4).

The key variable in insertion, other than common-sense precautions relating to antisepsis, is the need to place the devices appropriately high in the fundus. Devices which are not inserted completely clear of the internal cervical os, or which for some reason are bunched up in the lower part of the uterine cavity, are more likely to be expelled, cause pain or be associated with pregnancy and probably give rise to more menstrual disturbances.

Time of insertion

It used to be recommended that devices be inserted at or just after menstruation, on the grounds that this excluded the possibility of an early pregnancy, instrumentation of the cervix was easiest and the small amount of traumatic bleeding following insertion was not so noticeable. However, as noted, the prime action of IUDs appears to occur after fertilization and there is no evidence to suggest that the effectiveness, safety or continuation rate of an IUD can be substantially improved by limiting insertion to the time of the menses. In 1978 the US Food and Drug Administration (FDA) acknowledged it as 'necessary and proper' to insert IUDs at times other than around menstruation. White *el al.*[94] found that women whose Copper T IUDs were inserted on days 1–5 of the menstrual cycle had a *lower* continuation rate in the first few months than did those whose IUDs were inserted at a later time. Edelman and co-workers found that Copper T and Copper 7 IUDs could be inserted at any time during the menstrual cycle without any increased risk of subsequent pregnancy, removal for medical reasons or expulsion during the first 12 months post insertion.[22] Pooled IFRP data (Table 11.3) indicate that there is no consistent pattern with respect to the time in the cycle that the IUD is inserted and later performance.

The woman who presents herself asking for an IUD is expressing a need for immediate contraception and saying that she has prepared herself for the necessary minor procedure. If this procedure is delayed she may well be disappointed and may possibly not return.

Careful studies have been done on post-abortion, postpartum and now also on post-coital insertion. In the past, expulsion rates of 20% and over at six months have been recorded in the case of immediate postpartum insertions. If the insertion is delayed for one or two days, the expulsion rate falls dramatically but the perforation rate rises. In Singapore, there were 11.8% perforations among 4371 IUD insertions performed at 8 weeks postpartum.[71] More recently, it has been found that careful fundal placement of an IUD *immediately* after delivery of the placenta,[96] by hand or using a small ovum forceps, greatly reduces the rate of postpartum expulsion. Devices which can anchor themselves by embedding a projection 1 or 2 mm into the uterine wall, such as the T devices, the Petal device[70] and IFRP Delta loops,[52] appear to perform best. The offer of an IUD to women who are still in the delivery room is a realistic possibility and does not appear to be associated with any increased risk of complications when compared with an interval insertion. In the developing world, particularly in rapidly growing cities where more and more women are being delivered in hospitals but may remain for only a few hours, this development is particularly welcome.

Devices inserted during lactational amenorrhoea are reasonably well tolerated. Some bleeding may occur following insertion but the menorrhagia commonly associated with an IUD is apparently less troublesome.

In the case of legal abortion, where the risk of infection is slight, post-abortal IUD insertion is often a welcome choice, and results are generally good (Table 11.4). However, for a long time doctors were afraid to use IUDs after an incomplete abortion[2, 17, 39, 89] in case they added to the risk of infection. Careful studies have now shown that post-abortal IUD insertion is responsible even where the risk of infection exists. Goldsmith and co-workers studied 205 women who received an IUD after the treatment of incomplete abortion and 289 who did not. The study was

Table 11.3. *Outcome of IUD insertion at different times of the menstrual cycle for selected devices (12-month gross life-table continuation rates)*

Day of cycle when IUD inserted	Lippes Loop ($n \div 4047$)	Copper T ($n \div 4959$)	Copper 7 ($n \div 1766$)	Multiload ($n \div 1179$)
1–5	74.1	80.9	82.9	86.0
6–10	77.5	78.1	88.3	82.4
11–17	66.6	85.4	90.7	87.9
18 +—	76.3	80.6	80.2	71.2

Source: Family Health International Data (formerly IFRP Data) (1982).

conducted on a double-blind basis and those women who had not received an IUD were offered one at follow-up one month later. No statistical differences were found between the two groups with respect to infection as measured by fever or the need for antibiotics. In Latin America alone, it is estimated that one million women a year are admitted to hospital with incomplete abortion, the great majority being the result of illegal operation. A vigorous policy of offering IUDs to such women could bring great health benefit to the individuals concerned and relieve the strain on hospitals from repeat abortions.

Personnel

Physicians, midwives, nurse practitioners and specially trained family planning personnel have all been successfully trained to insert IUDs and to supervise further care.[44, 72, 95] It is possible to insert IUDs single handed but where the woman is nervous, or there are complicating factors, an assistant is of great value. Training is essential, whatever the person's background qualifications and when non-doctor personnel are used, there must be an appropriate system of supervision as well as the opportunity to refer problem cases.

Insertion techniques

The equipment needed for inserting an IUD is a speculum, a volsellum (ideally a single-toothed tentaculum), sponge forceps, scissors (to cut threads), kidney dishes and utensils for holding sterile instruments, and cotton wool and sterilizing solution for cleaning the cervix. A uterine sound and small cervical dilators up to 5 mm in diameter are also required.

A bimanual pelvic examination and speculum examination are made noting the position and flexion of the uterus and any evidence of pelvic infection, such as tenderness in the fornices, or pain on moving the cervix, the presence of fibroids and any evidence of vaginal or cervical infection.

Table 11.4. *Two-year cumulative life-tables rates per 100 women for Copper / 220 interval insertions and after therapeutic abortion*

Events	Interval insertions[a]	Following therapeutic abortion
Pregnancy	3.6	2.0
Expulsion	5.4	3.9
Removals for medical reasons	21.3	11.2

[a] Parous women only.
Source· Population Council and WHO data.

A firm couch at a convenient height for the operator and a good adjustable light are essential. Insertion can easily be performed with the woman in whatever position the operator commonly uses for bimanual vaginal examination. In the US this will usually be the lithotomy position but in the UK the left lateral may be chosen. The hands are scrubbed, sterile gloves should be used but a mask need not be worn. A sterile speculum is passed and the cervix clearly illuminated. It is useful to hold the cervix with a single-toothed tentaculum although in many cases the more experienced operator will not find this necessary. Cervical stabilization is particularly important where the uterus is retroverted or the cervix relatively inaccessible. A sterile uterine sound is passed in order to discover the direction of the cervical canal and to measure the uterine cavity. There is a good deal of variation in the anatomy of the cervical canal, which may not be centrally placed to the external os, and occasionally there may be blind passages so that the sound must be partially withdrawn and reinserted before it will enter the cavity. It is essential that the sound should be passed with minimal force letting it rest between the finger and thumb like a loosely held pencil. If the sound can be passed into the uterus but some tightness of the cervix is felt, it is useful to pass cervical dilators to the same size as the IUD introducer.

Flexible plastic devices must be left in their introducer for the minimum interval, or they will fail to return fully to their original shape after insertion. Some devices are picked up by their tail and pulled into the introducer while others are inserted by manipulation through the transparent sterile pack. Lippes loops must be fed into the proximal end of the introducer and then pushed along until the tip (opposite threads) almost protrudes from the distal end. A no-touch technique is advisable.

When the introducer has been passed along the cervical canal it is important to rotate it so that the device is expelled in the transverse plane of the uterus. The device should be inserted slowly over a few seconds, and the woman's face, rather than her perineum, should be observed to watch for any signs of discomfort or shock. In the case of the Lippes loop, the plunger should be withdrawn before removing the introducer, or the threads may become caught and the devices pulled out again. The threads should be trimmed to about 2 or 3 cm from the external os. In the case of postpartum or late post-abortion fitting, the threads should be left long at insertion and will require shortening at a follow-up visit, after full involution of the uterus. The art of inserting the IUD is to ensure that the device is an appropriate one for the size of the uterine cavity and that it has been carefully placed so that it is in contact with the fundus but without perforating the uterus.

If pain occurs, the woman should be asked if she wishes the procedure to continue or if she would rather return for another attempt. If there has been considerable manipulation of the cervix, it may be best to postpone the operation until another occasion when the woman will be more familiar with the procedure and the operator with her cervix. The next menstrual period may well be appropriate.

The insertion of an IUD is a stressful experience for some women even though pain may be a minor feature. Syncope or vaso-vagal attack is by far the most common complication of the procedure.[1] Spontaneous recovery is virtually certain though women who have become deeply unconscious may possibly vomit when consciousness returns and are therefore at risk of inhaling fluids. Careful positioning of the unconscious woman may prevent this potentially serious complication; ideally, a prone position with head turned to one side is desirable but since the procedure will probably have been undertaken in a lithotomy or at least supine position this may be impractical and bringing the legs down from the lithotomy position can actually worsen the circulatory collapse. Conversely, a patient in syncope lying flat can be helped by simply raising the legs through 90° or by tipping the couch to a steep head-down position. In clinical practice a vaso-vagal attack is most frequently encountered during actual stimulation of the cervix and further stimulation should be discontinued until the woman has recovered and been reassured. If a device has already been inserted and is known to be within the uterine cavity its removal will not aid recovery and it should be left in position. An intravenous injection of 0.4 mg atropine sulphate will reverse vaso-vagal reactions but is rarely needed.

Anxious women may occasionally overbreathe during IUD insertion: this phenomenon is sometimes triggered by the advice 'just take lots of deep breaths and relax'. Overbreathing expels all carbon dioxide and causes alkalosis which results in carpo-pedal spasm resembling an epileptic fit but without tongue biting or voiding of urine. Treatment is reassurance, sedation and, with a conscious patient, instruction in breathing in and out of a paper bag. Very occasionally IUD insertion may precipitate a severe asthmatic attack in an asthmatic woman. She will usually be carrying an inhalent and this will generally control the attack, otherwise a *subcutaneous* injection of 1 ml of adrenalin 1:1000 solution is almost invariably effective. Grand mal seizures have been reported at insertion but occur in less than 1 in 200 insertions.

Parasympathetic stimulation from manipulation and dilatation of the cervix during IUD insertion, in exceedingly rare cases, causes cardiac arrest. This grave condition is recognized by cessation of respiration, absent heart beat and pulses (best sought at femoral and carotid positions) and widely dilated, non-reactive pupils. Treatment is to restart the heart by rhythmic sternal compression and to give mouth-to-mouth artificial respiration, preferably using a simple airway in the woman's mouth to hold her tongue forward. Those who have immediate access to a laryngoscope and endotracheal tube and who have been trained in their use, can pass such a tube and then maintain forced respiration with an anaesthetic machine. Those lacking the skill to use a laryngoscope will do better to carry out mouth-to-mouth respiration, secure in the knowledge that this simple technique is highly effective even if needed for quite a long period of time.

There has been speculation concerning the mechanism of delayed perforation, or so-called translocation of an IUD. It has been argued that, normally placed, a device will not spontaneously perforate the uterus and most observers believe that perforation either takes place at the time of insertion or part of the device enters the myometrium at the time of insertion and the rest is slowly extruded through the uterine wall as a result of uterine contraction. Nevertheless cases are encountered where the device would seem to have been properly inserted and functioned well for several years; the woman then develops pain and the device is found to have partially or wholly perforated the uterus.

Follow-up visits

Good follow-up is as important as a good insertion technique for good IUD use. When possible, the woman should be seen in the next menstrual cycle and asked about her last period (which she will probably say was heavier than usual); occasionally massive flooding will be reported, perhaps with clots, and it may be necessary to remove the device, but usually menorrhagia is not too excessive and women will persevere for one or two more cycles to see if the loss gets less. In these cases, oral iron should be prescribed and another appointment made for the following month. More than usually careful supervision is necessary when the woman herself is particularly anxious to persevere with the technique, lest she does so by ignoring health-threatening menorrhagia.

The timing of long-term follow-up is determined by the woman's age, whether she considers her family complete, her intelligence and the resources of the family planning services. Some women can be left for a year after the first check visit and perhaps even longer. In general, an annual check-up is performed but few professionals carrying out such checks can give convincing reasons why they are especially needed for IUD users. On the other hand, it is important not to lose contact with the IUD wearer although the task may be a considerable burden. The success or failure of widespread IUD use invariably comes back to the quality and consistency of follow-up. Adequate follow-up can be arranged in situations with weak health services, as has been done in the island of Bali, Indonesia, where village workers have been the main source of reassurance and referral for IUD users. However, sooner or later somewhere along the line, there must be access to experienced individuals who can deal with any problems that may arise.

Follow-up should include a pelvic examination seeking any evidence of infection. If the strings of a tailed device cannot be seen or palpated the uterus may be sounded to feel the device and distinguish between a possible perforation and simple withdrawal of the threads into the uterus. The use of a MR syringe (Chapter 13, Menstrual regulation) is a simple way of recovering the threads without removing the device.[32]

Side-effects
Death

IUDs can cause death as a result of pelvic inflammatory disease (PID), perforation, peritonitis, intestinal obstruction, ectopic pregnancy with a device in place and infected spontaneous abortion of an intrauterine pregnancy with an IUD in situ. Cardiac arrest at insertion has occurred but to our knowledge the women have survived. Of course, if failure occurs and term delivery supervenes there is also a risk of maternal death. The risks of infection or ectopic pregnancy leading to death are greater where medical attention is not readily available.

In a survey of 8506 North American physicians in 1967, 10 deaths were reported in IUD users although a direct correlation was only established in seven cases.[76] As more information became available it was apparent that one cause of death to IUD users was the association between sepsis and spontaneous abortion late in pregnancies in women where the device had remained in place after conception had occurred.[47] The sepsis was severe and the clinical cause rapid.[16] Septic complications of pregnancy have been reported with most types of IUD, but appear to have been most common among Dalkon Shield users.[14] The Centre for Disease Control in the US estimated that about 15 deaths occurred for every 1000 pregnancies with an IUD remaining in place. Of the 50 US deaths associated with spontaneous abortion during those years, 23 were of IUD users. While the death to case rate for IUD users was more than 50 times higher than for non-IUD users during the same period the figure makes it clear such deaths, in absolute terms, were rare.

Any woman who falls pregnant with an IUD in place should be advised to have the IUD removed, even if probing for a device hazards the continuation of the pregnancy. Any woman with a device in situ and signs of a spontaneous abortion must receive prompt treatment. These precautions, together with the withdrawal of the Dalkon Shield, have almost (or probably completely) eliminated the syndrome of septic abortion and death with an IUD in place. In the 17 months following the adoption of new clinical policies in the US no deaths due to septic abortion occurred.[15]

Infection

In the absence of an IUD, the incidence of PID varies more than 10 fold between the Far East and parts of Europe and America. Some of the range is accounted for by sexual lifestyles, but other less understood factors may also be involved. The vagina, like the skin, has its own bacterial flora and the cervical canal is 'infected' in up to 80% of normal women. Such cervical infection is not relieved by swabbing the cervix with antiseptic solutions. It is for this reason that many operators using a 'no-touch' technique make no attempt to sterilize the cervix before inserting a device. The uterine cavity is normally considered to be sterile unless there is some predisposing factor to infection such as cervical cancer. The only reliable method of obtaining material for culture from the uterine cavity is by a transfundal approach at laparotomy or laparoscopy. When this method is used in the case of IUDs, infection is almost always found immediately following insertion but the uterus appears to become sterile again during the next cycle.[61, 66, 69]

It must be concluded that it is impossible to avoid carrying infection from the cervical canal into the uterine cavity at the time of insertion, but in nearly every case the uterus is able to deal with this infection. The view has even been put forward that IUDs, by mobilizing leucocytes and macrophages, could help to cure chronic infection. There are objective data which show that the presence of an IUD does not affect progress of infection following abortion.[26] It has also been demonstrated that prophylactic antibiotics do not affect the resolution of mild post-abortal infection with an IUD in place. It is a common observation that more serious infections occur some months or even years after insertion.[12, 21]

In practice, it is generally agreed that an IUD should not be inserted in the presence of known intrauterine or serious pelvic infections. On the other hand, cervicitis or an erosion is not normally considered a contraindication, although if a heavy vaginal discharge is found, insertion should be postponed until its cause has been identified and treated.

There is no doubt that in some women the use of an IUD is associated with serious intrauterine infection leading to PID and even death. PID is an

important but poorly defined condition.[24] Broadly, it denotes acute or
chronic infection of the Fallopian tubes and includes such conditions as
tubal ovarian abscess. It is suspected more often than it is proved. Lippes
found that when 23 cases of suspected pelvic infection in 1673 patients
fitted with loops were investigated, the diagnosis was confirmed in only
nine cases.[58] Tietze reported a 2% infection rate per year.[88]

Today, more than 10 epidemiological studies have investigated a
possible relation between PID and IUD use. The largest is that by Vessey
and his colleagues in Oxford, involving more than 20 000 woman-years of
exposure to IUD use compared with over 65 000 woman-years of non-IUD
use.[92] Among current IUD users there were 1.5 definite diagnoses of acute
PID per 1000 woman-years of exposure. Among ex-IUD users there were
0.48 definite diagnoses of acute PID. Among women using oral contraceptives and barrier methods there were only 0.14 comparable diagnoses per
1000 woman-years of exposure. There was no control group of non-users of
any method. Findings from other selected studies are given in Table 11.5.
Weström found a three-fold increase in reported PID among IUD users[93]
and Gray,[29] using the same data, found that the risk was concentrated
among younger nulliparous women, reaching perhaps times 8 in women
under 20 years of age. Beral and Guillebaud found an equally high risk.[10]
Neisseria gonorrhoea is found to be present in about one-third of PID cases

Table 11.5. *Pelvic inflammatory disease and IUD use*

Number of Women	Comparison groups	Relative risk
United States		
1447 with PID	IUD : non-users	1.6
	IUD : oral contraceptives	4.5
3454 controls	IUD : barrier	3.3
Sweden		
690 with acute salpingitis	IUD : non-users	2.1
690 controls		
Finland		
144 with acute salpingitis	IUD : non-users	2.0
229 controls		
Multicentre trials		
262 with PID	IUD : non-users:	
524 controls	Developed countries	6.7
	Developing countries	3.1

Source: Edelman, D. A., Berger, G. S. & Keith, L. E. (1979). *Intrauterine Devices
and their Complications.* Boston, Massachusetts: G. K. Hall and Co.

and chlamydia is also being increasingly recognized as an important causative organism.

Pelvic actinomycosis, a fungal infection, has now been reported in a number of IUD users.[3, 83] These cases include both women with severe pelvic infection and others in whom the evidence of the disease was found only at the time of IUD removal. In the presence of partial or complete perforation intra-abdominal actinomycosis may develop with grave consequences such as intestinal obstruction or development of multiple bowel fistulae. Recommended treatment is large and prolonged doses of penicillin. The risk of actinomycosis infection may be less in the case of copper devices. If asymptomatic infection is diagnosed then treatment is unnecessary, although the device may be removed.

Insertion is always associated with some bleeding from the cervical canal, and in theory it is possible to transfer infective hepatitis between women when a non-disposable IUD introducer is used. Although the sterilization of an introducer by cold-soaking techniques is widely considered inadequate to deal with viral agents, no proven case of transmission is known.

There is considerable speculation that IUD tails predispose to PID. Several small studies have been unable to demonstrate any increased risk of infection between tailed and non-tailed devices,[11] but larger numbers are required before a definitive conclusion is reached. Elstein found, when multiple uterine biopsies were taken at laparotomy, that 15 out of 17 users of tailed devices were suffering from demonstrable bacteriological infection but that there was no infection in five cases with tailless devices.[81]

While the role of the IUD tail remains debated, it does seem likely that multifilament tails predispose to a greater risk than monofilament tails.[86]

Intrauterine pregnancy

Most intrauterine devices are associated with a pregnancy rate of about two per 100 woman-years of exposure in the first year of use but a lower rate beyond this point, so that in 10 years of use a woman's cumulative risk of pregnancy is about 6%. Where uterine pregnancy occurs with an IUD in place spontaneous abortion is high and in a large number of study series a mean value of 30% spontaneous abortions has been reported. This is three to eight times the rate of miscarriage for women without an IUD and, as noted, women aborting with an IUD in place are about twice as likely to develop fever at the time of the spontaneous abortion as are non-users. Removing the IUD will cut the risk of spontaneous abortion in half. There is some evidence that the continued presence of an IUD may increase the risk of premature delivery. Although isolated cases of congenital abnormality have been reported with IUD use, there is no evidence that pregnancy associated with an IUD is more likely to result in an infant with congenital abnormalities[53, 92] Edelman, Berger & Keith[21] point out that in the US over 15 million women have now used IUDs and even if four out of five pregnancies occurring to IUD users are aborted, between 150 000 and 450 000 IUD-associated pregnancies will have occurred and it seems unlikely that an increase in abnormalities in this group would have gone unnoticed. The device, of course, remains trapped *outside* the fetal membranes and stories of new-born babies holding their IUDs are the stuff of cartoons not anatomy.

Progesterone and copper-releasing devices need to be evaluated separately in relation to the possibility of congenital abnormality but insufficient data are available for definitive conclusions at present.

Ectopic pregnancy

The possible role of IUDs in ectopic pregnancy is debated.[5] It is certain that an IUD grossly alters the relative ratio of intra- to extrauterine gestation, but less certain whether the *absolute incidence* of ectopic pregnancies is changed, particularly by the hormone-carrying devices. The topic is an important but difficult one to study because for a number of reasons, ectopic pregnancy has become more common in recent decades in many countries, especially the US and parts of Europe.[23] Has the increasing use of IUDs over approximately the same time interval been a cause or a coincidence?

The purpose of an IUD is to prevent intrauterine pregnancy and if it succeeds in doing this, but has less effect on ectopic pregnancies, then the ratio of the two events will change. Extrauterine pregnancy is a phenomenon limited to menstruating animals and, in the case of an ectopic pregnancy, it is not impossible that the blastocyst had a brief sojourn in the uterine cavity. Even so, it seems that the ectopic pregnancy rate is not reduced as much in IUD wearers as is the intrauterine rate,[55] so that in the US for example 2–5% of all pregnancies in IUD users are ectopic compared with 0.5% in non-users. A meeting called by the US FDA in 1978 concluded that copper IUDs are associated with the least risk of ectopic pregnancy and progesterone-releasing IUDs with the highest.[21] The latter finding also appeared to be confirmed by British data.[78] However, a US study by Ory of ectopic pregnancy in 615 women and 3453 controls found *no* difference in the risk of ectopic pregnancy between copper-loaded and inert devices.[63] The study confirmed a reduced risk of ectopic pregnancy in IUD users and no difference in risk in women who had used a device sometime previously and those who had never used one. Both US and

British studies have confirmed an *increased* risk of ectopic pregnancy with duration of IUD use: the relative risk triples after the first two years of use and also appears to be higher immediately after discontinuation. In view of these findings the question needs to be asked whether the higher rate of ectopic pregnancy suggested for progesterone-loaded devices is a genuine biological effect or an artefact of introducing a new device at a time of rising incidence of ectopic pregnancy. It is a fact that reported ectopic pregnancy rates for the same device for different geographic areas more than overlap those for different devices. The low rate of ectopic pregnancies in the Orient is noteworthy.

Perforation, translocation and embedding

The risks of perforation at IUD fitting have already been discussed. Lippes has commented: 'IUDs do not perforate. For this to happen we need a practitioner.' Tatum[85] lists four variables that influence the risk of fundal perforation:

(a) The size, shape and consistency of the device.
(b) The status and configuration of the uterus.
(c) The insertion technique.
(d) The skill and experience of the operator.

He comments that the last factor is crucial (Table 11.6).[71] As noted, perforation is more likely if an IUD is inserted in the puerperium at any time (except within a few minutes of placental delivery) or more than two but less than 40 days post-abortion.[71]

Fundal perforations are usually the result of improper insertion. Cervical perforations are commonly due to the phenomenon of translocation whereby a device is moved within the cavity after insertion under the forces of uterine contraction. Cervical perforation is often totally asymptomatic.

Where perforation is total and the device is lying in the peritoneal cavity,

Table 11.6. *Variation with individual operator in the risk of uterine perforation with an IUD*

	Insertions	Rate per 1000 insertions
Physician A (House officer)	1948	6.2
Physician B	429	11.7
Physician C	342	2.9
Physician D	789	2.5

further management is controversial. Lippes has pointed out that at least two deaths have been reported in the US as a result of surgery to remove an asymptomatic device but that there were no reports of deaths caused by linear devices remaining in the peritoneal cavity after perforation.[56] IUDs which have partially or totally perforated through the uterus can usually be removed by laparoscopy[65] but facilities for immediate laparotomy are mandatory. Closed devices have been associated with internal intestinal hernia into the device itself.[76]

Pain

Uterine cramp at the time of insertion is common and there may be some dysmenorrhoea if the device provokes a heavy flow, but pain at other times in the cycle is unusual. Those analgesics which act primarily as prostaglandin inhibitors, such as aspirin, seem to be particularly effective at relieving the pain. Soluble aspirin has long been recognized as useful and drugs such as mefanemic acid (250 mg every 4 h) can be helpful. Some practitioners suggest the taking of such a drug about 1 h before fitting an IUD.

Bleeding

A woman's subjective description of her menstrual loss is not always correlated with quantitative measurement. The most objective method of estimating blood loss is to collect used tampons, float them in a measured volume of fluid and measure the iron content.

Mean blood loss at menstruation totals about 45 ml and the loss is highest in women nearing the menopause. Loss is less in oriental women than western women.[45] A loss of 60–80 ml will be ultimately associated with a low haemoglobin level and must be considered pathological. The mechanism of IUD-induced bleeding is disputed. At insertion there is, of course, trauma to the endometrium and there may be increased myometrial contractions. Increased fibrinolysis has been demonstrated[8] and the use of anti-fibrinolytic agents such as E-aminocapronic acid has been shown to be effective when used orally or in bioactive devices.[90]

Menorrhagia is the most common and troublesome side-effect of an IUD and IUD use often increases the duration of loss so that about 1 in 5 users have menstrual loss lasting for seven days or more for up to six months after insertion.[31] The haemoglobin content and haematocrit also tend to fall with time.[74, 84] The exception to this generalization is the progestogen-releasing IUD which is frequently associated with a reduction in menstrual loss. Between 5 and 15% of IUDs are removed because of excessive bleeding or pain (see Table 11.1). Persistent heavy blood loss, particularly if accompanied by pain, requires treatment. X-ray or preferably ultrasound examination may demonstrate that the device has been badly fitted or is too large for the uterine cavity.[48] In either case its removal and appropriate reinsertion may cure the bleeding. A decline in haemoglobin levels can be pre-empted by prescribing oral iron and this may be particularly important in developing countries.

Expulsion

Over the first year after insertion between 3 and 24% (see Table 11.1) of women are liable to lose an intrauterine device by expulsion. About one-fifth of women who experience expulsion do not notice it at the time and for this reason about one-third of pregnancies among IUD users occur after unnoticed expulsion. IUD expulsion is less common in older women.[30] Among nulliparous women expulsion is about twice as common under the age of 30 as over that age. The highest incidence of expulsion occurs in the first three months of use. Lippes found that after three years no expulsions at all occurred among his patients.[58]

Expulsion is not a serious clinical problem if it is discovered and reported promptly. More often than not, another device can be readily reinserted and is usually retained. Complete expulsion exposes the user to the risk of pregnancy but incomplete expulsion can increase the risk of pregnancy and also be associated with an increased risk of infection. Usually the patient or her sexual partner is aware of partial expulsion of the coil.

Long-term effects

The long-term presence of a foreign body in animal uteri can lead to keratinized metaplasia of the endometrium but such changes have not been found in the human situation.[20] Copper IUDs are associated with minute traces of malonaldehyde, a possible carcinogen, in the cervical mucus,[7] but again no adverse human effects have been demonstrated. Changes in the histology of the human endometrium can be detected at light and electron microscope level and vary from mild to moderate trauma and inflammation.[9, 43, 91] Possibly the human uterus is partially protected against severe long-term changes by the fact that the epithelium is only in contact with the device for not more than 20 days and is then cast off at the time of menstruation.

Subsequent fertility

Following removal of a device one in every three women becomes pregnant in the next succeeding cycle, three-quarters within six months and seven out of ten in one year. The duration of IUD use does not influence the time taken to conceive. The proportion of premature deliveries *falls* with the duration of IUD use.[4] This is almost certainly a consequence of adequate pregnancy spacing rather than a direct effect of the device.

Unfortunately no data are available on the pattern of conception after an episode with an IUD present. It is possible that subsequent fertility could be adversely affected in those groups most at risk of infection, such as the young nulliparous user. However, any theoretical risk in some of the most disadvantaged groups must be set against the hazards of abortion, especially if illegal.

Evaluation

Theoretically an IUD should be an ideal form of contraception: its use requires a single decision and its insertion one clinical initiative; it is coitally independent, without systemic hazard, has a low failure rate and its effect is reversible. In practice, its use can be marred by expulsion, infection, pain, heavy uterine bleeding, (Fig. 11.5) perforation and even death. IUDs are like girls with curls in the middle of their foreheads, when they are good they are very very good but when they are bad they are horrid!

It is this balance of satisfied users and complaints which has given rise to, and continues to stimulate, strongly divided views about IUDs. Moreover the defects of the method tend to be more visible to the medical profession. People do not usually complain to the doctor if pregnancy occurs when they are using the condom, but they do complain if an IUD fails. However, as with many other methods of contraception, adequate training, appropriate selection of users and good follow-up are essential ingredients of successful use both for the provider and for the woman.

In many ways IUDs can play a complementary role as a reversible method to the Pill. While the advantages of the Pill are concentrated in younger women, particularly in the twenties, the advantages of IUDs increase in older women. Expulsions are less common in the parous than in the nulliparous and even if parity is controlled for, are less frequent for older than for younger women.

Like steroidal contraceptives (see Chapter 10, Peri-coital steroids) IUDs can be used post-coitally.[6] The advantages of using IUDs instead of hormones are absence of nausea, no possible risk of thrombosis, no risk of adverse effects on the fetus if pregnancy persists and the fact that the woman will be left with an effective method of contraception once the device has achieved its effect. The only situation where steroids may have an advantage is in the case of the young nulliparous woman where the risk of infection must be weighed seriously.

IUDs have been used in young and nulliparous women with apparent success,[77, 87] but the risk of PID must be taken seriously, especially in the US and Europe where it has become frighteningly common. The risk of contracting PID with an IUD is a more important risk from the point of view of the user's health than some more widely published risks of contraception such as cardiovascular disease among women using oral contraceptives. Weström estimates that among US women born in 1950, 1 in 28 will fail to achieve a wanted pregnancy because of PID.[93] A single attack of PID is associated with over 10% bilateral tubal occlusions and three attacks will leave more than half the victims permanently sterile. In addition PID is a major predisposing factor to ectopic pregnancy and following one ectopic pregnancy only, about one-third of women can expect to deliver a term intrauterine pregnancy. If, as noted under

Fig. 11.5. Discontinuation of IUD use for various reasons (1126 Ota ring users in Japan). (Modified from Muramatsu, M (1973). *Statistical Analysis of Long-term Wearers of Ota Ring*. Tokyo: Department of Public Health Demography, The Institute of Public Health.)

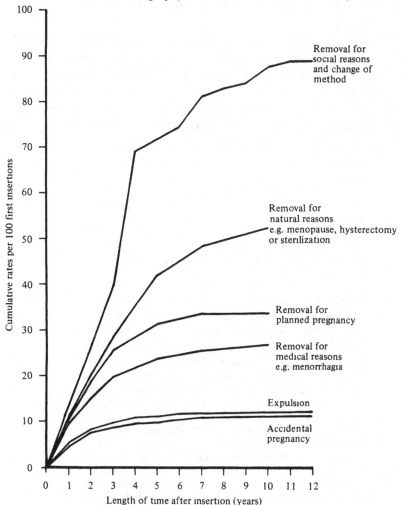

infection, the relative risk of PID among IUD users is between 2 and 5 times that of non-users (and may be even higher in women under 20), then in a society such as that of the US, 1 in 14, or possibly even 1 in 7, IUD users may become infertile. Other variables, such as frequency of intercourse and variety of sexual partners, have a large, or even larger, effect (Table 11.7). Conversely, for the older woman in a stable partnership, the IUD can be a satisfactory method of contraception with a low pregnancy rate, which becomes even lower with duration of use.

Spontaneous abortion with the possibility of severe infection and in rare cases death, is about three times as common with an IUD in place but this rate is halved if the IUD can be removed when pregnancy is diagnosed. The role of the IUD in the aetiology of ectopic pregnancy is still in dispute. No significant long-term effects among IUD users, such as cancer or teratological effects on a fetus conceived with an IUD in place, have been demonstrated.

The overall mortality rate associated with the use of IUDs is probably about 3–5 per million per year and the morbidity rate is approximately 3–5 per thousand. This is much lower than for the Pill in older age-groups and, even though these rates may be higher in developing countries with weak health services, the IUD offers positive health advantages to the individual user. IUD services are an important part of preventive medical services as well as a sound contraceptive choice for many couples.

Table 11.7. *Risk factors for pelvic inflammatory disease*

Risk factor	Relative risk
More than one sexual partner	2.6
Intercourse more than 5 times per week	1.9
Age less than 25	1.9
Black race	1.8
Current use of an IUD	1.6
Current use of a barrier contraceptive	0.5
Current use of oral contraceptives	0.4

Data assembled by Stewart, F. (1981) from: Eschenbach, D.A., Harnisch, J.P. & Holmes, K.K. (1977). Pathogenesis of acute pelvic inflammatory disease: role of contraception and other risk factors. *Americal Journal of Obstetrics and Gynecology*, **128**, 838; Kaufman, D.W., Shapiro, S. & Rosenberg, L. (1980). Intrauterine contraceptive device use and pelvic inflammatory disease. *American Journal of Obstetrics and Gynecology*, **136**, 159; Weström, L. (1980). Incidence, prevalence and trends of acute pelvic inflammatory disease and its consequences in industrialized countries. *American Journal of Obstetrics and Gynecology*, **138**, 880.

12

Voluntary sterilization

Introduction

In 1881, an Ohio surgeon performed what is believed to be the world's first tubal ligation.[48] Sir Astley Cooper[7] performed the first experimental vasectomy on dogs in 1823, and at the end of the nineteenth century (1899) Harrison[36] recommended vasectomy in men as a supposed cure for prostate enlargement. Other ethically reprehensible and biologically irrelevant motives for a vasectomy included its enforcement upon 'habitual criminals', 'compulsive masturbators' and as a supposed mechanism of male rejuvenation.

The unhappy link between sterilization and the 'eugenic' movement, the gross and inhuman abuses by Nazi doctors and the recent excesses of the Ghandi government in India are an unfortunate starting-point for an operation which, when wisely used, enhances human freedom.

Today on a world level, sterilization prevents more pregnancies than any other contraceptive method.[68] By 1980 it was estimated that approximately 100 million couples were using sterilization as their selected method of fertility control. The largest number, perhaps around 40 million, are in China. Approximately 24 million men and women have been sterilized in India and 13 million in the US. A further 4.5 million are thought to have had sterilization operations in Latin America and more than double this number in Europe.

Surgical services are now required to meet a backlog of sterilizations which could have and should have been performed many years ago but did not take place because of confused thinking by decision-makers and uncertainty within the medical profession. Once this backlog has been cleared there will be an ongoing maintenance level of sterilization to be performed. Kessel and Mumford have estimated that 180 million sterilizing operations may be required annually in the 1980s. It remains to be seen if the world has the will and the realism to set up this service.

The spectacular popularity of voluntary sterilization is a phenomenon of the 1970s and it is likely that more voluntary sterilizations were performed in those 10 years than in the preceding 90. Between 1971 and 1975 the number of couples using voluntary sterilization in the US increased from an estimated 3.6 million to 7.6 million and more than a million women had hysterectomies during the child-bearing years.[89,90] By 1975, 31.3% of US couples using any form of family planning were using sterilization (16.3% female; 15% male, whereas 10 years earlier the rate had only been 8%. For women aged 15–44 in Britain and the United States, voluntary sterilization is now the third most common operation performed, exceeded only by dilatation and curettage and induced abortion. In 1975 56% of all female sterilizations were interval operations, just over a quarter were performed immediately postpartum, 1 in 10 with Caesarean section and 1 in 20 after an induced abortion.[90]

The rapid rise in voluntary sterilization in the 1970s was almost certainly due to changed attitudes among those providing the operation and to the development of outpatient laparoscopy, rather than to alteration in attitude by users and potential users. In western countries the change of attitude among doctors towards sterilization is as dramatic as towards abortion. Younger members of the profession have grown up accepting abortion and sterilization as licit procedures falling within the normal ambit of medical practice whereas the more senior members of the profession were trained in days when neither procedure was performed by a reputable doctor unless there were exceptional indications. Baird has described how, in Aberdeen, postpartum tubal ligation was first offered in 1930 to women between 35 and 40 years old with eight or more children. Over the years, the criteria relaxed and by 1966, 7.2% of women over 30 had been sterilized and 12.6% of those over 35.[8]

Contrary to popular expectations, sterilization has proved popular from tribal societies with a shifting agriculture, such as the hill tribes of Burma where women will walk two or three days to obtain a sterilization, to the modernity of the US. There is no reason to assume that voluntary sterilization would not have been widely used 50 or even 100 years ago, particularly in developed societies when fertility was falling rapidly; the barrier to acceptance has been primarily on the side of the providers.

The sterilization programme in Puerto Rico began in the 1930s when Ernest Greeting, the then Governor, created liberal policies. Over the years sterilization became increasingly popular. Today, approximately one-third of all women have a sterilization operation in this poor country, and the median age for operation is below 30 and the median duration of marriage at the time of operation is six years. By contrast, across the Caribbean on the mainland of South America at the Maternidad Concepcion Palacios in Caracas, the busiest maternity hospital in the world, social indications for sterilization are not recognized. In the decade of the 1960s only 1 in 500 women received a postpartum tubal ligation. The mean age was 34 and the mean parity 10.1. Twenty-one women had 20 or more pregnancies. No doubt medical practice will change, but at present the restraining factor is not lack of demand, which may well be as high in Venezuela as in Puerto Rico, but patterns of medical practice.

In China a cumulative total of 34 million sterilizations is reported to have been performed between 1971 and 1978 and the number still seems to be rising. The proportion of vasectomies to tubectomies varies between provinces (for example vasectomy is popular in Sichuan Province) but for the nation as a whole there have been approximately 1.5 female steriliz-ations for every male operation.[12]

Nearly all medical communities appear to go through the same evolution of attitudes towards sterilization. Initially, sterilization is approached with extreme caution and considered a treatment for disease. This is the situation, for example, in contemporary Brazil, where, among women who can afford to pay, 75% of all deliveries are performed by Caesarean section in order that, after three babies, 'therapeutic indications' exist for sterilization.[39] At a lesser extreme, doctors apply rules of age and parity. This was common in Britain before the Second World War, almost universal in America until the 1960s and continues to apply in countries such as Indonesia. However, with the passage of time and experience, the medical community eventually discovers that voluntary sterilization is not a cure for over-fertility but a choice which mature and informed adults have a right to make and where their decisions are likely to be more reliable and easier to live with than when taken by contrived medical paternalism.

Counselling

As with the acceptance of any other contraceptive technique, it is imperative that the couple, and especially the member who elects for sterilization should be fully informed of the nature and consequences of the proposed operation. As sterilization is likely to be an irreversible process (even reversal of vasectomy has a high failure rate) such counselling is far more important than where a temporary, reversible form of contraception is being sought. The less educated the patient, the greater the importance of discussion and explanation. The basic questions everyone needs answered are 'Will I be the same afterwards?' 'Will I still be like a woman?' 'Will I behave like a man?' It is common to equate sterilization with castration and even those who realize that the two are different may still need reassurance. The doctor can explain that the testes or ovaries are left behind and that they make the hormones which are responsible for sexual behaviour. Some kind of illustration or model may be helpful. At an individual level, discussion with others who have been sterilized is the most helpful and emotionally informative thing of all. Men will need reassurance that they will continue to have an orgasm and that the ejaculate comes mainly from the accessory glands so that they will notice no difference in the amount. Women may be puzzled about the fate of ripened ova. Normally a couple will be counselled together and all possible alternatives, including choice of which partner is to be sterilized, will be discussed and plenty of opportunity given for a change of mind.

Subsequent regret concerning sterilization appears to be slightly more common if the operation is performed postpartum or at the time of abortion. Sterilization may well be a common-sense choice at such a time, and to withold it may indeed by counter-productive, but the surgeon should be aware that the heightened emotional states common at childbirth or abortion may make these times unsuitable for such important decision-making.

Legal aspects of sterilization are considered in Chapter 15.

Male sterilization (vasectomy)

Before vasectomy is undertaken the man's general health should be assessed. Diseases such as haemophilia or diabetes are relevant to the risk of bleeding or infection at operation. The presence of a varicocele, a hernia, a hydrocele or a cyst of the epididymis may well suggest that the vasectomy should be combined with a more major procedure designed to treat the condition.

Usually vasectomy is undertaken as an out-patient procedure. The operation is eminently suitable for local anaesthesia except in the most nervous of men. Inexperienced surgeons may wish to persuade their clients into accepting general anaesthesia until they have sufficiently improved their expertise.

Methods

It is easiest to ask the man to shave his own scrotal and pubic hair. Ideally this should be done about 12 h before the operation so that any concomitant minor skin trauma will have settled. Self-shaving is most easily performed in the bath. Abstention from food or drink is imperative if a general anaesthetic is to be given.

Variations in technical details of vasectomy are possible[25] (Fig. 12.1). Most surgeons make two scrotal incisions, each about 1 cm long. Some experienced surgeons prefer to make one mid-line incision manoeuvering each vas through it in turn, but this is technically more difficult. One or two per cent lignocaine (xylocaine) with or without adrenalin (1 part in 200 000) can be used as anaesthetic and only a very fine gauge needle is necessary. The scrotal skin is sensitive and most men are somewhat apprehensive so it is imperative to allow adequate time (60 seconds timed by a watch) for the anaesthetic to take effect before making the incision.

The vas is palpated under the skin and gripped firmly against the skin between the finger and thumb. Local anaesthetic is inserted into the skin over the vas and the surgeon's left hand being Immobilized by holding the vas, he or she works only with the right hand in making the incision, identifying the vas and delivering a small loop through the incision. Once the vas has been grasped with a tissue forceps the surgeon has both hands available for completing the separation of the vas from its sheath, a procedure which should be carefully performed with meticulous attention to haemostasis. The injection of a little local anaesthetic into the sheath of the proximal part of the vas is advisable to obviate discomfort in handling such a sensitive tube. The three muscular layers of the vas deferens have a rich sympathetic and parasympathetic nerve supply and contract in response to noradrenalin (norepinephrine) via sympathetic fibres from the hypogastric plexus. During ejaculation, the full length of the vas contracts, expelling some of the contained sperm. It is relatively easy to separate the vas from the fibrous coats surrounding it and a careful operator can usually ligate the vas leaving the artery to the vas deferens intact; this may, in some cases, also preserve the nerve supply.

Most surgeons are interested in using a technique which allows the

Fig. 12.1. Vasectomy.

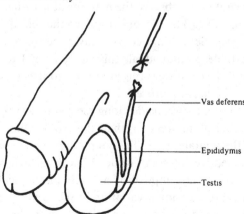

greatest possibility of reversal should the man's circumstances change in the future, and the removal of several centimetres of the vas as a protection against re-canalization is no longer recommended. Some operators will remove a very small segment solely for medico-legal purposes so that histological examination can confirm that what they have divided was indeed the vas. Probably the most commonly accepted technique is simple division with crushing of the vas a few millimetres from the cut ends and ligation at the site of crushing, sometimes with turning back of the cut end so as to fold over the crushed portion and double ligation of both ends of the divided structure. Non-absorbable ligatures are generally preferred because most surgeons believe they are less likely to allow re-canalization. The aim of ligation is to destroy the epithelium of the vas and induce fibrosis. The vas is a thick-walled tube so loose ligation may have no effect, while if the ligature is tied too tightly it can cut right through. Electrocautery can be used as an alternative method of destroying the vas epithelium.[73] Interposing facia between the cut ends of the vas prolongs the operation but does not seem to increase efficiency.[70]

Not only is the vas itself extremely well supplied with blood vessels but the scrotal skin is similarly endowed and the laxity of the tissues in the area means that unless very careful attention is given to haemostasis the whole of the scrotum on the one side or other may fill with blood and occasionally it may be necessary to readmit the man for evacuation of such a haematoma. Scrotal incisions are usually closed with a single cat-gut or other absorbable suture. Small dressings may be placed over the incisions, if non-adhesive they can be kept in place with a suspensory bandage or other athletic-type support. Such scrotal supports are helpful in preventing discomfort associated with movement of the testes during the first 24 or 48 h after operation.

It is a wise precaution to observe the man for at least half an hour and preferably for as much as 3 h after operation, so that bleeding if it occurs, can be detected early. Sexual intercourse may be resumed as soon as the man feels comfortable. In individuals this varies from 1 h to one month after completion of the operation. It is important to stress that intercourse is not harmful to the healing process.

Some surgeons inject a spermicide along the distal vas prior to ligation, but there is a clinical impression that this sometimes gives rise to inflammation of the genital tract.[55] The couple are recommended to use an alternative contraceptive for some while. Following ligation, the sperm which remain in the vas are emptied by a purely mechanical process, but there is a great deal of individual variation in the total number of sperm stored in the reproductive tract on the penile side of the ligation. The first ejaculate may contain from 10 to 100% of the sperm remaining. One masturbatory semen specimen free of sperm at six weeks post operation is commonly taken as a criterion of operative success in the US. In Britain it is normal to ask for two specimens at 10 and 12 weeks. The presence of a few non-motile sperm at such examination is almost certainly of no real significance but the presence of motile sperm, even in small numbers suggests that re-canalization may have occurred or that one vas was not adequately ligated and a second specimen should be examined two weeks to one month later. If follow-up is not possible, as in some developing countries, the man should be told to use a condom for 12 consecutive intercourses. Giving Depo-Provera to the wife is a practical alternative.

Vasectomy has been competently performed by medical auxiliaries and doctors in training in Thailand and a group of inexperienced medical students each performed 20 vasectomies with a surgeon available if any emergency arose. In 463 volunteers randomly allotted to surgeons and medical students there was no significant difference in bleeding occurring at the time of operation, post-operative infection or failure to occlude the vas in operations performed by the medical students compared with those done by qualified surgeons.[67] The fact that the success of the operation can be checked, and that it is performed on basically healthy men and that it teaches both gentleness and good haemostatic and sterile technique makes vasectomy an ideal basic teaching operation.

Female sterilization

The human Fallopian tube consists of three morphologically histologically and physiologically distinct parts, the fimbriae, the ampulla and the isthmus (Fig. 12.2). The fimbriae are essential to fertility and can even pick up the egg from the pouch of Douglas. Fertilization takes place in the ampulla and the ensuing transport of the egg to the isthmus is slow in humans, taking some 72 h. Passage of the morula from the isthmus into the uterine cavity is relatively rapid and takes only 3 to 4 h.

A wide variety of surgical approaches to the tubes is possible[41] and more than 200 methods have been described. A number of occlusive mechanisms can be employed including ligation, use of a clip, a variety of surgical techniques or heat coagulation. The technique chosen will depend upon the facilities available, and most particularly upon the attitude of the surgeon towards allowing for reanastomosis should the woman's circumstances change dramatically.

Female sterilization is simple to perform postpartum, and can be done literally within minutes of delivery. A small incision can be made below the umbilicus, the uterus rotated so that each tube in turn presents at the incision and the tube ligated and/or divided. The large size of the uterus immediately after delivery combined with the laxity of the abdominal wall makes the procedure simple but the tissues are somewhat more vascular and slightly more failures will occur than with interval sterilization. There are, however, many parts of the world where women come to hospital for only one or two days to have their children and where this immediate sterilization is acceptable and highly effective. Similarly, sterilization can be readily combined with therapeutic abortion[13, 42] or with evacuation of the uterus after an incomplete spontaneous abortion; once again the increased vascularity must be taken into account, although the tubes are less enlarged and failure less likely than with postpartum operation. Complications of abortion and sterilization combined are less than for the aggregate of the operations separately. It may be wise to combine interval sterilization, especially if performed late in the menstrual cycle, with vacuum aspiration to avoid the risk of a luteal phase pregnancy, something which accounts for approximately one-quarter of all pregnancies occuring after sterilization.

Fig. 12.2. The uterus, Fallopian tubes and ovaries.

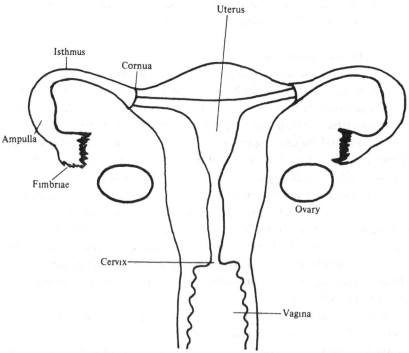

Unfortunately, from the point of view of surgeons, administrators, students and textbook writers, there are a multitude of methods of female sterilization which can be categorized in many overlapping ways. Such a diversity generally means that no one method is outstandingly satisfactory and this is certainly true of present techniques for female sterilization.

Methods of approach to the Fallopian tubes

Conventional laparotomy. Conventional laparotomy is the oldest and simplest approach to the Fallopian tubes. It is something any general surgeon can do and requires no special equipment. As an interval procedure it is invariably performed under general anaesthetic. The woman needs to stay in hospital for at least two days before she is fit to return home. A visible abdominal scar remains though a low transverse incision below the pubic hairline is usually chosen.

The advantage of conventional laparotomy is that all the abdominal organs can be inspected or palpated to check for unsuspected disease. Any foreseeable complications can be dealt with at the time of operation. In a woman who is known to desire sterilization, tubal occlusion can be offered at the time of some other operation and general surgeons should keep this option in mind. Conventional laparotomy is particularly straightforward immediately following delivery and can be done under epidural (possibly already administered for the relief of pain at childbirth), spinal or even local anaesthesia if preferred. If regional or local anaesthetic is utilized the normal inspection of all the abdominal contents to exclude or detect abnormality is not feasible.

Minilaparotomy. Interval and postpartum sterilization by laparotomy allow the use of a very small incision which can be carried out under local anaesthesia and on a day-stay basis. The bladder is first catheterized and an assistant uses his or her hand[60] or a specially constructed uterine elevator inserted into the uterine cavity to manipulate the uterus and thus present each tube in turn at the small abdominal incision made by the surgeon. This incision is normally a small transverse supra-pubic one and access is improved by the use of a special retractor, a small vaginal speculum or even a protoscope. Local anaesthesia is effective right down to and including the abdominal peritoneum but minimal handling of the tube is essential and some surgeons deliberately inject or spray the tube with a small quantity of 1% lignocaine. The actual occlusion of the tube is by any technique at the surgeon's preference, but gentle handling is imperative to avoid pain. The use of an analgesic and a tranquillizer for nervous women accepting local anaesthesia is often advisable.

The technique of minilaparotomy was first used by Palmer in France[61] and Uchida in Japan in the 1960s. It was adapted and proved to be highly successful in health centres in Thailand in the 1970s. It is the most appropriate method for interval sterilization in developing countries.[52] The equipment needed is cheap and robust. The surgeon need not be a specialist and in one large series of cases in Bangladesh, illiterate medical auxiliaries performed minilaparotomy as successfully as doctors, while in Thailand nurse midwives do the operation.[58] After delivery the enlarged uterus is appropriately placed for easy access to the tubes. At the time of very early abortion or interval sterilization the technique cannot be used if the woman has a fixed retroverted uterus, something which can be detected by a vaginal examination at the time of counselling. Dassenaike has described a modification of interval minilaparotomy under general anaesthesia in which the uterus is manipulated to bring each tube in turn to the incision.[24]

Colpotomy (vaginal sterilization). Colpotomy can be carried out under general, spinal or epidural anaesthesia but local anaesthesia is not feasible. The woman is placed in the lithotomy position, preferably with her buttocks at a higher level than her head so that the abdominal contents tend to fall away from the pelvis. After catheterization of the bladder, the vagina is cleansed thoroughly and the posterior fornix is picked up between two tissue forceps. The fold defined is cut with scissors and the peritoneum of the pelvic cul-de-sac boldly opened. Then, using non-tooth forceps, the tubes are sought for, grasped and delivered through the incision. The technique is most easily accomplished on women who have a retroverted uterus or in whom the uterus can readily be retroverted. Obesity is irrelevant. Initially, this operation was developed by Punrandrae in Bombay, and Soonawala[79] has used it in conjunction with first-trimester termination. The technique has been used on a large scale in camp situations in India, far removed from the resources of fully equipped hospitals. The main complication is post-operative infection and intercourse should be avoided for at least two weeks. The technique works best in highly parous women.

Culdoscopy. The posterior vaginal fornix is used to gain access to the abdominal cavity for the technique of culdoscopy also, but a smaller incision is used than for colpotomy and a culdoscope inserted. During the operation the woman must be in the knee-chest position and usually has to be anaesthetized in this position. The culdoscope reverses left and right in the field of vision and familiarity with the instrument is therefore necessary.

The instrument is dangerous in the presence of even mild pelvic adhesions. The use of the culdoscope for sterilization is diminishing.

Laparoscopy. In 1901 the Russian physiologist Ott first demonstrated in animals that endoscopic visualization of the abdominal cavity was feasible. Jacobeaus in Stockholm, using an instrument he called a laparoscope, applied the principle to humans for the first time in 1910. The technique was greatly developed by Palmer during the Second World War using a modified urological instrument. It was Palmer who first performed a laparoscopic sterilization in 1962 using electrocoagulation to destroy a segment of the Fallopian tubes. Steptoe helped to popularize the method in Britain.[81]

In the 1970s the use of laparoscopic sterilization increased enormously in developed countries. It is particularly acceptable from the woman's point of view because it can be performed on an out-patient or day-stay basis with reduced cost, it involves only minute scars, which are cosmetically acceptable, there is minimal discomfort and rapid recovery with a quick return to normal activity, including sex. The surgeon is able to take a panoramic view of the entire abdominal cavity, although this examination is far less reliable from the diagnostic point of view, as well as being somewhat more dangerous, than a full laparotomy.

Normally, good anaesthesia with full relaxation of the abdominal muscles and control of respiration is a prerequisite for laparoscopic sterilization using any form of heat coagulation but the use of the laparoscope under local anaesthesia with occlusive rings or clips is increasingly common. About 1 in 500 laparoscopies requires a laparotomy to complete the procedure[16] and the chances of proceeding to an open operation are greatest among those who have had a previous operation. The immediate availability of a general anaesthetic is always desirable and laparoscopy is both easier and safer with a general anaesthetic giving control of the patient's respiration.

The key to successful and safe laparoscopy is the establishment of a satisfactory pneumoperitoneum, preferably with the introduction of carbon dioxide or nitrous oxide though room air has been shown to be safe.[27] A small skin incision is made in the lower border of the umbilicus and a special needle, with a spring-controlled blunt cannula passing through its lumen is used (the Palmer or Verries needle). The cannula protrudes once the needle enters the peritoneal space and so prevents the bowel from contact with the sharp point of the needle. To introduce the needle the operator holds up the abdominal wall and inserts the needle in a controlled manner through the fascial planes, recognizing the different feeling and increased freedom of movement as it enters the peritoneal space. With the needle in position 2.5–3 litres of gas are passed and then a valved trocar within a cannula of a diameter which fits the chosen laparoscope is introduced into the space well above the bowel in a similar manner. The cannula has a fitting to allow the continuous introduction of gas and there are various specialized delivery units which ensure that the pressure and volume of the gas in the abdominal cavity are maintained constantly, something a good surgeon and anaesthetist are in fact equally competent at doing. Illumination of the laparoscope is provided by a fibre-optic source. With most fine-bore laparoscopes a second trocar within a cannula has to be introduced into the abdominal cavity (this time, of course, under direct vision through the laparoscope) so as to introduce the instrument designed to perform the actual tubal occlusion. Some laparoscopes, necessarily of a rather larger bore, have a narrow channel through which operating instruments such as electrocoagulating forceps, clip applicators or tubal rings can be passed. Laparoscopic vision is monocular and for this reason the two-entry-points technique allows the surgeon much greater manipulative control.

Laparoscopy inevitably requires a higher degree of surgical skill and specialization than does laparotomy or the use of minilaparotomy. It has been estimated that it costs approximately US $10,000 to train and equip a surgeon in laparoscopic techniques. This sum of money in a developing country would provide, for example, an additional room for four or five primary health centres thereby increasing their ability to perform minilaparotomy. Laparoscopes are difficult to maintain and auxiliary workers must be specially trained in their repair. In summary, laparoscopy is a valuable option offering considerable advantages to the woman and is a challenging and satisfying operation to the specialist gynaecologist, but, like other difficult techniques, the procedure should not be performed without adequate back-up facilities, which in this case would involve the skills and facilities for laparotomy, and, if necessary, for vascular surgery.

Hysteroscopy. The development of the hysteroscope (a telescope carrying its own illumination introduced through the cervical canal into a uterine cavity distended by fluid) has allowed the direct visualization of the tubal orifices and various experimental techniques have been used to block them[23, 74] Electrocautery has proved dangerous and various attempts to use metal, ceramic, silastic or other plugs have shown varied but, on the whole, low success rates. The technique remains experimental and its complexity means that future applications might only be applicable in countries with high technology.

Hysterectomy. Gynaecological practice varies widely between different countries. Estimates made in 1973 suggest that approximately 6% of American women of reproductive age had undergone hysterectomy whereas the British figure was only 2%.[28] In countries where sterilization is either not available or not readily accepted by the medical establishment, for example in Ireland or in the Philippines, women are often subjected to hysterectomy when all they really wanted was sterilization.

Techniques for occluding the Fallopian tubes

Several techniques exist for occluding the Fallopian tubes and the choice will be greatly influenced by whether or not it is important to leave a potential for reversal.

Bilateral total salpingetomy with fulguration and oversewing of the corneal ends of the tube is the most secure operation. It takes a few minutes longer than some other techniques. Reversal is impossible.

Until the last decade, the most commonly used technique was that associated with the name of Pomeroy in which the middle third of the tube is grasped with forceps, a loop is raised and ligatured with fine cat-gut and excised. Usually about an inch and a half (4 cm) of tube is sacrificed. In the Madlener technique, the tube is picked up at its mid-point as before, the two limbs are crushed with a cramp and the crushed areas are ligated firmly with non-absorbable suture. In the Irving technique, which is a modification of Pomeroy's developed over 50 years ago as a means of sterilization at Caesarean section, a loop is picked up in the centre and divided, the resulting ends are ligated and then the proximal end (the end attached to the uterus) is brought backwards, buried into a small incision in the peritoneal covering of the uterus and oversewn. The Uchida method, first described in 1961, involves the separation of the peritoneal covering of the tube from the tube itself for a distance of a few centimetres in the middle third.[85] This is done by injecting saline immediately under the peritoneum. Once ballooning has occured, the peritoneum is incised to expose the denuded tube. A segment of tube is removed and the end ligated. The proximal end of the tube is then buried, complete with its peritoneal balloon ahead of it, between the two layers of the broad ligament. At the end of this procedure, the two cut ends of the tube are not only ligated but are firmly separated by the peritoneal layers of the broad ligament and by ligated peritoneum covering the proximal end of the tube. The failure rate is exceptionally low but the operation takes considerable time.

From the mid 1960s electrocoagulation, initially by unipolar techniques but more recently using short-wave diathermy between small bipolar electrodes, has been widely used to occlude the tubes. Coagulation is usually repeated at two or more points along the tube. Sometimes a considerable length is totally destroyed. The unipolar technique may accidentally burn adjacent organs, particularly the bowel; this presents a considerable risk when the technique is used via the laparoscope because of its monocular vision. Short-wave diathermy is far safer, though even here, direct heat burns of adjacent bowel can occur.

Sterilization by local heating, particularly unipolar diathermy, may cause local burns to adjacent viscera when used laparoscopically, so safer techniques were sought. In 1970 Hulka in the United States produced a plastic clip which is hinged at one end, and, once in position around the tubes, locked by a stainless-steel spring.[38] A special laparoscopic applicator is required so the two-puncture technique is usual. Several other clips (Filshie, Blier, etc.) have been developed but reliability is still being assessed.[30] In 1974 Yoon introduced a method which applies a silastic band over a knuckle of tube using a single-puncture laparoscope.[91] This method has been evaluated in over 10 000 women and is safe and effective.[54, 84] The major advantages of clips and rings are the low morbidity, the feasibility of application as an out-patient procedure and the fact that since only a small area of tube is crushed, reversibility may be possible. The disadvantages are in some cases a higher failure rate than for ligation or cautery, the need for special applicators and the high cost of the clips. In addition, mechanical devices are associated with more abdominal pain post-operatively.[14]

Ideally, each woman should be able to make an informed choice about the method used, taking into account such competing factors as reliability, length of stay in hospital, post-operative discomfort and morbidity and potential reversibility. In practice the place where the operation is to be performed and the facilities available are commonly the determining factors. In a busy, well-staffed maternity hospital rapid postpartum sterilization by minilaparotomy under general anaesthesia may be the method of choice. In parts of the world where facilities are poor and anaesthesia less safe, and certainly in travelling or 'camp' situations where the operator is not a specialist gynaecologist, then minilaparotomy under local anaesthesia is unquestionably the best method. Under optimal conditions, with a trained gynaecologist doing interval sterilizations, laparoscopy is likely to be the procedure chosen and occlusion will be by a technique selected for high security, in which case bipolar (short-wave diathermy) heat coagulation will probably be selected; alternatively, clips or rings may be used, since they offer the best prospect of reversal.

Reversal

When counselling the couple or individual seeking sterilization it should always be stressed that the procedure is likely to be permanent and irreversible. Nevertheless, the operator should always bear in mind that circumstances may change and reversal become desirable. As a generalization, the more secure the technique, the more difficult is reversal. When operating on a young person it is wise to consider a technique which allows an increased chance of reversal. In vasectomy on a young man one can cut the vas, crush and turn back the ends but remove nothing, in an old man removal of a few centimetres of vas reduces the chance of operative failure. For the young woman the Uchida method of sterilization combines a high degree of security with good prospects for reversal but requires a laparotomy under general anaesthesia with its necessary hospital in-patient stay and potential morbidity.

Reversal of female sterilization

Repair of the Fallopian tubes is most easily accomplished if the occlusion has been in the isthmus or ampullary-isthmus junction.[10, 56] The tube here is least vascular, most uniform in diameter and has the best developed muscular coat, all of which are favourable factors for resuturing following removal of the blocked portion (Table 12.1).

Experience in reanastomosis is still limited, and many series of cases are so small that it is difficult to determine to what extent the results depend upon the practice of the surgeon as opposed to the mechanics of the technique or of pure chance. Varying criteria are used by different surgeons

Table 12.1 *Efficacy of tubal repair*

	Site of occlusion			
	Cornu	Isthmus	Ampullary-isthmus junction	Salpingetomy (after fimbriectomy)
Number of operations	19	8	10	4
Intrauterine pregnancies	12	5	3	0
Ectopic pregnancies	1	0	0	0

Source: Brosens, I. & Winston, R. (Eds.) (1978). *Reversibility of Female Sterilization*, London: Academic Press.

for accepting a woman for reanastomosis and the surgeon who rejects as unsuitable for his technique all but the simplest cases with the best prognosis can, and unfortunately does, publish results showing success rates far better than those of his or her contemporaries. A reanastomosis operation using simple naked eye 'macro-surgery' is associated with approximately a one-third chance of the woman conceiving a baby. Some series of reanastomosis using microsurgical techniques have been reported as yielding restoration of fertility in two-thirds or even three-quarters of patients, but for reasons given above, direct comparison between different series is impossible. The superiority of microsurgery over more conventional techniques is probable, but is not yet satisfactorily proven. Whatever technique is used, ectopic pregnancy is likely in about 10% of conceptions occurring after tubal repair.

At the moment, it seems that expertise and extensive experience is more important than the exact technique used in reanastomosis and repair operations should be in the hands of relatively few surgeons who are well practised in the technique and who work with the best possible equipment and anaesthetists. From the point of view of the couple, a check should first be made on the man's fertility if not already proven, and they should fully understand the risks of ectopic pregnancy. Broadly, women over 35 are not usually considered promising candidates. Above all, the couple must be thoroughly counselled to accept a good deal of tiresome clinical investigation and surgery with attendant risks and the discomforts and no promise of success.

Reversal of male sterilization

Vaso-vasectomy or reanastomosis following vasectomy is sought in something between 1 in 100 and 1 in 500 men who have had the operation. The vas, being a thick-walled tube, is easier to repair than the Fallopian tube. Shrikhande has described a simple technique for restoring vasal patency[76] and most surgeons following this technique will achieve a success rate of approximately 50%. As surgeons gain considerable clinical experience and if microsurgery is available, more encouraging results may be obtained.[47,59,77] F. Soonwalla, in a series of approximately 200 splinted operations, obtained sperm in over 70% of the cases and pregnancies in 40%. When he turned to microsurgery, in similar series, he had sperm present in 88% of cases and pregnancies in 65–70%. The maximum time between the original vasectomy and repair with the reappearance of sperm was 24 years and between vasectomy and repair, followed by pregnancy, 13 years. It is sometimes recommended that repair be attempted on one side only: if successful, a perfectly satisfactory sperm count from one testicle will result and if unsuccessful the opposite side remains undisturbed for a further attempt. Restoration of a fairly normal sperm count is not always followed by pregnancy.

The possibility of storing sperm by freezing has been known since the work of Mantegazza in 1866. The first conceptions with frozen human sperm were achieved in 1950. A sperm bank was opened in Philadelphia in 1962, storing human semen in liquid nitrogen at $-196°C$. The idea of storing semen from men who have had a vasectomy is at first sight obvious and attractive but nowhere has it become a routine. Sperm have been stored for up to eight years in the Philadelphia Bank but motility declined with time.[80]

Side-effects
Mortality

Death following vasectomy in an advanced country would almost certainly be due to anaesthetic catastrophe and to our knowledge no such reports have yet been published. In under-developed countries where large numbers of vasectomies are carried out in 'camp' conditions with primitive facilities and poor local hygiene, serious infections have been reported and deaths from tetanus and from gas gangrene infections have occurred. Under normal circumstances, and even in a poor country, the mortality for vasectomy operation is negligible.

Mortality in the US for tubal sterilization was reviewed by Peterson and colleagues of the Centre for Disease Control, Atlanta, Georgia in 1981. It was estimated that the risk of death was 1 per 10 000 procedures.[62] In developing countries the risks of surgical sterilization have proved to be considerably greater than in the West. In Bangladesh the death to case rate of 21.3 per 100 000 female sterilizations was reported in 1979. Among 22 526 vasectomy cases, there were seven deaths (death to case rate 31.1 per 100 000). These rates need not necessarily be representative of the risks involved. Those associated with vasectomy can be considerably reduced with improved supervision of surgery and greater adherence to sterile techniques. However, where surgical services are grossly overburdened and supplies of materials as essential as cat-gut are often short, it is unlikely that western levels of mortality will be achieved. Despite these disappointing results, voluntary sterilization offers marked benefits in relation to the risks of maternity. Assuming a mean age of sterilization of 30, it has been calculated for Bangladesh that tubal ligation in 100 000 women averts approximately 178 000 births over the next 15 years. The maternal mortality is thought to be about 570 per 100 000 and therefore this number of operations would avert more than 1000 deaths due to childbirth.

Morbidity

Immediate complications: male. Reactions to lignocaine may occasionally occur: collapse with peripheral blood vessel dilation can be severe but is usually short lived and spontaneous recovery is virtually certain. Some degree of post-operative discomfort is felt once the effect of the local anaesthetic has worn off, but severe pain is very rare in the absence of haematoma formation. The main immediate complication of vasectomy is bleeding into the scrotal tissues and, since these tissues are very lax, bleeding may continue for a long time and one side of the scrotum may completely fill with blood to a total volume of 500 ml or so. Such a complication requires hospital admission and evacuation of the blood with location of the bleeding point and arrest of the bleeding. Superficial infection of the skin wound is rarely serious, although if there is a large haematoma present superficial infection may spread and an abscess develop. Gas gangrene and tetanus have been reported with infected vasectomy wounds in India. Shrikhande[76] has pointed out that antibiotics give a false sense of security to some doctors. In one centre the incidence of infection was controlled not with antibiotics but by attention to appropriate hygiene in the surgery itself and a previously high infection rate declined when a more responsible doctor took charge of the centre.

Immediate complications: female. The need for an intra-abdominal procedure, whether by laparotomy, laparoscopy or by vaginal approach inevitably involves higher risks than for the male. Anaesthetic complications are more frequently encountered than with vasectomy because general anaesthesia is more widely used and because any abdominal procedure inevitably inhibits the full return of normal respiratory function. Haemorrhage, infection and accidental damage to other abdominal viscera are all possible complications of female sterilization. As with other forms of pelvic manipulation, temporary retention of urine is theoretically a complication but in practice is very rarely encountered. Temporary menstrual irregularities are common, particularly if the procedure has involved intrauterine manipulations. Tubal ligation in the first weeks postpartum has no immediate effect on lactation but may cause a reduction in milk output some days later.[57] Local endometriosis at the site of artificial occlusion, often leading to fistula formation, is a fairly common finding after female sterilization and may be the basis of failure in some cases.

Pregnancy after sterilization is more common among women under age 35 at the time of sterilization and those who were not breast-feeding. Such failures occur more frequently in the early experience of a centre or an individual surgeon and failure is more frequent with clips and rings than with electrocautery.[15,18,19,20]

There are a number of surgical hazards associated with laparoscopy itself. The peritoneum is punctured blind and injuries to the bowel or other viscera may occur at this point, particularly if there are pre-existing adhesions. Secondly, the laparoscope may be inadvertently introduced through the mesentery of some portion of the bowel and since only monocular vision is feasible operators may not appreciate this unless they are very experienced. Tearing of the mesentery with contained blood vessels can lead to severe and continuing haemorrhage. Direct puncture injuries of a large blood vessel such as the aorta or vena cava have been reported but are very rare. The most feared complication of unipolar high frequency tubal coagulation is electrical burning of intra-abdominal viscera, the bowel being especially vulnerable. The American Association of Gynecological Laparoscopists published a retrospective survey for the year 1975 showing major complications of laparoscopic sterilization at 3.7 per 1000 cases with 5 deaths in a total of 200 879 operations.[37,66] The defect of this American survey was that it was a retrospective one and clearly complications and deaths might well have been missed. The British Royal College of Obstetricians and Gynaecologists carried out a *prospective* survey in 1976–77 and the incidence of serious complications for sterilizing procedures was 31 per 1000 cases with a death rate of 1 in every 15 000 cases.[69] It will be appreciated, therefore, that even with highly trained and skilled surgeons, laparoscopic sterilization carries an appreciable risk of morbidity and mortality.

Long-term complications: male. Following vasectomy, luteinizing hormone, testosterone and oestradiol levels are unchanged.[78] In experimental animals there are considerable species differences in response to vasectomy. Differences in the amount of connective tissue probably determines this. In rodents the epididymis simply goes on enlarging while in monkeys there is local rupture of the epididymis at a number of sites.

Electron microscopical examination of testicular biopsies taken at the time of reanastomosis of the vas have demonstrated that the blood supply to the seminiferous tubules is unaffected by the operation, the Sertoli cells are intact and functioning and the germinal epithelium has a normal ultrastructure.[34] However, the maturing sperm tend to be closer to the basement membrane after vasectomy.[33]

It might truly be said that the main long-term complication of vasectomy is either failure of the operation at the time with persistent sperm count 10 or 12 weeks later or else spontaneous re-canalization of the vas occurring months or even years after operation. Both are rare. Very occasionally a discharging sinus may develop in the scrotum, particularly if non-absorbable sutures have been used to ligate the vas. Sperm granuloma occur when sperm leak into a tissue setting up a sterile inflammatory reaction. They give rise to complaints of pain and swelling and may occur as late as 25 years after operation.[29]

The body has the capacity to remove sperm from the vas deferens and the epididymis but how it deals with the sudden load that follows total obstruction of the vas is unknown although there is a massive influx of mono- and multinuclear macrophages.[65, 72]

Although there are still several weak links in the chain of evidence, leakage and destruction of sperm are probably the basis of the immunological changes which occur in man and other mammals. There is a good deal of variation between individuals and in the same individual over time. Sperm antibodies cross-react with other tissues and long-term autoimmune disease is a biological possibility although as yet there is no epidemiological evidence of such a complication in man. Sperm agglutination can be found in the presence of normal testes. Cytotoxic antibodies arise in the presence of testicular lesions or cause such lesions. Additional and deeper studies of the immunological consequences of vasectomy may well follow further refinements of technique and more accurate identification of antibodies and antigens.

Approximately two-thirds of men develop sperm-agglutinating, and about 40% develop sperm-immobilizing, antibodies following vasectomy. Ansbacher has demonstrated that about half of the men with sperm-agglutinating antibodies can father children, but the possibility of pregnancy when immobilizing antibodies are present is remote.[1, 6, 64]

In five cynomologus monkeys, which were caged and fed a cholesterol-rich diet, vasectomy appeared to be associated with more arteriosclerotic disease when examined post-mortem.[4] It was postulated that immune complexes formed following vasectomy damaged the endothelium of blood vessels, precipitating arteriosclerotic changes, and subsequent observations on several groups of rhesus monkeys appeared to confirm this hypothesis.[3, 21, 22] Fortunately, however, several epidemiological studies in men have shown no evidence of increased cardiovascular disease after vasectomy.[31, 32] Wallace and colleagues[88] studied the prevalence of vasectomy in 55 men with coronary disease and found the prevalence to be identical with that in non-vasectomized controls. Workers in the Boston

Collaborative Drug Surveillance Program conducted a historical prospective case-control study on 4830 vasectomized men in the Group Hospital Cooperative of Puget Sound, Seattle, Washington, and found 0.9 cases of non-fatal myocardial infarction per 1000 man-years among vasectomized men and 1.0 per 1000 man-years in the controls.[86,87] In a similar study using health data from the Kaiser Health System in San Francisco, Petitti and colleagues found no increased risk of cardiovascular disease or alteration in blood chemistry in vasectomized men. Each of over 4000 vasectomized men were matched with three controls and blood pressure, blood count and serum sodium, potassium, calcium, cholesterol, glucose, uric acid, blood urea, nitrogen, creatinin, total bilirubin, alkaline phosphatase, lactate dehydrogenase and transaminases were all compared. There were no biologically significant differences.[63]

Long-term complications: female. The only predictable long-term effect of tubal ligation which has received serious attention is the possibility of alterations in menstrual patterns after operation. Biologically, it is possible that surgery might affect the ovarian blood supply, more hypothetically, prevent the passage of prostaglandins from the uterus along the tubes and on to the corpus luteum. Epidemiologically, it is a difficult field to study because menstrual bleeding and cycle length normally change with age, because different surgical procedures might have different effects and because many women coming to sterilization have previously used Pills or IUDs which themselves alter blood loss. Bhiwandiwala *et al.* have recently reviewed reports of changes in menstruation in more than a thousand cases of electrocautery (which is the method giving the greatest tissue damage) and find no alteration in overall patterns (Fig. 12.3).

Psychological factors

The study of dissatisfaction after sterilization is a methodological and philosophical minefield and not surprisingly reports in the literature of regret after sterilization vary from 0% to 40%.

The nature of the sample, cultural background, time elapsed since operation and technique of evaluation all influence the outcome. Even more important is the nature of the question being asked. Careful psychiatric tests and semi-directive interviews are most likely to elicit reports of regret after sterilization. In one sense regret is inevitable and regret about sterilization may be no more than regret about aging. The natural or artificial termination of childbearing, like other aspects of growing old such as the wearing of false teeth, is bound to be the subject of ambivalence.[35] The key question is not 'Do you regret being sterilized?', which is analogous to asking 'Do you regret going bald or wearing false teeth?', but 'Would you have the operation again?' or 'Were you appropriately informed to make a satisfactory choice?' In answer to the latter type of question only 2–5% report regret.[2, 11]

The great majority of men and women report unchanged or improved health after sterilizing operations and many have better marriages.[71] In a follow-up of vasectomized men Ferber, Tietze and Lewit (Table 12.2) found that 70% claimed to be happier than before the operation and less than 2% claimed to be less happy.[29] For many there is an improvement in

Fig. 12.3. The effect of sterilization on menstrual loss. (From Bhiwandiwala, P., Mumford, S. & Feldblum, P. J. (1982). Menstrual pattern changes following laparoscopic sterilization: a comparative study of electrocoagulation and tubal ring in 1025 cases. *Journal of Reproductive Medicine*, **27**, 249.)

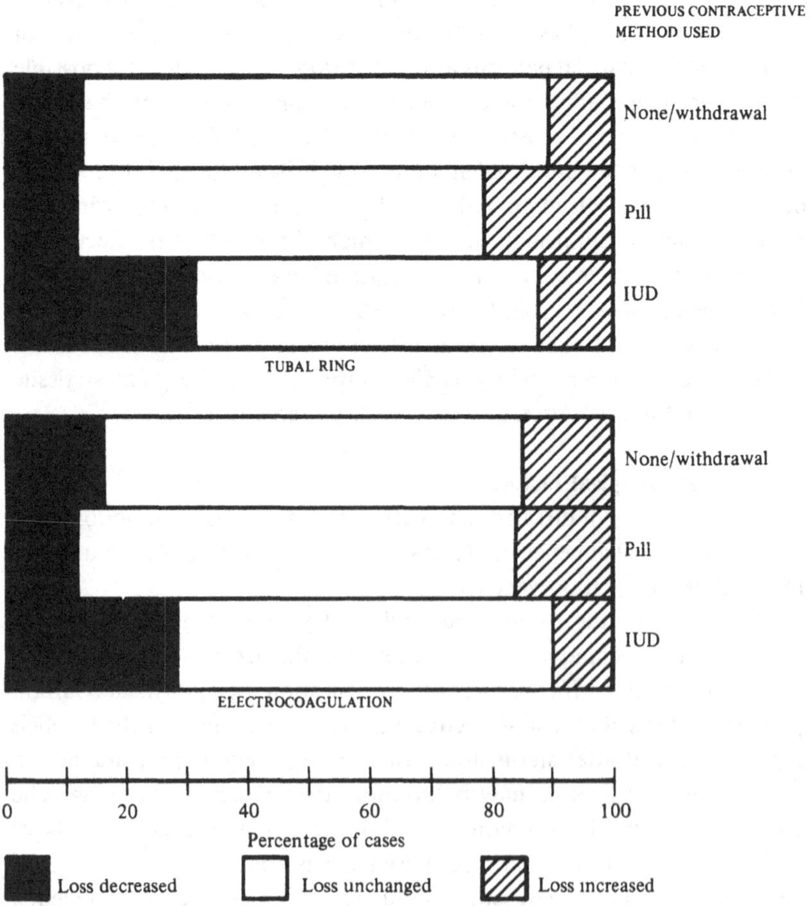

PREVIOUS CONTRACEPTIVE
METHOD USED

None/withdrawal

Pill

IUD

TUBAL RING

None/withdrawal

Pill

IUD

ELECTROCOAGULATION

0   20   40   60   80   100

Percentage of cases

Loss decreased   Loss unchanged   Loss increased

their sexual life and, in the above study, mean coital frequency per month rose from 8.4 before the operation to 9.8 afterwards. Adams,[2] Lu & Chun[49] and Thompson & Baird,[83] in surveys of patients coming from very different cultural backgrounds, have reported similar findings in women after tubal ligation. Those who are most disturbed by sterilization are often men or women with a history of previous psychiatric instability[40] although there is no evidence that severe psychiatric disturbance after the operation is any higher than among the population as a whole. There is a group of men and women who, after having obtained sterilization, will rapidly weave the operation into the fabric of their emotions. One such group of women has been described as having 'feeling of inferiority, weakness, emptiness, being torn up inside, and being a changed person'. All subsequent misfortunes of life such as accidents, obesity, frigidity, marriage failure or new physical illness were blamed on the operation.[9] Regret is less likely if the woman requested the operation than when the physician suggested it and less likely when done for reasons of family size than for organic disease or previous Caesarean section. Sterilizing operations are more likely to have an unsatisfactory outcome if the couple were in disagreement about the need for operation: the two worst results in one follow-up occurred in the only four cases where the wife has disagreed with the husband's wish to be sterilized.[29] Sterilization is a powerful weapon which men and women can use to hurt others and/or themselves.

Emotionally, it is difficult to avoid equating sterilization with castration. Using interviews and self-administered psychological tests Ziegler and his co-workers[71,92] in California have been able to demonstrate such an attitude among a number of vasectomized men, and the proportion rises among those who were psychologically unstable before the operation. Only 50% of men are willing for those around them to know they have been sterilized and less than one-third recommend the operation to other men.[29]

Table 12.2. *Sexual satisfaction after vasectomy (73 cases)*

	Much more	Little more	No change	Little less
Husband				
Feeling of freedom and decreased inhibition	10	40	2	1
Satisfaction with coitus	6	49	15	3
Husband's report on wife				
Feeling of freedom and decreased inhibition	13	14	15	1
Ability to reach climax	8	28	35	2

Sometimes humour can defuse uninformed but deep-rooted fears. One surgeon in Korea found farmers particularly liable to confuse vasectomy with castration. He gave lectures and drew diagrams, but to no avail until one day he thought of an agricultural analogue. 'Vasectomy', he said 'is like a water melon! Sex is something juicy and enjoyable and if you remove the seeds it is even better!'

There is widespread fear that a sterilized couple may later want more children if there is a family death or divorce or remarriage, but in practice it is uncommon. In over 800 tubal sterilizations in the US only three women wanted more children.[9] While voluntary sterilization among couples of low parity in their twenties is more likely to be regretted than in older couples,[5] the reverse situation is also possible with older women or men regretting they were not sterilized earlier.[49] Among high parity women sterilized in Hong Kong, dissatisfaction was more common because of operative failure leading to unplanned pregnancy than because of a desire for more children.

Some side-effects are culturally determined, for example, the Chinese believe sterilization makes the memory worse, but religion has little influence on the demand for voluntary sterilization. Sterilization appears unassociated with marital infidelity and in one follow-up a respondent said 'I think less about other women than I did, I guess it's because I'm more satisfied now'.[29]

Future developments

Vasectomy is a simple operation which is difficult to improve. The Chinese have experimented with percutaneous injection of the lumen of the vas with phenol and Davis in the US has developed a clamp to localize the vas under the skin in an attempt to develop a percutaneous method requiring less dexterity. Experiments in fitting 'taps' into the vas have not been successful and seem unlikely to be so. Probably the most effective method of reversing male sterilization will continue to be straightforward reanastomosis.

In women, several experimental methods have attempted to produce temporary sterility, including the introduction of notched plugs made of teflon, silicon and other substances. Laufe has experimented with a fimbrial hood made of silastic which would require a minilaparotomy to apply, and, if necessary, to remove.[45] It has been demonstrated that the hood is unassociated with any morphological damage to the tube or fimbriae. So far, restoration of function is a theoretical matter and there are inadequate data to confirm or deny the reliability of any technique.

Attempts to block the tube by instilling a variety of chemicals into the uterine cavity have been made since work by Froriep in 1849. The Chinese have extensive experience with 0.1 ml of a mixture of phenol, mucilage and barium sulphate injected through a cannula passed through the cervix into the ostia of the tubes. The procedure is undertaken blind using a curved metal cannula containing a soft plastic tube passed into the uterine cornu. The plastic cannula is manipulated and placement in the isthmus confirmed by the passage of 8 ml of saline (cervical reflux is taken as evidence that the cannula has *not* entered the tube). The placement of the phenol mixture is usually checked by X-ray. The World Health Organization is working on the use of methylcyanoacrylate (MCA or 'crazy glue') delivered to the ostia with a special instrument which allows the solution to polymerize and form an obstruction in the intramural portion of the tube.[75,82] A single procedure blocks about 80% of tubes. Family Health International (formerly the International Fertility Research Program (IFRP)) is working on delivering pellets of quinacrine into the uterine cavity by a simple, blind technique.[43, 44, 50, 93, 94, 95] The placement of a quinacrine solution in the human uterus can produce toxic systemic effects but in a pellet form appears to be without serious hazard and animal studies appear to confirm safety. Gross life-table rates per 100 women at 12 months after three treatments with quinacrine in consecutive months are 9.9 for quinacrine solution and 3.1 for pellets.

Evaluation

Voluntary sterilization is common, popular and easy. It is essential to remember that for the individual it will always remain a profoundly important decision. Whenever the operation is undertaken, those responsible have an obligation to ensure that the candidate understands fully the risks and benefits of the procedure, accepts it as probably irreversible and has been appropriately informed about all alternative family planning choices. For example a 23-year-old woman who requests sterilization may do so only because she is afraid to take the Pill and suitable information may leave her using this, or some other contraceptive method, satisfactorily and happily.

Observation shows a marked variation in the incidence of voluntary sterilization in different countries and a dramatic variation in ratio of male to female operations. Do these differences represent true variations in the cultural acceptability of the two operations? It is often assumed that macho men in Latin America will not accept vasectomy, that the operation will be rejected on religious grounds in Muslim countries or that villagers living in areas with high infant mortality will be afraid to accept sterilization because their existing children may die. However, a detailed look at specific situations suggests that the attitudes of those who make sterilization available or choose not to make it available, are more important in determining the prevalence of the operation than are cultural variations.

Vasectomy services in Colombia, Latin America, have existed long enough to show that the operation can be a reasonable choice. Several hundred vasectomies have been performed in Yemen although most observers previously believed the operation would be totally unacceptable. This is not to say that cultural determinants are non-existent. For example, the demand for voluntary sterilization appears to be much lower in Africa than in South East Asia. However, from the point of view of those who provide family planning services it is essential not to allow cultural differences in acceptability to become barriers to making the operations available because such judgements may become self-fulfilling prophecies.

As a generalization, it appears that in nearly every society there are women who are burdened with too many children and would accept the option of female sterilization, in some cases almost as an act of desperation. This same pressure does not exert itself as forcefully in the case of the male operation. Therefore, in most countries where male and female sterilization have been made available there has been a rapid climb in the number of tubal ligations performed but often a longer, slower climb in the use of vasectomy. In fact, from a pragmatic point of view it is reasonable to argue that where vasectomy is likely to receive least acceptance, services should be made available as early as possible. Put another way, it is unlikely that a great number of West African or Brazilian men will accept vasectomy, but it is certain that a small number would and that the total number of men selecting this choice in 1990 could well be dependent upon how early in the 1980s the service is introduced.

Perhaps the single most practical contribution that can be made to family planning in the 1980s would be the development of a simple non-surgical method of female sterilization which medical auxiliaries could perform safely in countries with weak medical services. Progress in this field will be watched carefully. In the absence of such a development female sterilization will remain technically more complicated than vasectomy and probably always carry a higher mortality. Vasectomy is, in one sense, a 'trick' operation in which standard surgical procedures for obtaining good exposure and identifying structures can be safely short-circuited because of the surety with which the vas deferens can be palpated and stabilized prior to operation. It has a second anatomical advantage over the female operation in that while neither procedure can be reasonably regarded as reversible, vasectomy repair is easier and safer than tubal reanastomosis and carries no risk of ectopic pregnancy. When services are equally available to both sexes, are there still sociological differences in those who choose vasectomy and those who choose tubal ligation, or is it a matter of which partner selects sterilization? Deys[26] has observed that many couples divide their sexual roles, and where the man has been dominant and previously used condoms and coitus interruptus, vasectomy is commonly chosen, presumably because the men maintain their decision-making role in fertility control and because they don't want their wives 'mucked about with'. Conversely, the wife often sees herself as having 'suffered enough' and a survey in Australia showed that following vasectomy 'over half the women's general health improved – *he* had the operation and *she* felt better'.[46]

The choice of technique for female sterilization is difficult. The multitude of surgical techniques available both to open the abdomen and to obstruct the tubes suggests that no one method is pre-eminently successful. To some extent, surgeons have followed their enthusiasm and used their own intuition and personal preference in selecting the method to use. However, with the growth in sterilization in the 1970s it has been possible to conduct a number of epidemiological studies and these are beginning to demonstrate important differences between methods.

The largest data set available for analysis is that collected from centres all over the world by Family Health International. In the developed world laparoscopic sterilization, with its need for only a brief hospital stay, can be an attractive method, although one requiring a great deal of specialist experience to conduct safely. In the developing world, laparoscopic sterilization has much less of a place, both because of the high expense of installing and maintaining the equipment and training the surgical team and because of the need for full operating theatre back-up in case vascular or bowel repair needs to be conducted. Minilaparotomy, on the other hand, can be taught to non-specialists and conducted safely in a wide variety of medical facilities.[53] In Thailand and the People's Republic of China theatre nurses perform the operation with a high degree of competence. Current experience with female sterilization also suggests that minilaparotomy has a greater potential in the developed world than was originally appreciated.[51]

Case-control retrospective studies allow some decisions to be made about the choice of method of tubal occlusion (Table 12.3).[18,19,20] Although the failure rate for electrocautery is least, mechanical occlusion still has certain advantages. Electrocautery destroys most of the tube making the possibility of reanastomosis exceptionally remote. In addition, ectopic pregnancy, in the IFRP series, was more common following electrocautery than following mechanical occlusion.[17] Finally, when electrocautery is performed with a laparoscope there are dangers of unseen burns to the viscera. Mechanical occlusion with the Yoon ring is now a well-proven, robust technique. However, it destroys more tube than does a clip. Research continues on tubal clips, which are more susceptible to small variations in engineering and design than the tubal ring.

Sterilization is the most negative and final form of contraception and it is remarkable that so many women and men express satisfaction with their operation. Intellectually, such an irreversible procedure, which deprives an individual of an important faculty, can never be wholly satisfactory but it seems certain that voluntary sterilization will remain a highly important family planning choice for the remainder of the twentieth century (Fig. 12.4). Modest improvements in the technique and perhaps a greater possibility of reversal are likely but training and objective selection of the most appropriate technique will continue to determine safety. Above all, the policy controlling availability of the operation must be to continue to offer voluntary sterilization as an informed choice to all who may want it, but to impose it on none.

Table 12.3. *Laparoscopy and minilaparotomy: complications and failure rates*

	Laparoscopy			Minilaparotomy	
Method of tubal occlusion:	Electro-cautery	Yoon ring	Hulka/ Clemens clip	Pomeroy	Yoon ring
Number of operations:	9811	4464	1517	3380	998
Operative injuries (%)	1.5	2.2[a]	0.7	1.1	2.3[a]
Laparotomy required (%)	0.3	0.2	0.5	0.1	0.0
Alternative technique required (%)	0.1	0.7	0.7	0.8	1.9
Twelve month pregnancy rate per 100 women	0.3	0.5	2.0	0.4	0.6

[a] The majority of injuries with the Yoon ring were to the tube or mesosalpinx.
Sources. Mumford, S. D., Bhiwandiwala, P. & Chi, I.-c. (1980). Laparoscopic and minilaparotomy female sterilization compared in 15 167 cases, *Lancet, ii*, 1066; McCann, M. F. & Bhiwandiwala, P. (1979). Is minilaparotomy appropriate to the United States? *Advances in Planned Parenthood*, **24**, 1.

Fig. 12.4. Annual estimates of male and female voluntary
sterilizations performed in the United States 1969–80.

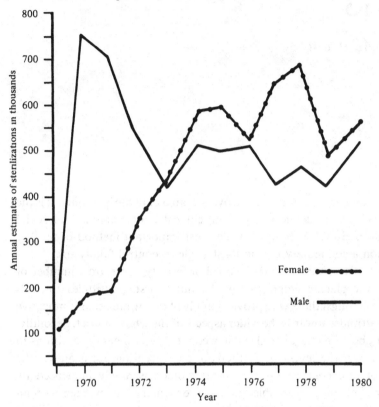

13

Abortion

Abortion is the most controversial area of family planning. It is the last to achieve academic recognition, clinical understanding and social acceptance. However, it is often the most important method of fertility regulation a community uses in its struggle to control family size.[98]

In reviewing options for the control of fertility, there are a number of reasons for placing emphasis on abortion. Firstly, attitudes towards abortion amongst those who provide family planning are usually indicative of their attitudes towards the wider aspects of the whole subject. Secondly, whether abortion is legal or illegal in a country determines the decisions to be taken over the reversible methods of contraception: for example, the choice of oral contraceptives in older women is highly influenced by whether abortion is accessible and legal, or whether the woman with an unwanted pregnancy is likely to be driven into the hands of an illegal abortionist. Thirdly, sociological and epidemiological evidence from many different localities and cultures demonstrates that abortion is often a first option that a community actually uses as it begins to control its fertility although it is the last which the medical profession and the providers of family planning normally make available.

This chapter documents the universal use of induced abortion, analyses the relation between abortion and contraception in fertility control, reviews legal and illegal techniques and sets induced fetal wastage in the context of reproductive loss as exemplified by spontaneous abortion. It is essential to remember that western medical practitioners are now divided by age into those who qualified when abortion was illegal and those who have only practised against a background of legal abortion. The overall picture of illegally- and legally-induced abortion must be comprehended if the consequences of possible future restrictions of liberal abortion laws are to be understood.

Definition

The medical and legal definition of abortion is the termination of pregnancy before the twenty-eighth week of gestation starting from the first day of the last menstrual period. In the eyes of the law a fetus is not viable before the twenty-eighth week, although there are now rare but recorded instances of survival earlier than this. Abortions may be either spontaneous or induced and induced abortions are subdivided into legal and illegal.

SPONTANEOUS ABORTION

Mammalian reproduction is an exquisitely complex but exceedingly wasteful process. For every oocyte which matures to ovulation there are many thousands which degenerate and die. For every sperm which fertilizes, hundreds of millions are lost. To what extent those two factors form a part of a 'survival of the fittest' process of natural selection is not known. After fertilization has occurred less than half of the gametes achieve implantation and delay the next expected menstrual period, so that for every known pregnancy there is at least one whose existence is totally unknown to the mother. It would seem that the very high wastage of fertilized ova is a continuation of a 'quality control' mechanism. Approximately 95% of all chromosomally abnormal conceptions among recognized pregnancies are spontaneously aborted.[71] Put another way, 5% or more of all human conceptions suffer a significant chromosomal abnormality but, owing to the selective effect of spontaneous abortion, the level drops to 2.4% at 12 weeks and 0.6% at term.[54] At a microscopic rather than chromosomal level, the American embryologist A. T. Hertig studied very early human development with great thoroughness. He found that about 15% of eggs which are ovulated either failed to reach the tube or were not fertilized, even under optimal conditions, and that of those fertilized eggs which implant in the uterus, only about 40–50% actually survive long enough to cause menstrual delay and lead to recognizable pregnancy.[50] Radioimmunoassays of urinary gonadotrophins have shown that over one-third of women fall pregnant in one cycle of unprotected intercourse, but that 43% of the pregnancies fail to progress as far as a delayed period or produce a recognizable spontaneous abortion.[79]

Apart from genetic causes of abortion, the developing gamete or embryo is subject to teratological factors which are as yet poorly understood. Even gross associations, as with the correlation between thalidomide and limb deformities, have not always been recognized immediately. Experimental findings in one species do not necessarily apply to another. Drugs and other teratological agents may act at one particular stage of development only. In general, the very early stage up to the conclusion of organogenesis, that is about the twelfth week of pregnancy, is the truly susceptible stage. Most teratogens cause a rise either in the abortion rate or in the congenital abnormality rate at birth, or in both, depending on the dose and on the time of pregnancy when they acted. There is a high incidence of spontaneous abortion among women who have a child with anencephaly or spina bifida, and possibly these miscarriages are of fetuses with neural tube defects that do not survive until birth.[58]

The range of potentially teratological agents increases with our knowledge and includes viruses (all of which pass the materno–fetal barrier), drugs and ionizing radiation. Cigarette smoking increases fetal loss and raises the prematurity rate at delivery, which in turn can give rise to mental retardation or other defects resulting from the unavoidable trauma of birth acting on the immature central nervous system.[79]

The effects of coital behaviour, namely the usage of periodic abstinence, have already been discussed (Chapter 7).

Maternal factors which contribute to spontaneous abortion include severe generalized diseases and virulent infections, especially those producing very high temperatures (e.g. malaria). These causes are far less common in both developed and developing countries than previously. Other maternal factors giving rise to abortion include local physical or physiological changes in the genital tract. Certain congenital abnormalities of uterine development predispose to abortion without preventing conception. Uterine fibroids and benign tumours, which are very common in certain racial groups during the second half of reproductive life, are an important cause of spontaneous abortion, especially in those societies where late marriage is the cultural norm. The role of hormone deficiency in spontaneous abortion is more controversial. Progesterone deficiency is responsible in only a very small number of cases and the routine administration of progesterone to women who have had a previous abortion is both illogical, unless deficiency has already been proven, and potentially damaging. It should be remembered that the administration in the 1950s of diethylstilboestrol to pregnant women with a previous history of abortion was responsible for many cases of vaginal cancer in girls of the next generation (see Chapter 10, Overall picture of neoplasia and Pill use).

All obstetricians can recall cases where spontaneous abortion followed a strong emotional shock. Sudden news of death or injury to a loved one in war, or a road traffic accident, may be followed within hours by the onset of abortion. The mechanisms by which such psychological factors work upon the pregnant uterus are of great theoretical interest but as yet they remain speculative. It is dangerous to argue from work in animals, but certain types of maternal stress predispose to spontaneous abortion, for example mares mated soon after foaling miscarry four times as frequently as those mated later. Serious overcrowding in rodent communities raises the instance of prenatal wastage. Estimates of early fetal loss under different conditions in cattle, horses, sheep and swine vary from 10 to 60%[88] In monkey colonies the probability of spontaneous abortion is partly related to the length of time that has elapsed since the last delivery. If conception occurs within one month, over one quarter of conceptions abort, but where the interval is over four months the rate falls to 7% of all pregnancies.[1] It seems possible that the same variable, whatever its mechanism, may also be relevant in cases of human abortion.

The epidemiology of spontaneous abortion
In the large majority of cases, it is impossible to distinguish clinically between induced and spontaneous abortion other than by relying on the history given by the woman herself. In one hospital on the outskirts of London serving 270 000 people in the early 1960s, between 375 and 400 cases of abortion were admitted annually out of a total of 1500 gynaecological admissions. At that time less than a dozen therapeutic abortions were performed each year.[25] On normal medical history taking and clinical findings, evidence of induced abortions was recorded for about 50 cases annually, but in 1965, out of 1384 gynaecological admissions, 397 were cases of abortion and each was interviewed by one person. After the woman's confidence had been gained, 241 actually admitted that the abortion was induced, either by themselves or by someone else acting illegally. Even so, during this period, one severely ill woman of 24 who had borne five children, four of whom were living, was admitted with a septic abortion and then developed renal failure, but maintained right up to the time when the last rites were administered by her priest that her abortion was spontaneous. Yet when the fetus was passed, and she began to recover, a rubber catheter appeared with it.

It is because of such difficulties that few reliable studies surveying the incidence of spontaneous abortion have been completed. In a prospective study on the Hawaiian island of Kauai, women were encouraged to report their pregnancies to study teams soon after missing a period.[40] Three thousand pregnancy histories were collected over three years and 24% of all pregnancies recognized at the end of the first lunar month of pregnancy ended in abortion. Monthly house visits to all women of reproductive age were made in a group of Punjabi villages in 1965 and 1765 pregnancy histories were collected; a spontaneous abortion rate of 10.5% was measured.[3] As elsewhere, retrospective studies collected in the same area revealed only one-fifth of the fetal loss detected in the prospective studies. Among 12 000 records of pregnancy taken from the Health Insurance Plan of Greater New York covering the years 1958 to 1960, pregnancy losses at differing stages of gestation were analysed.[104] The Plan mainly covered married women of above average income and it was thought that the induced abortion rate was probably lower than average although this assumption must be accepted with caution. The data were analysed as specific abortion rates for each week of pregnancy (Fig. 13.1).

Fig. 13.1. Risk of spontaneous abortion at various stages of pregnancy (12 000 women surveyed, Greater New York 1958–60). (Redrawn from Shapiro, S., Levin, H. S. & Abramowicz, M. (1971). Factors associated with fetal loss. *Advances in Planned Parenthood*, **6**, 45.)

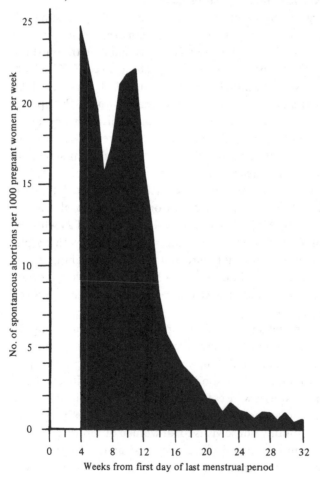

No. of spontaneous abortions per 1000 pregnant women per week

Weeks from first day of last menstrual period

In general, a figure of 10–15% spontaneous abortion is widely accepted in clinical practice.[71, 90, 117, 134] Maternal age is important and spontaneous abortion is most common among the very young, in women over 30 and in women of high parity. Ethnic, nutritional and other variants may be significant but are particularly difficult to analyse statistically.

INDUCED ABORTION

Traditional abortion practices

Abortion is as old as legend. However ancient the civilization, if we have evidence about everyday people, we nearly always have evidence of abortion. Certainly, it was used as long ago as Middle Kingdom Egypt (2133–1786 BC) and excavations at Pompeii yielded a form of vaginal speculum suitable for its performance. The Roman poet Ovid lamented: 'There are few women nowadays who bear all the children they conceive.'[85] There is only one reference to abortion in the Bible:

> If men strive, and hurt a woman with child, so that her fruit depart from her and yet no mischief follow: He shall be surely punished, according as the woman's husband will lay upon him; and he shall pay as the judges determine.

> And if any mischief follow, then thou shalt give life for life,
> Eye for eye, tooth for tooth, hand for hand, foot for foot,
> Burning for burning, wound for wound, stripe for stripe.[32]

This can only be interpreted as indicating that induction of abortion must be regarded as a crime but not as murder.

Among over 300 tribes or cultural groups reviewed by Devereux[23] only one denied using induced abortion as a method of birth control. We cannot know the frequency of induced abortion amongst women in primitive tribes but anthropologists suggest that it is used for social reasons, as by Hottentot women where frequent pregnancies would endanger their ability to work and their mobility, and for personal reasons, such as those of Chagga women who tend to seek abortion when they consider themselves 'too old to continue reproducing' or of Masai women who are said to seek abortion if they find themselves pregnant by an old or unfit man because they fear giving birth to an unfit child. These examples neatly illustrate the difficulty in differentiating between social and personal motivation. Abortion was certainly well known in pre-industrial England.[75]

Traditional abortion practices fall into three categories: medicinal, mechanical and massage. The pattern of traditional abortion practices existing in the developed world today, especially in countries where abortion is illegal, is similar to that which obtained in Europe and north America in the nineteenth century and first half of the twentieth century.

Medicinal methods

Most societies have, or have had, a range of drugs and herbs which it is hoped will end an unwanted pregnancy. Emmenagogues are substances which are intended to bring on a delayed period and abortifacients are materials which will terminate an established pregnancy.

In Britain both types of medicine were sold until the 1960s and even today remain available in European countries, such as Spain, where abortion is still illegal. In the developing world widespread sale continues from Peru, through Africa and Asia, to the Philippines. Sometimes, emmenagogues are explicitly labelled, but often their purpose is so well known that no explanation is needed. It is probable that most preparations are ineffective and the frequent appearance of beetroot, raspberries and potassium permanganate in emmenagogues may be for no better reason than that they are red. Belief in sympathetic magic must account for the fact that solutions of gunpowder have been drunk as abortifacients. Preparations containing ergot, quinine and lead may all have had some genuine effect as abortifacients but they also caused many cases of maternal death (lead poisoning acquired in this manner was a common phenomenon in nineteenth century England) and fetal damage such as blindness and deafness.[98] Savin, or oil of juniper, was a well-known abortifacient to the Greeks and Romans and Nicholas Culpeper (1616–1656), writing in *The Complete Herbal* says 'to describe a plant so well known is needless, it being in almost every garden'; he adds that 'inwardly it cannot be taken without manifest danger, particularly to pregnant women and to those subject to flooding'.[98]

> Help her make manslaughter, let her bleed,
> Never want for savin for her need.[26]

The use of emmenagogues and abortifacients continued in Britain until recent times. In a love-letter to Prince Edward, later to be King Edward VIII, the actress Lily Langtree wrote: '. . . my own darling, I am not sure yet . . . there must be something wrong or what I took would have made me . . . please go to the chemist and ask how many doses one ought to take a day as I must go on taking it . . .'[105]

In 1965 Cole conducted a survey of abortion drugs on sale in herbalists, chemists and rubber goods shops in Birmingham and found that of 40 randomly selected outlets investigated, no less than 31 sold preparations for facilitating abortion.[13] It was concluded that most of these preparations had 'no effective abortifacient function' but that there was some risk of the drugs taken by the mother damaging the fetus in addition to the risk of poisoning the mother herself.

Mechanical methods

Where abortion is illegal, surgical services still exist. Indeed, there are usually meaningful and accessible services for each socio-economic group. The wealthy can afford the high fee which physicians charge where abortion is illegal. The poor go to traditional midwives, slum doctors or lay people who have developed an appropriate technique.[57] For pregnancies around and after the third month the intrauterine introduction of a urinary catheter or similar flexible device is the technique used in most places. In Latin America it is called the *sonda*. It has the advantages of only involving one operator and of not producing, at any single moment in time, so much pain that local or general anaesthetic is necessary. It almost invariably produces the desired result and it is readily and cheaply available. The catheter technique has the disadvantage that abortion takes 1–2 days to occur once the foreign body has been inserted and that infection is common during this interval, particularly in circumstances encountered by most illegal operators. The separation of the placenta and the delivery of the fetus can be slow and haemorrhage is the second great risk of the method.

Practices in the contemporary developing world mirror those which were used in the West during the century prior to abortion law reform. Van de Warkle described curettage and intrauterine injection of fluids in New England in the 1870s. One practitioner charged US $10 and, complained van de Warkle, 'takes his pay in instalments'.[128]

A sample of illegal abortion techniques which had been used upon or by women admitted to a hospital on the outskirts of London immediately before the liberalization of the British Abortion Laws is illustrated in Table 13.1.[25] Of the 734 patients who admitted illegal abortion, 381 were married. Just over 10% claimed that they had induced the abortion themselves but possibly some of these claims were false and made in order to protect a husband or a lover. A large number of the women had also tried various advertised tablets or potions without success and these were not recorded.

In the 1970s, Gallen interviewed 106 illegal abortion practitioners in the Philippines. Most of their clients were young married women (average age of 29 years) and whenever possible they patronized the services of a practitioner in their own community.[57] Over 75% of the abortions were performed within the first trimester. In the majority of cases the abortion was not a secret: other people knew about it, her husband as well as relatives and friends. Few women appeared to suffer shame or guilt. The vast majority were Roman Catholics who attended church regularly but religion apparently had little influence on their decision. Up to the time of the abortive pregnancy 68.5% of the women were using no form of

Table 13.1 *Techniques of illegal abortion in one London Hospital 1964–68*

Technique	Number of patients
Drugs alone	(17)
Quinine Tablets with purgatives	9
Ergot extracts with purgatives	3
Purgatives alone or with alcohol	5
Vaginal Douching only (all self-administered)	21
Transcervical injections	(218)
Soap solution	36
Potassium permanganate solution	30
Utus paste	24
Toothpaste	18
Hypertonic saline (Brine)	16
Whisky	4
Boiled water	14
Solution or paste unknown to woman	76
Intrauterine instrumentation	
A. Sharp	(86)
Deliberate rupture of membranes at 16 weeks or more	6
Crochet hooks	12
Uterine sounds	4
Thin lead pipe	1
Surgical artery clamps	2
Fine ovum forceps (cord cut)	21
Unknown to woman	40
B. Introduction of soft foreign bodies into uterus	(116)
Male rubber catheter	31
Nylon cord	20
Plastic-covered curtain cord	2
Multiple IUDs	10
Other soft tubing	38
Material unknown to woman	5
Dilatation of cervix and curettage	(6)
With general anaesthesia	5
Analgesics only	1
Technique totally unknown to woman	270
Total	734

contraception but after the abortion 61.3% did so. The majority of the abortion practitioners were Roman Catholic women (mean age 47 years) and all were, or had been, married and most had large families (average 4.5 children). Less than one-third of these practitioners had attended college and a fifth had received no formal education at all. They each performed an average of 12.7 abortions per month. Despite the fact that they were well known as practitioners of abortion less than 1 in 5 had ever been harassed by the police. Only one woman had ever been imprisoned and this was simply overnight. She was released the following morning for lack of evidence.

In the Philippines now, as in western countries in the past, the majority of women first try to abort themselves, or at least try to induce delayed menstruation, using one of many medications that are widely available, including hormonal 'pregnancy tests'. It is suggested that at least 100 000 induced abortions occur in Manila alone. The situation is similar in other developing countries. In Seoul, the capital of Korea, which has a population of about 5 million, there may be as many abortions annually as in the whole of England and Wales with a population of 50 million. In Mexico, in 1978, there were 2.5 million births and an estimated 0.6–0.7 million induced abortions.[57]

In Britain at the turn of the century, the use of a crochet hook manoeuvred inside the uterus to disrupt the embryo was a common method of abortion. This technique is still much practised in the Howrah district of Calcutta. The preferred instrument is identical in all respects because crochet work is one of the cottage industries of the city. In rural India, abortion by the insertion of a fire-hardened straight twig is commonly practised. The introduction of foreign bodies such as the rolled bark of trees is also commonly used in India, and was the technique in Europe 50 years ago, the bark of the slippery elm being most used.

The transcervical intrauterine injection of fluid is a fairly recent form of abortion because it requires a suitable form of syringe or water pump. The rubber-ball 'enema' syringe was commonly used in Britain and the United States until very recently. In the Caribbean, Coca Cola is the preferred liquid.

Massage abortion

Massage abortion (Fig. 13.2) is a procedure well known in the Orient from Burma to the Philippines and south to Indonesia,[51] though it is virtually unknown in the West. In these countries, massage is a traditional treatment for many illnesses and is also used after delivery. The pressure applied to the abdomen to procure abortion is very much greater than normal and may involve literally stamping on the woman's abdomen as she lies on the floor. Pain is commonly a limiting factor in a procedure which may need repeating on several successive days. Haematuria, malaena and an appendicitis-like syndrome of fever, abdominal pain and board-like rigidity have been described as complications. Sometimes hysterectomy is necessary to deal with uterine damage.

Nearly 50% of all abortions in the Philippines are procured by abdominal massage, though the introduction of a catheter into the uterine cavity is used by about one-third of practitioners, plant preparations by 5% and surgical dilatation and curettage by 5%: various combinations of methods account for the remainder. Gallen concludes that in the Philippines 'abortion is a drastic, commonly expensive, sometimes dangerous event of great personal significance, but it is largely invisible to society'.[57]

In both urban and rural Thailand, induced abortion appears to be common, readily available and an open procedure.[120] Most of those who perform abortions are respected members of their local community. Eighty per cent of induced abortions in the survey conducted by Tongplaew were done by massage, which is almost universally known to village women. It is estimated that a quarter of a million massage abortions are performed annually.

The number of women who resort to abortion, even when it is illegal, is a

Fig. 13.2. Massage abortion.

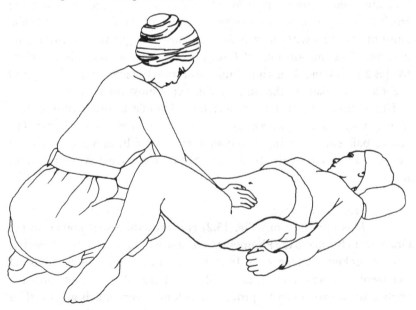

powerful demonstration of the popular demand for fertility control worldwide.

Consequences of abortion legislation
Incidence of illegal versus legal abortions

Liberal abortion laws (discussed in Chapter 15) are nearly always associated with a rising number of legal abortions and this often continues for several years.[8, 17, 18, 84, 93, 116, 126] There is strong evidence, from statistics on births and registered abortions relating to residents of New York State following a total repeal of previously restrictive abortion law in July 1970, that the *total* number of abortions did not change greatly, while the use of contraception actually *improved*.[114] For the most part, the rise in legal abortions after the introduction of liberal legislation appears to be a process of transferring previously illegal operations to the legal sector. The situation in England and Wales, following the implementation of liberal legislation in 1968 supports this picture. The birth-rate is accurately reported and although no reliable statistics on the number of illegal or *legal* abortions prior to 1968 is available, good data exist from that year onwards because notification of abortion is compulsory and failure can lead to prosecution. The number of known abortions performed on residents of England and Wales therefore rose by at least 80 000 between 1967 and 1970 but this had a minimal effect upon the birth-rate, which was already declining, and unless 80 000 criminal abortions were being performed in England and Wales immediately prior to the change in the law, the only other possible explanation is a sudden nationwide alteration in sexual habits accurately synchronized to the legal change. Clearly, Mr Roy Jenkins, the Home Secretary in 1967 when the Bill was being debated, was essentially correct in his estimate of 100 000 illegal abortions occurring annually in Britain. In a similar way, in 1965 the birth-rate in the Northern Italian province of Piedmont was 13.4 per 1000 total population, almost exactly equal to the Hungarian birth-rate of 13.1 per 1000 total population for the same year, although contraceptives at that time were even less readily available in Italy than in Hungary. The marriage rate and age structures of the two societies were comparable and therefore it seems likely that the illegal abortion rate in North Italy paralleled the legal abortion rate in Hungary, which at that time exceeded the live birth-rate by a factor of 1.35.

The total or partial reversal of a previously liberal law does not immediately mirror the change from illegal to legal abortion, because while women can transfer from back-street operators to legal clinics rapidly, it takes some time for illegal networks to re-establish themselves and become known. In October 1966 Rumania tightened up its law, which had permitted abortion on request, and the number of legal operations fell to one-twentieth of that found earlier while, nine months later, the birth-rate doubled. However, as illegal abortionists set themselves up, so the birth-rate fell: and the number of women dying from abortion rose[20, 93, 116, 126] (Fig. 13.3).

All the evidence suggests that social and economic factors primarily determine the number of induced abortions occurring in a society at any specific time, while the law determines how these abortions shall be performed and consequently the death rate to women. A simple law allows most terminations to occur early in pregnancy, a complex law, and especially one requiring committee decision, delays operation. Whatever the law, some groups, especially young teenagers, seek abortion later than more mature women. Menopausal women are also likely to seek abortion late because they may have failed to recognize that they are pregnant (see Fig. 13.4).

How many abortions are done?

The abortion *rate* per 1000 women is usually highest in the years of highest overall fertility (18–24) while the abortion *ratio* per 1000 preg-

Fig. 13.3. The effects of abortion legislation in Rumania. (After David, H. P. & Wright, H. H. (1972). Abortion legislation: the Rumanian experience. *Studies in Family Planning*, **2**, 205.)

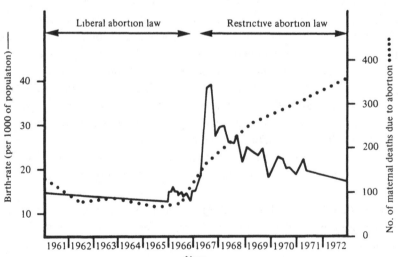

nancies is greatest at the extremes of fertile life, that is amongst young teenagers and women over 40 (Fig. 13.4).[116, 123]

Abortion is common: more than 7 million legal operations were performed in the US between 1973 and 1981. In 1979, 1 560 000 abortions were performed; 35% of the women were aged 20–24 and 30% were 19 years old or less. More than half the women were nulliparous and only 6% had three or more children. The legal abortion rate of the black population is approximately twice that of the white population.[115]

In 1979, 120 611 legal abortions were performed on women resident in England and Wales. More than half the women were unmarried, a quarter were between 20 and 24 years old and 27% were 19 or younger.

Important differences exist in the pattern of legal abortion, and, by inference, of illegal abortion, in different countries and at different times in the same country (Table 13.2). When a society begins to control its fertility (as happened in Korea and Taiwan in the 1960s or England and the US during the period 1880–1900), both the use of contraception and the resort to abortion appear to rise. As the birth-rate falls further, so abortion levels appear to peak (as happened in Japan after the Second World War or is

Fig. 13.4. The relation between the proportion of pregnancies ending in legal abortion and the age of the pregnant woman (US data). (Data from Tietze, C. (1981). *Induced Abortion. a World Review, 1981.* New York: Population Council.)

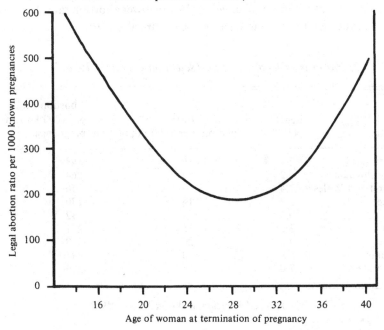

happening in some parts of contemporary Latin America). Finally, when the demographic transition is fully established (as in contemporary Europe, the United States and Japan), contraceptive practice continues to rise and abortion rates fall, but the need for abortion is never eliminated[98, 126] (Fig. 13.5). The rate at which society passes through this 'hump' is greatest when contraceptive services are readily available and is probably assisted by liberal laws which enable women who have abortions to be immediately offered contraceptive services. In Tunisia, the total number of abortions may have declined since abortion was made legal and contraception (including sterilization) was made available.[82] In Russia, however, contraceptive services are practically non-existent and as a result abortion rates continue to be persistently and exceptionally high. In countries with poor contraceptive services and illegal abortion (for example Burma and Peru), the suffering associated with abortion and the total loss of fetal life remains greatest.

Subgroups within society may behave in much the same way as larger groups such as countries. Requena demonstrated that throughout Latin America it is not those totally lacking education but those with an elementary school background who have most abortions.[100, 129] They are the groups where fertility first begins to decline rapidly, and they are the groups who adopt contraceptives but make many mistakes. Those with the privilege of at least high-school education enjoy a further decline in fertility but use contraceptives more effectively so have a lower abortion rate (Table 13.3). The young unmarried in western society are also learning to control

Table 13.2. *Patterns of legal abortion (selection countries 1978–79)*

Country	Legal abortion rate per 1000 population	Birth-rate per 1000 population	Abortion ratio per 1000 known pregnancies
Canada	2.7	16	148
Czechoslovakia	6.2	19	264
England and Wales	2.4	12	156
France	2.9	14	170
India	0.5	34	12
Japan	5.3	16	271
Poland	4.2	20	179
Romania	18.8	20	498
United States	7.0	15	303

Source: Tietze, C. (1981). *Induced Abortion: a World Review, 1981.*
New York: Population Council.

their fertility for the first time, and, like their married grandparents or women in contemporary Latin America, they are experiencing a high abortion rate while striving to improve their contraceptive practice. The number of woman having legal abortions appears to be determined not by the availability of abortion but by the pre-existing cultural norms of the

Table 13.3. *Induced abortion by educational level in three Latin American cities. (Figures show the percentage of women reporting one or more illegally-induced abortions)*

Education	Santiago, Chile	Bogota, Columbia	Mexico City, Mexico
None	27.3	26.0	29.6
Elementary only	39.3	28.0	34.2
High school and beyond	24.3	19.1	24.8

Source: Requena, M. B. (1971). The problem of induced abortion in Latin America. In *Proceedings of the International Population Conference of the IUSSP*, vol. 3. Liege, Belgium: International Union for the Scientific Study of Population (IUSSP).

Fig. 13.5. Abortion during the demographic transition.

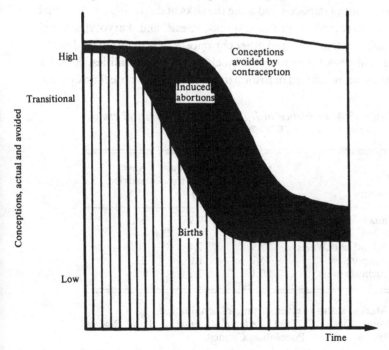

country (Table 13.4): the abortion laws in Singapore and England and Wales are virtually identical, yet abortion rates for young women are very different, reflecting different patterns of chaperonage. In addition, the earning power of the young and parental expectations are very different in the two societies.

Who has abortions?

Most women seek abortions because they feel that they cannot give a child, if born, the love and care they believe it deserves. Abortion is a private act and in many ways an altruistic one, even if it can still arouse dismay in others and sometimes shame in the woman concerned. Most abortions represent a woman's desire to control her own fertility.

Few abortions are carried out because continuation of the pregnancy might threaten the pregnant woman's life since with technical improvements in obstetrics this dramatic situation becomes rarer each year. Young unmarried girls, particularly Roman Catholics from well-to-do areas, are sometimes at higher than average risk of suicide.[28] A small number of abortions are carried out because of rape or incest and an increasing, but still small, proportion because of evidence that the fetus may be abnormal.[47]

Recent advances in fetal diagnosis coupled with elective abortion are making a substantial impact in reducing the risks of delivering an abnormal baby in industrialized countries. Amniocentesis and karyotyping can detect Down's syndrome[111] and other chromosomally determined defects. Other tests will detect a number of biochemical abnormalities. Routine amniocentesis is now offered in Britain to those women whose fetuses are at

Table 13.4. *Incidence of legal abortion by marital status (selected countries 1978–79)*[a]

Country	Currently married (%)	Previously married (%)	Never married (%)
Canada	26.0	9.9	64.1
United States	26.4	—— 73.6 ——	
England and Wales	37.9	11.4	50.7
Singapore	75.7	1.0	23.3
Czechoslovakia	80.1	7.3	12.6

[a] Marital status is given at time of termination.
Source: Tietze, C. (1981). *Induced Abortion: a World Review, 1981.* New York: Population Council.

particular risk of genetic abnormality, to virtually all women pregnant for the first time at the age of 35 or over and all pregnant women over the age of 40. Neural tube defects, including anencephaly and spina bifida, occur at a rate of 1–3 per 1000 births. In 1972 Brock & Sutcliffe reported increased amounts of α-fetoprotein in amniotic fluid from pregnancies with neural tube defects.[7] Subsequently, raised α-fetoprotein in maternal serum was shown to be a satisfactory preliminary screening test for the abnormality. During screening for raised serum α-fetoprotein in 12 000 women in Scotland, 75 were selected for amniocentesis and as a result 34 were aborted. In every case the aborted fetus had major defects.[124] The quality control in the testing laboratories must be high.[133] The confirmatory amniocentesis carries a small risk of inducing miscarriage, tests can only be done after about the sixteenth week of gestation and second-trimester abortion must be ethically acceptable to the woman and the obstetrician.[43] Nevertheless, such developments are a natural extension of the process whereby spontaneous abortion screens out abnormalities and will become increasingly significant. Already, current techniques have the potential of reducing the risk of an older woman (aged 35–44) bearing an infant with a severe birth defect to a level comparable with that of a younger woman. For a woman over 45, screening can reduce the risk of abnormality, but it will still be higher than that of a younger woman.[41] In the future, transcervical methods of diagnosis which can be done earlier in pregnancy may be developed and the range of detectable defects (e.g. sickle-cell disease and thalassaemia) will continue to expand. Hysteroscopy and direct visualization of the fetus is already a useful tool in technologically advanced centres.

Techniques of abortion
Post-coital and menstrual therapy

The post-coital use of steroids is reviewed in Chapter 10 and of IUDs in Chapter 11.

Several chemicals may act as emmenagogues although only prostaglandins (PGs) have reached the stage of clinical trials for the medical induction of a late period. The presence of PGs in menstrual fluid was demonstrated by Pickles in 1957[91] and in 1971 Karim showed that menstruation can be induced by the vaginal application of PGs[61] though the quantities required are large and the side-effects unacceptable for routine use. Prostaglandins also make the smooth muscle of the gut and bronchi contract, so side-effects include vomiting, diarrhoea and asthma-like attacks. The earlier in pregnancy that PGs are used, the higher is the dose required and the worse the side-effects.[62] Despite these disadvantages, because of their effectiveness, PGs do open up the possibility of eventually becoming what Ravenholt defined in 1968 as the most essential missing element in fertility control, namely: 'a non-toxic and completely effective substance or method which when self administered on a single occasion would ensure a non pregnant state at completion of a monthly cycle.' To achieve that goal the desired uterine effects must be separated from the unwanted and burdensome side-effects.

Csapo suggested that a double-impact dose of PGs was particularly effective in early pregnancy[15, 16] and several clinical trials using PG $F_2\alpha$ derivatives have been conducted with the PG $F_2\alpha$ being administered in the form of vaginal pessaries and intramuscular injections.[8, 76] Usually the procedure is successful but occasionally the surgical evacuation of the uterus is also necessary to complete the abortion. The use of prostaglandins to induce menstruation is not yet a routine, service procedure. On the one hand increasingly effective analogues are discovered every year.[31] On the other hand major manufacturers are increasingly afraid of pursuing research in this field and there is a serious danger that one of medicine's greatest immediate needs at global level will go unfulfilled, not because of lack of scientific know-how, but because of protests by a vocal minority in certain western countries.

Surgical techniques

Historical development. Dilating the cervix and scraping the uterine contents in early pregnancy has been practised since pharaonic times. There have been three fundamental improvements in techniques over the last one hundred years or so. From the time of Lister aseptic technique has greatly reduced the risk of infective complications. The introduction and improvement of anaesthetics, first general and then local, has meant not only that the woman is relieved of severe pain but also that the operator is able to proceed slowly and calmly, dilating the cervix in a gentle and as far as possible atraumatic manner, thus enabling full removal of the uterine contents and reducing the likelihood of cervical damage. Recently, the technique of vacuum aspiration (VA) has made uterine evecuation simple and remarkably safe.

In 1863 James Simpson, who introduced chloroform to Europe and gave it to Queen Victoria during childbirth, described a technique of 'drycupping' the interior of the uterus to bring on menstruation during early intervals of amenorrhoea.[106] This suction technique was rediscovered by the Russian Bykov in 1927 but its use disappeared when the Russian law was made more stringent in 1936.[9] In 1958 Wu and Wu in China reintroduced vacuum aspiration, which spread to Japan, China, Russia and parts of Eastern Europe by the late 1950s and the 1960s.[135] In 1967 Dorothea Kerslake began to use suction termination in Britain and by 1969, 45% of all early terminations were being performed in this manner.[65] The advantages of suction over the more conventional curettage or scraping of the uterus are now firmly established, not only for early termination of pregnancy but also for the treatment of incomplete abortion.[98] The technique is more gentle, thereby less damaging, and more thorough because the suction is effective even if the operator has failed to approximate the suction curette closely to every part of the uterine cavity.

Anaesthesia. Termination can be performed under local, spinal or general anaesthesia. Before 8 weeks since the last menstrual period, when VA can be completed without cervical dilatation, it can be conducted without anaesthesia at all if the women and the surgeon so wish, or with sedation such as intravenous (5–7.5 mg) diazepam. About 30% of western women who had menstrual regulation (see below) without anaesthesia rated it a painful procedure and pain was most likely in the nulliparous and particularly in those who proved not to have been pregnant.[112]

In a high volume clinic, with a specialist anaesthetist present, rapid general anaesthesia (with facilities for resuscitation and tracheal intubation if needed) has been safely used in hundreds of thousands of cases. Anaesthetics, including halothane and trichloroethylene, which relax smooth muscle are best avoided.

Local anaesthetic by paracervical block is simple, safe and satisfactory for vacuum aspiration and for dilatation and curettage (D and C) when these methods are used simply to terminate a pregnancy. Injections whould be given at the reflexed vaginal epithelium, that is at the junction of the cervix and vagina, and a total of 10 ml of 1% lignocaine should be given in two or four doses at 1 cm depth at the 4 and 8 o'clock or 2, 4, 8 and 10 o'clock positions respectively (Fig. 13.6).

Five deaths due to local paracervical anaesthesia were reported in the US between 1972 and 1975 and most or all involved overdose or hypersensitivity.[44] Care must be taken to determine that the woman is not allergic to lignocaine and to avoid injection into a blood vessel by drawing back the plunger before each injection. It is essential to wait at least 2 min by the clock for the anaesthetic to work.

Cervical dilatation. Most of the immediate and some of the long-term risks associated with abortion derive not from emptying the uterus but from entering it. When dilating the cervix rapidly with metal dilators, Pratt or

Hanbin Ambler dilators, which are tapered, are preferable to Hegar dilators, which require greater pressure for equal dilation.

For well over a century, laminaria (compressed stem of the seaweed *Laminaria digitata*) tents have been used by surgeons to dilate the cervix slowly. (In parts of Yugoslavia dried asparagus used to be used for the same purpose). Their use is widespread in Japan and Korea, and they have a long history in Britain[99] and are becoming increasingly well known in the US for the induction of abortion (and also full-term labour[119]). Tents are inserted under sterile conditions 6–12 h before surgery and secure a slow, largely painless, even dilation so that on removal a 10 mm cannula or metal dilator can be inserted easily. Infection is a danger if the tents are left in situ for too long. For more advanced pregnancies the cervix can first be dilated to 12 mm and then packed with tents which will slowly dilate it much further and are unlikely to tear it.

It has also been observed that although laminaria tents swell, they exert little external pressure and the process of dilatation is not comparable to expanding a wooden wedge with water to split off stone in a quarry, but rather to the slow driving out by pressure of interstitial fluid. With this in

Fig. 13.6. Injection sites for local anaesthetic in termination of pregnancy. (Woman in lithotomy position.)

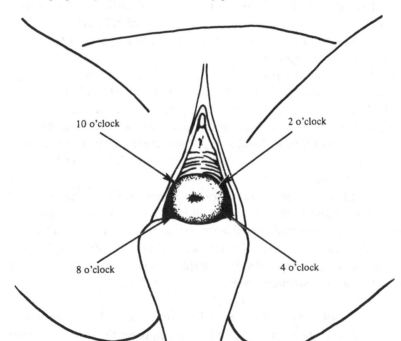

10 o'clock

2 o'clock

8 o'clock

4 o'clock

mind, the International Fertility Research Program (now Family Health International) has developed an osmotic dilator of a cellular plastic inpregnated with 0.7 g of magnesium sulphate. This performs better than conventional laminaria, is cheaper, quality control is simpler and it may be applicable to brief (2–4 h) use, so that it can become part of a day-care service (see under Day-care abortion).

Menstrual regulation. Menstrual regulation (MR), menstrual aspiration, very early suction abortion and pre-emptive uterine aspiration are all terms used to describe suction aspiration of uterine contents when the first missed menstrual period is less than 14 days overdue. This arbitrary definition was accepted because the routine diagnosis of pregnancy cannot be established with certainty and this has considerable medico-legal importance in some parts of the world, particularly in Latin America and several Commonwealth nations where definitive abortion procedures still fall under restrictive statute laws (see Chapter 15).

In 1961, Harvey Karman, a Californian lay psychologist who was appalled by the misery he found amongst the unwillingly pregnant, began to abort women entra legally. Not being conditioned by a formal medical training, he approached the problem of abortion with an open mind, and, lacking the facilities to give general or even local anaesthetics, he sought to apply the principles of vacuum aspiration using a very small-bore tube to avoid dilating the cervix.[98] He choose soft and pliable tubing for curettes and a hand-held syringe to form the vacuum. Up to this time all suction curettes had single openings, which often became blocked. Karman introduced two openings (Fig. 13.7) in his curette and so overcame this problem. An additional advantage is that the pliable tubes tend to be deflected and to curl up inside the uterine cavity rather than to perforate the wall of the uterus as any rigid instrument may do. Thus, as far as very early pregnancy is concerned, Karman's ingenuity solves three problems at one stroke: the need for anaesthesia to dilate the cervix (this being the painful part of dilatation and curettage), the problems of blockage of small-bore tubes and the danger of perforation with a fine instrument. The technique was first published by Karman & Potts in 1972.[63] Menstrual regulation is quick and simple.[66, 70, 127] Anaemic women and women with a known blood coagulation disorder should only be operated on in a hospital.

Fig. 13.7. The Karman curette.

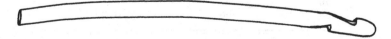

Careful pelvic examination is necessary to check the history of amenorrhoea and exclude fibroids, gross uterine abnormalities or pelvic inflammatory disease. The equipment is cheap and robust[37] and does not require
elaborate facilities or specialist operators. Paramedical workers or even
traditional midwives can perform MR safely after adequate training and so
long as they refer any doubtful, complicated or potentially difficult cases to
a gynaecologist. The greatest danger of MR is over-confidence in an
operator who has neither the skill nor the facilities to cope with a surgical
complication or who lacks the experience and confidence to estimate the
duration of a pregnancy.

For carrying out MR, a good light, a clean room and a firm table are
necessary. With the woman in the lithotomy position, a speculum is passed
and the cervix cleansed with a suitable disinfectant. She need not be draped
nor the operator gowned but a no-touch technique is essential. The cervix
must be stabilized, if possible with an atraumatic instrument. The syringe is
drawn back and the valve closed and set aside before a 4- or 6-mm cannula
is passed gently through the cervix: the larger the cannula that can be used,
the less the chance of a failed procedure. The cannula should be used to
sound the uterus, once again checking the duration of pregnancy. (Table
13.5). Sounding to an excess depth should suggest an error in dating the
pregnancy, fibroids or uterine perforation and it may be necessary to refer a
woman receiving MR in a simple facility to a better-equipped institution.

With the cannula in the uterus (often liquor will begin to drain) the
charged syringe is attached with a firm twist to ensure an airtight lock, and
the valve opened. The products of conception rapidly enter the syringe and
the walls of the uterus should be gently curetted by 'in-and-out' stroking
motions accompanied by rotation of the syringe and attached cannula to
ensure that all parts of the uterine cavity are curetted. If the syringe fills or
the vacuum is lost, the syringe should be detached, emptied and recharged.

Table 13.5. *Assessment of the duration of pregnancy:*
clinical findings and embryonic growth

Days since LMP	Length of embryo (mm)	Uterine length (sounding) (cm)
28	<1	7
42	4–5	7–8
56	15	8–9
70	30	9–10
84	60	10–11

If the cannula blocks it should be removed and cleaned with a sterile swab or instrument. No additional instrumentation is necessary and MR can usually be completed in 3–5 min. Discomfort varies from little to moderate,[112] and cramping pains may be severe towards the end of the procedure. Local anaesthesia, if needed, is given in the same way as for routine vacuum aspiration. The fine-bore aspiration technique can be used to treat incomplete abortion, for endometrial biopsy and for routine curettage for dysfunctional bleeding.

Uterine perforation is rare and excessive blood loss requiring transfusion was not encountered in closely monitored series (Table 13.6).[36] Pregnancy can continue after any abortion but the risk is slightly greater in the case of MR than in routine first-trimester procedures and it is essential that the woman clearly understands the need to return if the signs and symptoms of pregnancy persist. Experience has shown that the use of a 4-mm cannula is particularly likely to end with a failure to terminate the pregnancy and it is recommended that 6 mm should be the smallest size used. The operator must also be alert to the risk of ectopic pregnancy.

A proportion of women who undergo MR will not have been pregnant.[6] Up to 14 days' menstrual delay nearly 30% of MRs may be unnecessary. However, even though the number of redundant operations is cut down by asking women with negative pregnancy tests to return some days later, it must also be recognized that any delay in operating produces a measurable increase in complication rates. The decision is likely to depend on the

Table 13.6. *Menstrual regulation (immediate and delayed complications reported from a 21-country multicentre study 1972–76)*

Complication	Number	Rate per 1000 operations
Immediate (112 888 cases)		
Uterine perforation (definite)	3	0.2
Uterine perforation (suspected)	1	0.1
Cervical laceration	2	0.2
Blood loss in excess of 100 ml[a]	51	4.0
Delayed (11 309 cases followed up 2–4 weeks after MR performed)		
Continuation of pregnancy (positive pregnancy test)	111	9.8
Fever (requiring antibiotics)	95	8.4
Repeat curettage for bleeding	101	8.9
Undiagnosed ectopic pregnancy	2	0.2

[a]No patient required transfusion.

country's law, medico-legal practices and the emotional choices of the woman and the surgeon.

In certain special circumstances, very early abortion may lead to a rushed and possibly incompletely-accepted decision. For example, single women with a good and stable relationship with the putative father may be ambivalent and adequate time for discussion and possibly counselling may not have elapsed; in such circumstances adequate time to decide is an essential part of good treatment.

Perhaps the main drawback of MR is its simplicity! Unfortunately, gynaecologists and those working in abortion clinics who acquire considerable expertise in first-trimester abortion rarely perform menstrual aspiration. In Britain it is rarely used because abortions are limited to defined clinical facilities and by the time women are referred it is too late to use the procedure. In the US a larger experience has been accumulated but prices have never dropped to the $25 or $50 that a 5-min procedure with a $15 piece of apparatus deserves. Globally, Laufe estimates, 5 million MRs may have been performed by the end of the 1970s.[73, 94] In Calcutta the procedure is offered for US $2–3 and in the Philippines, Indonesia and parts of Africa and Latin America it is beginning to be used widely. The technology is appropriate to the developing world as it is cheap, safe, simple and robust. In Malaysia one practitioner performed 5000 consecutive MRs with one syringe and with only one woman requiring hospital admission (for perforation). Paradoxically, MR has still to reach its full potential in western countries where abortion is legal.

Emptying the uterus before the woman knows for certain that she is pregnant profoundly changes the emotional, legal and ethical aspects of early abortion. Gynaecologists investigating involuntary infertility frequently perform a diagnostic curettage of the uterus during the 10 days before the next expected period and all will recall having inadvertently performed an early abortion when it was least desired. It is known that many seemingly normal menstrual periods are in fact very early abortions. Using the name 'menstrual regulation' alters the rules of the game which people play in relation to abortion. To describe such an important human problem in terms of a game may seem out of place but neither the general public nor the medical profession are logical in their attitudes to abortion. Politicians, lawyers, doctors and women in need all distort reality. It is not practical to write about abortion in a Bangladeshi newspaper in a straightforward way, but it has proved acceptable to hold a much-publicized conference on menstrual regulation in Dacca and MR is now counted as part of the government family planning programme. It is not prudent to have even a whispered discussion of the role of abortion in family planning in the Philippines or Latin America, but it generates immediate and widespread interest to discuss menstrual regulation.

Vacuum aspiration. Dilatation of the cervix and vacuum aspiration (VA) in early pregnancy (under 12 weeks from last menstrual period) is now accepted worldwide as the optimum technique for early abortion.[22, 30, 53, 67, 68, 97] Women with renal, cardiac or other serious disease, fibroids, uterine anomalies, pelvic infection, *severe* cervicitis, anaemias and blood coagulation disorders can all have VA, but require specialist treatment and full hospital facilities.

Careful pelvic examination is essential and is probably the most important step in the whole procedure. By about 40 days after the last period, the fundus of the uterus may be palpated as being more globular in shape. When the firmness of the cervix is traced upwards with the internal examining hand and the uterine isthmus is passed prior to slight palpable enlargement of the fundus, this is known as Hegar's sign and is valuable in diagnosis of early pregnancy.

The woman should be counselled so that she understands the nature and possible implications of abortion and makes a free and informed choice. Enquiry should be made about post-operative contraceptive choices and the option of inserting an IUD at the time of abortion considered. The possibility of a technical failure and continuing pregnancy should always be emphasized and also the need to return if signs of infection or undue bleeding occur.

Most operators find that the cervix is best exposed with a short-bladed, bivalve speculum (warmed to body temperature if local anaesthesia is used). After cleansing (as for MR) the cervix should be immobilized and the uterus sounded. If, after bimanual assessment and uterine sounding the pregnancy is found to be very early, say under 7 weeks from the date of the last menstrual period (LMP), it may be possible to introduce a 6-mm cannula without having to dilate the cervix. At a later state, or when a nulliparous cervix is unusually tight, dilatation will be required but should always be done to the smallest degree consistent with full uterine evacuation. Up to about 9 weeks from LMP, soft cannulas with outside diameters up to 8 mm are suitable and add to safety. After 9 weeks semi-rigid cannulas allow the aspiration of fetal and placental tissues more readily. The technique is suitable in the hands of most operators up to about the fourteenth week but the cervix should never be dilated beyond 12 mm if further childbearing is contemplated. Electric vacuum pumps are convenient and efficient, a negative pressure of 600 mm (30 inches) of mercury is desirable and 500 mm (25 inches) essential. Where facilities are lacking, suction produced by an assistant-operated reverse action bicycle pump is perfectly satisfactory.

When the vacuum is switched on and the cannula begins to 'grip' it should be moved inwards and outwards in the direction of the uterine axis and also rotated about its own axis. Aspiration is continued until the uterine wall can be felt all round. Signs of completed evacuation are (a) the appearance and amount of the evacuated products, (b) the presence of a slight froth in the aspiration bottle and (c) most significant of all, a gritty feeling of the suction curette being gripped by the walls of the empty uterus.

The advantages of vacuum aspiration over cervical dilatation and uterine curettage are that it is quicker, more complete in removal of tissue, involves less blood loss, results in fewer complications and is more easily performed with local anaesthesia.

It is unwise to prophesy future developments in medical technology but there are some surgical procedures, such as appendicectomy, which appear to have reached an end-point and where further technical improvement seems unlikely. Such a procedure is vacuum aspiration for the termination of early pregnancy.

Dilatation and curettage. Dilatation of the cervix and curettage of the uterine cavity (D and C) was for generations the accepted way of treating incomplete abortions and of performing first-trimester therapeutic abortions in centres where these were done. Local anaesthesia can be used but a very gentle technique is needed. The diagnostic potentiality of examination under anaesthesia is sacrificed, so the method is suitable only when the diagnosis and duration of pregnancy are certain. When terminating a pregnancy by this technique, particularly in very early pregnancy (8 weeks or less) it is essential to curette methodically the *entirety* of the uterine cavity otherwise a small piece of placental tissue may be left behind and a further curettage may later become necessary for continued bleeding and/or pain. It used to be taught that a blunt curette should be used for fear of perforation. In practice, uterine perforation almost invariably occurs as the instrument, be it sound, dilator, forceps, or curette is being introduced. Perforation almost never occurs during the return or truly 'curetting' action and therefore a sharp curette, which is lighter, more sensitive and more efficient than a blunt one, is actually safer for these very reasons. Similarly, experienced operators will rarely utilize oxytocic drugs because they know that good uterine contraction with full control of bleeding will occur spontaneously when the whole of the conceptus has been removed and this very typical contraction, occurring without the use of an oxytocic drug, is a useful indicator that the procedure is complete. Oxytocic drugs also cause post-operative pain.

Day-care abortion

Until the recent world revolution in abortion legislation the subject of abortion was medically taboo. No ambitious young doctor seeking advancement published papers of his experience or of an innovatory technique in abortion. There were, of course, doctors all over the world who specialized in doing abortions clandestinely, sometimes illegally and sometimes stretching the existing laws so as to be at least quasi-legal. There was, therefore, an almost total lack of information about abortion morbidity and mortality. The medical establishment in western countries believed that abortion was a dangerous operation, although their colleagues in Russia, Japan, China or Yugoslavia could have easily reassured them. When abortion first became legal in the West it was entirely an inpatient hospital procedure performed under the control of, and often personally by, a specialist gynaecologist. In practice the performance of abortion under general or local anaesthesia calls for specialized training and for constant awareness of potential risks but does not require the skill of a fully trained gynaecologist. Indeed, because of its repetitive nature, the operation may not hold the full attention of a highly skilled specialized surgeon (Table 13.7).

In the late 1960s the British Government set up an impartial committee

Table 13.7. *Incidence of complications in high and low volume abortion facilities*

Complications	Day-care abortion unit (US 1970–72)		Specialist hospital care (UK 1968–70)	
	Number of cases	Rate per 1000	Number of cases	Rate per 1000
Perforation (without sequelae)	36	1.4	14	12.0
Perforation (needing laparotomy)	13	0.5	6	5.0
Hysterectomy	1	0.03	2	1.6
Infection (temperature of 38°C or more for 24 h)	391	15.0	321	270.0
Total number of abortions	26 000		1182	
Percentage performed at 12 weeks and less	100		78	

Sources. Stallworthy, J. A., Moolgasker, A. S. & Walsh, J. J. (1971). Legal abortion: a critical assessment of its risks. *Lancet,* ii, 1245; Nathanson, B. M. (1972). Abulatory abortion experience with 26 000 cases. *New England Journal of Medicine,* **291,** 1189.

under a High Court Judge, Mrs Justice Lane, to examine the workings of the Abortion Act in Britain.[136] One of the recommendations of this committee was that abortion counselling and the performance of simple early abortion were tasks admirably suited to the specially trained general practitioner. The committee also recommended that day-stay, ambulatory operation facilities be provided rather than women be admitted to hospital for in-patient treatment. Unfortunately these recommendations have never been implemented in Britain, where more than half of all abortions are provided by the private sector which, with minor exceptions, is still prohibited from day-stay abortion care. In the United States a totally different situation developed. Here, for financial reasons, out-patient care was adopted from the very beginning and, similarly, local anaesthesia has been very widely used, certainly throughout freestanding abortion clinics. These clinics, staffed by personnel specializing in abortion have produced excellent and relatively cheap abortion services with extremely low morbidity and mortality rates.[78, 81, 96] Highly successful out-patient abortion clinics have been established in the Netherlands where they flourish despite a restrictive law.

Fig. 13.8. The risks of induced abortion at varying stages of pregnancy (US 1970s). (Modified from Tietze, C. (1979). *Induced Abortion: A Fact Book*. New York: Population Council.)

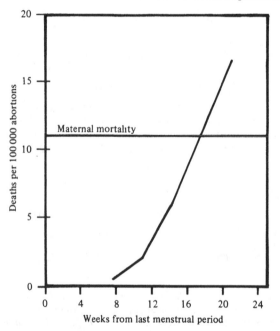

Out-patient abortion facilities are particularly applicable to the developing world, but within that world there is such a shortage of medical services that it is to be hoped that paramedical staff and perhaps traditional practitioners will be utilized after a short course of training. Several experimental schemes have shown such staffing to be safe and efficient.

The key to safe abortion is early operation (Fig. 13.8) and services should be established with this in mind. For example, the Nordic countries were early in legislation for abortion but the bureaucratic system forcing the woman to appear before an abortion committee (often on at least two occasions) led to inordinate delays with high mortality and morbidity simply because operations were being performed far later than need have been the case. To a lesser extent the British situation is similar except where, on local initiative, special abortion units have been set up within the National Health Service, thereby avoiding the delay usually associated with referral by the family doctor to the hospital specialist.[2] In Kingston, on the outskirts of London, approximately 5000 day-stay abortions have been done by family practitioners working in a special unit, but, although successful, this remains unusual.

Day-care or out-patient abortion requires selection of patients. Physically or psychiatrically ill patients should be excluded because they need longer post-operative care, support and observation. Each day-care unit needs access for back-up to the facilities of a fully-equipped gynaecological department. With these two provisos the concentration of facilities within one unit ensures that all members of the team are sympathetic to abortion and experienced in the handling of women at risk of emotional trauma. Abortion counselling and future contraceptive help should be a routine part of the work of such a unit. Experience has shown that the complications of abortion occur either during the operation itself or are those of secondary haemorrhage or infection which manifest themselves some days later and therefore would not, in any case, be detected by routine 24-h hospital in-patient stay.

Mid-trimester abortion

Late abortion can be dangerous and is always disagreeable. Surgical risks rise steeply after the twelfth of thirteenth week and psychological or emotional trauma to the woman is very much increased. In addition, medical and nursing staff associated with abortion invariably find late abortion to some degree stressful. The management of late abortion can be divided into one-step and two-step procedures.

One-step procedures

Uterine evacuation (dilatation and evacuation (D and E)) by the vaginal route is feasiole until about the twentieth week of pregnancy. It requires a high degree of surgical skill, adequate anaesthesia (usually general) and full operating room facilities. Laminaria tents reduce the risks of excessive force needed to dilate the cervix but there remains the danger of tearing the internal sphincter, with a risk of cervical incompetence and a threat to future fertility. The extent of this danger calls for assessment by prospective trials; none have yet been reported.

Dilatation and evacuation was used in Britain[33] for many years before it was tried in the US. In 1977 Grimes and colleagues from the US Center for Disease Control demonstrated, in a pruspective study of 6213 mid-trimester curettages and 8662 abortions performed by intra-amniotic injections, that the former had less short-term, major complications (0.69 per 100 versus 1.78 per 100).[10, 46, 113] It also has less complications than the intra-amniotic use of prostaglandins.[45]

Two-step procedures

Induction of late abortion by amniocentesis involves the introduction of a needle via the abdominal wall into the uterine cavity and the drainage of amniotic fluid. In modern practice the technique is not usually attempted before the fifteenth or sixteenth week of pregnancy.[64] Local anaesthesia only is required. The patient must fully empty her bladder before the procedure is attempted. A needle encased in a piece of fine-bore plastic tubing is introduced and once the amniotic cavity is entered amniotic fluid escapes. At this point the needle is withdrawn and the operator is left with a fine-bore plastic tube leading into the amniotic cavity. Such a tube, not being rigid or sharp, is not likely to perforate the uterine wall or cause damage to the placenta which might lead to mixing of maternal and fetal blood. Once the tube has been introduced the amniotic fluid inside the uterus is drained as fully as possible. At about 16 weeks it is normal to be able to remove about 200 ml and usually 200 ml of a selected solution is then injected.

The instillation of hypertonic saline into the intra-amniotic cavity to induce abortion was first reported by Aburel in 1939 and widely used in Japan between 1946 and 1952; it then fell into disrepute because of high complication and mortality rates.[131] Nevertheless, saline replacement after amniocentesis continues to be widely used in the US. The method is contraindicated for women suffering from cardiac or renal disease.

Hypofibrinogenaemia is always a risk. The introduction of saline usually kills the fetus and is followed by a drop of serum progesterone levels.[122] A live fetus is very much less likely to be delivered following saline induction than with some other two-step methods of abortion.

Because of the mortality associated with hypertonic saline, instillation of hypertonic glucose solutions was tried in many parts of the world but has been largely abandoned because it is associated with increased infection rates. A replacement solution that is free from serious sequelae, even if injected into the wrong place or if it is for some reason rapidly absorbed, is urea. It has been widely used in England and Wales since its introduction in 1971.[43] So far there have been no reported deaths with urea or urea and prostaglandins, although non-fatal complications including a ruptured uterus following urea and prostaglandins have been reported. Amniocentesis, inevitably, is associated with delay between replacement of the amniotic fluid and expulsion of the fetus and placenta. This delay can be shortened by using an oxytocin or prostaglandin intravenous drip.[14] The latter is about as effective as the former but more toxic.

Extraovular injections of soft soap pastes have long been known for both legal and illegal abortion, but were often associated with infection.[5, 108] Irritants such as rivanol (ethacridine lactate, a yellow dye and antiseptic) have been used as alternatives in some countries such as Russia, Japan and Israel. Recently such irritants have been supplanted by prostaglandins, with or without intra-amniotic urea. The extraovular introduction of prostaglandin $F_2\alpha$ for the induction of abortion, or even for the induction of pre-term labour is now commonly used.[98] Either a very fine-bore polythene tube is introduced for a considerable distance through the cervix, or else a self-retaining bladder catheter ending in a balloon is passed through the cervix, the balloon is inflated with sterile water to hold the catheter in place and an extra-amniotic injection is made either continuously using some form of drip or pump, or intermittently as a bolus delivered by a syringe.

Davis has used a method where, under sterile conditions and with local or general anaesthesia, the cervix is dilated to approximately 10 mm, a small-bore vacuum aspiration cannula is inserted into the uterine cavity, rupturing the membrane, and, with a low vacuum, the cord will adhere to the cannula and can be pulled down and divided. As with other two-step procedures, the aim is to destroy the placental function; once this is achieved, uterine contractions leading to expulsion of the products of conception will follow. An oxytocin drip can be used.

Hysterectomy is a miniature Caesarean section, and can be done vaginally or by the abdominal route. Abdominal hysterotomy is very much more dangerous than simple early abortion (Table 13.8). Vaginal hysterotomy has no advantages over D and E because once the cervix has been cut, resuturing rarely restores functional competence. Unlike abdominal hysterotomy, it cannot easily be combined with sterilization.

During 1972–73 in England and Wales, 15 244 cases of hysterectomy or hysterotomy were performed with 8 deaths, a mortality of 52.5 per 100 000 operations. Hysterotomy is rarely if ever indicated as an operation designed primarily for the termination of second-trimester pregnancies.

Hysterectomy, the total removal of the uterus, is even less frequently indicated for abortion. The dangers of hysterectomy are greatly increased when it is undertaken during pregnancy. Where there is a double indication for a termination of pregnancy and for hysterectomy on other grounds, it is safer first to terminate the pregnancy and later to perform the hysterectomy.

It seems that neither man nor nature wants to perform second-trimester abortions. Those methods which involve a short interval between induction and abortion are associated with a high incidence of incomplete procedures requiring a second, surgical emptying of the uterus, while those which involve the misery of slow effect tend to require less surgical intervention. These correlations apply to prostaglandins, which have a relatively quick effect, but may be associated with incomplete procedures, and saline or urea, which have a slower but more often complete effect, as well as to the

Table 13.8. *Mortality of abortion by method (England and Wales 1969–77)*

Year	No. of vaginal terminations	No. of deaths	Rate per 100 000 procedures	No. of hysterotomies and hysterectomies	No. of deaths	Rate per 100 000 procedures
1969	38 948	4	10.3	12 845	11	85.6
1970	68 703	7	10.2	14 159	6	42.4
1971	110 498	5	4.5	12 482	6	48.0
1972	132 819	8	6.0	9 203	6	65.2
1973	134 069	1	0.7	6 041	2	33.1
1974	150 004	5	3.3	4 098	1	24.4
1975	127 281	2	1.6	2 481	0	–
1976	117 761	1	0.8	1 940	0	–
1977	121 165	3	2.5	1 560	4	256.4

Source: The Registrar General's Statistical Review of England and Wales – Supplements on Abortion for the years 1969–1977. London: HMSO.

addition of oxytocin, which also speeds up the abortion but tends to result in the procedure being incomplete with retained products needing surgical evacuation.

Complications of abortion
Illegal abortion
Mortality. Speculations about the numbers of illegal abortions performed are always open to error, so the relevant morbidity and mortality rates must involve guesswork. However, better than usual estimates can be made from England and Wales because since 1952 every death of a pregnant or recently pregnant woman in England and Wales, has been automatically scrutinized by the Registrar of Deaths and made the subject of confidential enquiries carried out by an appointed group of gynaecologists who collaborate with the local community physician and make enquiries of every doctor and professional worker who had contact with the woman. An assessment is made of what are termed avoidable factors, these being errors of judgement either by the woman herself or by any of her medical or nursing attendants. The value of these reports depends upon the fact that every such enquiry is totally protected and its findings cannot be used in a legal action under any circumstances. It is possible to admit errors as well as challenge the wisdom of others in the management of the case without fear of damaging a colleague or of reprisal.[12] The system works well and reports are published every three years (Table 13.9). Although these reports are comprehensive, it is still possible that some criminal abortions may have been recorded as spontaneous, because once the woman has died, the secret of interference has died with her.

Table 13.9. *Deaths from abortion in England and Wales 1952–54 to 1976–78: abortion deaths in Triennial Reports on Confidential Enquiries into Maternal Deaths*

Type of abortion	1952–54	1955–57	1958–60	1961–63	1964–66	1967–69[a]	1970–72	1973–75	1976–78
Illegal	108	91	82	77	98	74	38	10	4
Spontaneous	43	50	52	57	25	25	6	5	2
Legal	2	0	1	5	10	18	37	14	8
Totals	153	141	135	139	133	117	81	29	14

[a] Liberal abortion legislation came into force on 27 April 1968.

Overall, in Britain as in other countries where abortion is legal, deaths due to illegal interference have been falling steadily over the past 30 years and, with the implementation of a liberal abortion law in 1968, the fall accelerated dramatically. Probably the fall between 1952 and 1968 was due to the fact that antibiotics had become available, not only to the medical profession but also to illegal abortionists, who were using them widely by 1965.

If we accept the estimate of 100 000 illegal abortions a year in England and Wales then the 74 deaths ascribed as criminal abortions over the period 1967–69 give a mortality rate of 24.7 per 100 000 abortions. If the number of abortions had been constant from 1961 onwards, then over the preceding six years 1961–66 (175 deaths) the rate would have been similar at 29.1 deaths per 100 000. These guesses seem reasonable because the sudden increase in the number of legal abortions performed after 1967 had little or no effect on the birth-rate, strongly suggesting that the increased number of legal abortions replaced an equal number of illegal abortions that were being performed before the reform of the law. Something over 100 000 therapeutic abortions were probably performed in hospitals and nursing homes during the years 1961–66, whereas between 1970 and 1975 the figure rose to 605 334. However, deaths believed to be due to illegal abortion fell from 165 in the first six-year period to only 48 in the second. Thus, transferring an estimated 500 000 abortions from the illegal to the legal sector appears to have saved 117 maternal lives.[25] Calculations based on this latter assumption give a mortality rate of 23.5 per 100 000 illegal abortions. Such a calculation is inexact, as it takes no account of possible improvements in contraceptive usage, but each of these approaches gives a consistent order of magnitude which suggests that the death rate from illegal abortion in England and Wales was probably about 25 per 100 000 during the 15 years 1961–75. Inevitably, in developing countries, illegal abortion will be associated with much higher risks.

Morbidity. Illegal abortion was, until 1968, the most common single cause of involuntary infertility in England and Wales[24] and the immediate complications of haemorrhage or infection were very common causes for hospital admission. Much chronic pelvic disease followed such abortions.

Legal abortion
Mortality. Abortion is not only one of the most common operations performed, it can also be one of the safest. In every country where abortion is legal and done on a large scale, first-trimester abortion has been associated with remarkably low mortality rates (Table 13.10). The statistical data are consistent and eloquent.[56, 98, 116, 123]

In most countries the mortality due to legal abortion declines year by year as the medical profession gains experience and as women gain access to the operation at ever earlier stages of pregnancy (see Tables 13.8 and 13.10). The death rate from legal abortion in the US in 1978 was 1 in 200 000 (1 409 600 legal abortions with 7 deaths reported). By contrast, the registered mortality for legal abortion in Denmark 40 years ago was 400 times as high and even in the US in 1970 it was 40 times the 1978 rate.

As death rates fall the proportion of deaths due to complications of anaesthesia, including local anaesthesia, rises. Based on US data, the death to case rate for legal abortions performed at 12 weeks' gestation or less for local anaesthesia is 0.15 per 100 000 while for abortions performed at the same stage under general anaesthesia it is 0.37 per 100 000.[89] The rate for general anaesthesia may have been inflated by an element of selection in that some women at particular risk may have been deemed unsuitable for local anaesthesia.

However low the risk to the woman, later abortions are always more dangerous than early ones (see Fig. 13.8). Abortions performed after 12 weeks of pregnancy carry more risks because at about that time the fetal head becomes too large to be safely extracted through a cervix dilated to the safe limit for a one-step procedure unless it is first crushed.

Table 13.10. *Mortality: abortion, delivery, surgery*

	Number of abortions	Number of deaths	Deaths per 100 000 operations or deliveries
Legal abortion (selected countries)			
England and Wales (1973–78)	874 000	31	3.5
D and C and VA:			
12 weeks or less	682 200	12	1.8
13 weeks or over	127 800	8	6.3
Amniocentesis	45 900	4	8.7
Hysterotomy and hysterectomy	17 700	7	40.0
Czechoslovakia (1973–79)	606 400	5	0.8
Hungary (1968–79)	1 682 500	22	1.3
United States (1978)	1 409 600	7	0.5
Maternal mortality (selected countries)			
United States (1978)			12.0
England and Wales (1980)			11.0
General surgery (US) (1969)			
Tonsillectomy and adenoidectomy			3.0
Partial mastectomy			74.0
Hysterectomy (not abortion)			204.0
Appendicectomy			352.0

The contrast between the risks presented by illegal and legal abortion – perhaps fifty fold in developed countries and a hundred fold or more in developing countries – is one of the most forceful in the whole of surgery and public health.

Rochat[101] and his colleagues interviewed over 1000 health workers in Bangladesh and estimated that they traced about 1 in 15 of all maternal deaths in that country. They suggest that, overall, about 21 000 women die each year from maternity-related causes and that one-quarter of these deaths are due to illegal abortion. This suggests that 2 out of every 10 000 women of fertile age die annually from abortion; the actual abortion mortality rate could not be estimated. There are 12 hospitals in Dacca providing services for at most a few million people and these hospitals report more deaths due to abortion than occur annually in the US.

Morbidity. By and large, operations which carry a low risk of death have relatively few complications and the complications of legal abortion follow the same distribution as the mortality, being least in operations performed early in pregnancy.[52, 87] However, failure to terminate the pregnancy is a relatively common complication of abortions attempted within 6 weeks of LMP as is incomplete emptying of the uterus. The latter complication may necessitate a further procedure.

Most uterine perforations probably occur at the time of cervical dilatation and are more likely in later abortions than early ones. Haemorrhage can occur at the time of operation, but the need for transfusion is rare and it is no longer routine to cross-match blood for first-trimester operations. Blood loss is slightly greater with general as opposed to local anaesthesia. Once the operation is over and the woman ambulant, there are few immediate risks and routine overnight stay has no logical place. Secondary haemorrhage and infection, however, can occur days, or even weeks, after surgery, the most common cause being incomplete uterine emptying at the time of operation.

The long-term consequences of abortion divide into the outcome of subsequent pregnancies, about which we have inadequate reliable data, and study of possible psychological sequelae. It has been suggested that induced abortions can lead to premature delivery, low birth weight and spontaneous abortion in later pregnancies.[101] The subject has proved difficult to study because of irregularities in reporting of prior abortions (whether legal or illegal), the presence of a number of confounding variables (e.g. smoking) and the extreme difficulty in achieving long-term follow-up of women who have had an abortion. Some studies show a small effect on later pregnancies when the woman's first pregnancy ends in abortion,[125] but it is possible that abortion merely shifts the proven risk associated with a first pregnancy to the first term delivery. Any effect that does exist is probably limited to those cases where there has been forceful rapid dilatation of the cervix and over-enthusiastic surgical curettage. The variation in the outcome of abortions performed in different centres as reported in the National Institute of Child Health and Human Development Multicentre study supports this hypothesis. A prior D and C abortion, under certain circumstances, can increase the risk of spontaneous second-trimester abortion in later pregnancies[77] while VA appears to have little or no effect.[29, 116, 130] One-step cervical dilatation should, if possible, be limited to 10 mm.[60, 83]

Illegal abortion is associated with subsequent infertility.[121] Undoubtedly, this also occurs with legal abortion (if only when an operation is associated with complications that lead to hysterectomy, something that occurred 24 times in 238 000 legal abortions in Canada) but the risk is too small to measure in epidemiological studies.[49, 74, 116]

An increase in ectopic pregnancies has been reported after abortion,[86] but again large-scale epidemiological studies, controlling for possible variables, have not substantiated such claims.[103]

The risks of Rhesus iso-immunization are small early in pregnancy but anti-D immunoglobulin (50 mg before 20 weeks and 100 mg afterwards) is recommended when available.

The literature on the psychological consequences of legally-induced abortion is rambling and sometimes contradictory. Poor sampling and absent or inadequate control groups plague many studies. However, a few careful studies were conducted in the 1970s and it is now accepted that severe depression, or other psychological disturbances which require treatment, are no greater than after childbirth.[42] Clearly, there is some short-term distress, but few women require in-patient care.[38] Among 73 000 abortions surveyed in the US, there were 16 major psychiatric complications, including two suicides. The psychiatric complication rate was 0.2–0.4 per 1000 abortions.[118] This compares with an estimated 1.0–2.0 major psychoses requiring hospitalization following childbirth. David, Niels & Holst conducted the most extensive study using computer-linked records of 71 000 term deliveries and 27 000 abortions among *all* women in Denmark for the year 1975.[21] The admission rate to psychiatric in-patient care was 1.84 per 1000 abortions within three months of induced abortion and 1.20 per 1000 deliveries within three months of delivery. Both rates were slightly higher than the 0.75 per 1000 calculated for all Danish women aged 15–49. It is important to note that separated, divorced or widowed women stood out as being at greatest risk of psychiatric complications, having a higher risk of admission following delivery (1.69 per 1000) and considerably higher risk following abortion (6.39 per 1000). It has also been suggested that the risk of distress is greater in repeat abortions.[39]

Abortion is as likely to alleviate as to precipitate psychiatric disorder, but the medical profession still views the risk of regret and emotional disturbance after abortion with more concern than experience documents. It is revealing of the attitudes of health workers, and of the lay public, that the possibility of psychological disturbance following a legal abortion was scored most highly by psychologists discussing psychoanalytic theories, less highly by health workers in a role-playing situation discussing abortion, more modestly still by those accompanying women having abortions or by the patient herself on the day *prior* to the operation and as least likely of all by the woman one day *after* her abortion.[4]

The interaction between the woman and the doctor is of critical importance in the assessment by the latter of the former's psychological reaction. The woman's emotional response to abortion is influenced by her doctor's reaction on the first occasion when she seeks advice about her unwanted pregnancy, and is further moulded by the response of all those in whose care she subsequently finds herself. Some doctors feel that the woman has sinned, but that they should extend charitable forgiveness and help her. Such doctors may well perform large numbers of abortions since they are overtly 'sympathetic', but women under their care tend to feel grateful but ashamed. Those physicians who expect abortion to be associated with guilt may indeed produce guilt in those they terminate and this may account for the fact that Simon & Senturia, surveying the literature in 1966, found that the incidence of severe guilt following hospital termination had been variously reported as being between 0 and 43% of all abortions.[107]

As experience of liberal abortion has spread, there has been an awareness that for many women termination brings genuine relief. The most fulsome rejection of traditional attitudes has come from the US.[11] Walter epitomizes the new viewpoint. 'A whole generation of professional health workers refuses to let the myth die out that abortion will irreparably harm a woman. Extensive review of the literature reveals that this has not been true. In fact, for the healthy woman with a happy marriage, abortion is most often truly therapeutic.'[132]

After an abortion the woman usually experiences a sense of relief and an awareness that many of her pressing problems have been solved (Table 13.11). She can face the future afresh and make new choices. In particular, the unmarried are now able to review their sexual reproductive attitudes and make positive decisions. This represents an important step forward because many have truly never considered their attitudes on these topics until they found themselves unwantedly pregnant. Many women make new and practical decisions about contraception.

No doctor enjoys performing abortions any more than he or she would enjoy carrying out limb or breast amputations. It is an appreciation of the improvement in the social and emotional health of the woman which can be expected to follow abortion that encourages him or her to operate, having taken account of the physical risks involved. The preliminary assessment and counselling of a woman before abortion, as well as the support of her during and after the procedure, bring the doctor into close contact with the woman and establish the same sort of link between them that is forged by a good obstetrician who cares for a patient throughout pregnancy and delivery.

Children born to women refused an abortion. 'Unplanned', 'unintended' and 'unwanted' are words to be used with care: a planned pregnancy is usually a wanted one but not all unplanned pregnancies are unwanted and a pregnancy that is unwanted at 8 weeks is not necessarily rejected at 8 months. Conversely, child cruelty can follow a pregnancy which was wanted by the parents as well as one that was rejected but where the woman had no access to abortion. Physically 'battered babies' are frequently children who were conceived premaritally[34] or are the last born. In addition, battering may begin when the mother falls pregnant again.

There is a wide no-man's land between the small minority of parents who ill-treat their children, or fail to care for them adequately, and the vast

Table 13.11. *Emotional benefits of legal abortion (360 women having first-trimester abortions in London)*

	Before termination	After termination (3 months–2 years)
Psychiatric symptoms requiring treatment	29%	19%
Depression (Hamilton rating scale)	11.67 ± 6.18	4.38 ± 3.95
Interpersonal relationship rated as satisfactory	62%	77%
Sexual adjustment rated as satisfactory	59%	74%

Source: Greer, H. S., Lal, S., Lewis, S. C., Belsey, E. M. & Beard, R. W. (1976). Psychological consequences of therapeutic abortion. *British Journal of Psychiatry*, **128**, 74.

majority who love and look after their children. But the small amount of objective study that has been carried out on women who were refused legal abortions appears to demonstrate that children whose mothers had sought unsuccessfully to have them aborted were disadvantaged when compared with other children. Forssman & Thuwe followed up for 21 years 120 children whose mothers had been refused a legal abortion in Sweden between 1939 and 1941.[35] They found a number of adverse outcomes when these children were compared with a control group. A more detailed study has subsequently been undertaken in Czechoslovakia of 233 children born to women who sought and were refused a legal abortion on *two* occasions in the same pregnancy, and compared with a control group born over the same years (1961–63) which was matched for sex, birth order and marital status of the mother.[19, 27] Over 400 physical and psychological factors have been compared. During childhood some differences emerged, with more frequent acute illness and poorer schooling performances among the children whose mother had sought but were refused an abortion. The two groups have now been followed up for 16–18 years and with the passage of time the differences between them have come to assume even greater statistical significance. Such studies provide comments on the aggregate but are of little predictive value for the individual. Overall, the children born to the women who sought abortion are more likely to consider themselves rejected by their mothers than those in the control group; they also believe their mothers are less satisfied with them. They had slightly poorer school marks and more hospital admissions. Their teachers rated them as less conscientious. The group is now on the threshold of its own reproductive life and interestingly, the boys in the group express more conservative views on such issues as unplanned pregnancies than those in the control group, while the girls born to women who sought abortion are more liberal. Overall, individuals, as we have always known, show a great ability to adjust to adverse circumstances, but in the aggregate never totally overcome the misfortune of being 'unwanted'.

ABORTION AND CONTRACEPTION

A woman who has an induced abortion demonstrates that she is fertile and does not want to have a baby. The time of an abortion, an MR or even a late period often becomes a turning-point in a woman's use of contraception, or in her decision to become sterilized. The relation is a two way one: women who use contraceptives are more likely than those who do not to seek abortion should their contraceptive technique fail, while those who have an abortion are often ready to adopt a contraceptive technique for the first time. The fact that a contraceptive user is more likely to resort to an abortion than a non-user appears to apply to all methods of contraception. In a study from Colombia it was found that, prior to adopting the rhythm method, 13% of pregnancies ended in spontaneous or induced abortion (the figure is consistent with the vast majority being spontaneous), while after using the method, 35% of pregnancies ended in abortion.[59] In Switzerland, in the 1960s, Catholics had slightly more abortions than Protestants,[110] possibly because they used less effective methods of contraception but felt the same need to control family size. In Korea, 80% of IUD users fell pregnant within six months of discontinuing use, but over 50% of those pregnancies ended in induced abortions.[48]

The relation between contraceptive practice and abortion has been clouded for social as well as academic reasons. Family planning in the West emerged against a background of controversy and the early pioneers were forced to separate contraception and abortion so that they could argue that contraception avoided the need for abortion. In real life they are complementary methods of fertility regulation. An observed change in the abortion rate may be associated with a change in the contraception rate in either the same or the opposite direction. Several factors influence such an apparent contradiction. These include: changes in the age distribution of women of reproductive age, the proportion of women who are sexually active, changes in contraceptive practice and switches from previously illegal (and therefore unrecorded abortions) into the area of legal (and therefore countable) operations.

Fortunately, a great deal of epidemiological and survey information is now available to document the rise and fall of induced abortion rates as societies pass through the major stages of demographic transition (see Fig. 13.4).[98] Both induced abortion and contraceptive practice are spreading through much of the developing world at the present time. In Korea, for example, the birth-rate fell by 30% between 1960 and 1968 and induced abortion is estimated to account for one-third of this decline, improved contraceptive use and a rising age of marriage accounting for the remainder.[97] It is probable that whether the operation is legal or illegal abortion rates will continue to rise in many places for the rest of the century, and perhaps most especially in the shanty towns of the Third World. However, this phase will not last for ever, as is illustrated by Japan, which, since the Second World War, has passed through a second stage where contraceptive practice has overtaken the resort to abortion (Table 13.12).[80]

Very few societies use only abortion to limit family size but when they do they have a great many abortions. For example, only 4.2% of Hungarian couples rely exclusively on abortion[72] for family planning, but they contribute disproportionately to the number of abortions taking place in the country. There are reports of women having 10 or even 20 abortions; this is because a woman who is not using contraceptives may have two, or even three, abortions in the same interval of time as it requires to conceive, carry and wean a baby (see Fig. 2.3). At the same time, modern methods of contraception also have their limitations and all have demonstrable failure rates. For example, data from Taiwan show that one insertion of an IUD does not avert one birth (Table 13.13),[92] yet even a poor method badly used will do a great deal to extend the interval between pregnancies.

The significance of abortion in family planning should come as no

Table 13.12. *Legal abortion and contraceptive practice in Japan (1955–65)[a]*

	1955	1960	1965
Legal abortions (reported)	1.17	1.06	0.84
Induced abortions (calculated total)	3.13	3.55	3.10
Number of births prevented by abortion	2.71	3.09	2.74
Number of births prevented by contraceptive practice	1.21	1.97	3.02
Ratio of births prevented by contraception to births prevented by abortion	100:256	100:180	100:104

[a] Millions of events.
Source: Muramatsu, M. (1970). An analysis of factors in fertility control in Japan. *Bulletin of the Institute of Public Health, Tokyo,* **19**, 97.

Table 13.13. *Limitations of an IUD in the perspective of a fertile lifetime*

	Additional births observed[a]		
Age of women	No family planning	IUDs[b]	Difference
22.5	7.14	6.48	0.66
32.5	3.10	2.24	0.86
42.5	0.38	0.31	0.25

[a] Based on programme data from Taiwan.
[b] Insertion and reinsertion in first pregnancy interval only.
Source· Potter, R. G. (1971). Inadequacy of a one-method family-planning program. *Social Biology,* **18**, 1.

surprise if the experience of contemporary western couples is considered. The present pattern of family building is such that most families have only two to three children, often borne while the wife is still in her twenties. Therefore, it is common for a couple to be faced with 10–15 years of fertile life following the last wanted child. Even with an effective method, such as the Pill or IUD, between a quarter and two-thirds of all couples will have one unplanned pregnancy during this interval and 3–5% of couples will have two.[55] Among women seeking a repeat abortion in the US, a quarter are using a reasonable method of contraception but have been unlucky enough to have a method failure.[102]

This should not be taken to deny that a great deal can and should be done to offer contraceptive advice following induced abortion. In the US 60% of abortion patients fail to adopt or use a method of contraception adequately and Rovinsky estimated that in 15% of abortion cases the institution performing the operation had failed to offer realistic contraceptive advice.[102] An IUD can be safely inserted at this time (see Chapter 11, Evaluation). Oral contraceptives or injectables can be dispensed before the woman leaves the facility. Voluntary sterilization can be a reasonable choice although care needs to be given to ensure an informed choice is being made and to certain technical aspects of the operation when performed at or around the time of abortion.

Illegal abortionists practically never offer contraceptive advice or referral. It is a reasonable hypothesis to suggest that the total number of abortions may be less in a legal service linked to the ready availability of contraceptives than in a situation in which abortion is illegal and in which those who are not ill enough to enter a public hospital will not be exposed to contraceptive or sterilization advice. Further, an open service, if unequivocally advertised is likely to result in an earlier operation than would a clandestine service.

The interwoven attributes of contraceptive practice and abortion are further illustrated by the way in which they complement one another in the effort to keep the risks of fertility to the user at the lowest level (see Fig. 16.1). A similar relation also affects the costs of health and family planning services. An aggressive service designed to meet the fertility goals of couples purely by extending the choice of contraception might result in few abortions but be so costly that it may be impossible to extend nationwide. For example, a Korean contraceptive project serving only 1400 couples required the part-time assistance of a physician and four full-time nurse-midwives in a country which at the time of the project only had enough midwives to serve 11% of the women in labour.[109] The same fertility goals can be reached more cheaply with integrated abortion and contraceptive services than with either alone. Invariably, there is a point on the graph of rising costs where providing contraceptives to 80% or 90% of couples, as opposed to say 50% or 60%, will exceed the costs of the extra abortions needed to reach the same fertility goal. There is always intense competition for health resources and, as any programme must rob competing areas, it is an ethical as well as an administrative problem to ask how hard a health service should strive in the difficult task of controlling fertility purely through contraceptive efforts when this investment begins to compete with other curative and preventive services.[95]

In a very real sense, both contraception and abortion are essential for controlling fertility and meeting the goals demanded of modern living. Put another way, a society cannot meet its fertility goals purely by the use of contraception, although many family planning programmes are promoted on this false premise. A society can, however, achieve any desired family size merely by using abortions but some women will need very large numbers and this is not ultimately good for their health; it is also a course which overburdens health services and is emotionally repellent to follow. Theoretically, it would be possible for every couple to accept sterilization as soon as they had the number of children they wanted, but this is unlikely to be acceptable without coercion and would inevitably be associated with disappointment and regret for many because of later changes in their circumstances. Therefore, the combination of reversible methods of contraception and induced abortion will remain necessary elements in fertility control for some while into the future.

EVALUATION

Throughout history, and with increasing force over the past one hundred years, societies have used a combination of contraception and abortion to control their fertility. However, this inescapable choice has not always been understood by academic commentators, administrators of health services, politicians or theologians.

Induced abortion appears to be particularly common in countries (for example those of contemporary Latin America) and groups (for example young unmarried women in Europe or North America) which are learning to control their fertility for the first time. In the early part of the twentieth century, and in nearly all countries, abortion was illegal, but since the middle of the century there has been a revolution in laws and medical practice relating to abortion and today abortion is legally available to almost three-quarters of the world's population; it is not easily accessible so widely.

In the late 1970s and early 1980s visible, passionate groups arose in affluent western societies who were seeking to reverse the liberal abortion legislation of the previous 10–20 years. Therefore, it is important to examine the choices that are, and are not, open for policy-making relating to abortion.

Policy choices

Experience shows that abortion laws have little direct effect on the total number of abortions taking place, but that liberal laws are associated with a dramatic and consistent reduction in deaths and ill health among women who have abortions. In other words, the law on abortion largely determines the number of deaths occurring among adult women having abortions, whereas the socio-economic circumstances and ease of access to contraception are responsible for the level of induced fetal loss.

At the very least doctors and all medical workers must recognize the existence of induced abortion and use its occurrence as an appropriate time to make contraceptive advice available. The International Planned Parenthood Federation (IPPF) unanimously resolved (1971) that 'in those countries in which abortion is legal to seek to maximise the provision of contraceptive services after an abortion' and 'in those countries in which abortion is illegal to seek . . . adequate and socially humane services to treat incomplete abortions and other complications of illegal abortion and that such services be linked with the provision of contraceptive advice'.[69]

Some liberal abortion laws (e.g. that of Britain) define the medical practitioners sphere of action, while others (e.g. that of the US) recognize the woman's need to make an informed choice. However the law is framed, it must permit decision-making, and operation if chosen, to take place as early as possible in pregnancy.

Early legal abortion can present no more risk to the woman than receiving an injection of penicillin. Yet whatever method of abortion is used the risks of operation increase with duration of gestation, rising particularly rapidly after 12–14 weeks. While early vacuum aspiration techniques are outstandingly safe, cheap and easy to provide, there is no pre-eminently satisfactory method of second-trimester abortion. The total number of deaths from abortion of all types has fallen dramatically in England and Wales in the last 50 years (Fig. 13.9) and the bulk of this saving of women's lives has been because fewer have died from illegal abortion.

Ethical choices

In the last analysis, abortion is a moral problem involving a wholly human judgement about the relative status of the embryo, which is on the threshold of human development, and of the mother, for whom the continuation of an unwanted pregnancy may have profound social consequences. Observation shows that nearly all pregnant women can find themselves in a situation where they will choose abortion as a preferable alternative to the continuation of pregnancy: this is borne out by the fact that virtually all women support the choice of abortion in cases where the fetus can be shown to be abnormal.

The decision of a woman, or a couple, to have an abortion is normally an expression of the fact that at this particular time in their life they feel that they cannot offer a child the love, security and physical support which would meet their ideals: the young unmarried girl feels that she cannot give a baby the life she sees as necessary for its proper happy development; the married woman often feels that another child would take away from her existing children too much of the physical and emotional resources available and would mean that in the future all her children would be to some extent deprived. Abortion is usually an altruistic decision.

Informed choice is essential to any responsible abortion service. Rather than asking, 'was the operation emotionally traumatic?' it may be more useful to ask, 'did the woman/couple make a healthy choice?' or 'did they have all the relevant information they needed to make their decision, in the context in which they found themselves?' or 'do they regret their decision or would they make the same decision again; were they using the decision to hurt themselves or other people: did they learn from the decision?'

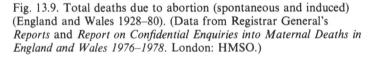

Fig. 13.9. Total deaths due to abortion (spontaneous and induced) (England and Wales 1928–80). (Data from Registrar General's *Reports* and *Report on Confidential Enquiries into Maternal Deaths in England and Wales 1976–1978.* London: HMSO.)

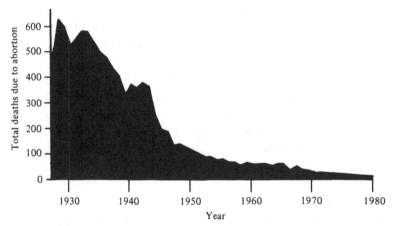

The moral and political attributions of abortion services outweigh such factors as proven mortality rates or the evidence of cost-benefit studies. There can be no doubt that abortion is an ethical problem on which opinions are deeply divided, and it is impossible to visualize any new piece of evidence that would unite opposing camps. There are deep and passionate divisions concerning what is meant by the sanctity of human life; the issues are often entangled with such emotive terms as 'innocent life' and 'the rights of the woman' so that it is difficult to see how such a fundamental conflict can be solved but such a situation is not unprecedented. The religious wars of the sixteenth century ended only when it became universally recognized that they could do so only through tolerance of differing viewpoints on fundamental religious issues. Ultimately this tolerance, born of necessity to stop bloodshed, gained recognition as a virtue which widened the horizons of all. So it may be that on both sides of the abortion debate the adoption of true tolerance might not only help to solve immediate problems but also yield a quantum leap forward in the acceptance of contraception in just those countries and communities where it is most needed.

Until such acceptance is attained, are there any areas of common ground on which reasonable people might agree? Possible there are, providing abortion and contraception are viewed as a totality. One approach is to acknowledge that abortions will occur in all low-fertility societies and are likely to be most common in those in which the birth-rate is falling in response to socio-economic pressures.

Most reasonable people would strive to keep abortion rates low, but would be realistic enough to appreciate that the need for abortion could not be eliminated in the foreseeable future. Everyone would prefer to see abortions performed early, rather than late, in pregnancy.

14

Medical aspects

Doctors and other medical workers who give family planning advice enjoy very special opportunities for practising preventive medicine because their work brings them into a close and trusting relationship with their clients and involves enquiries and concern about a large number of medical and social factors. They meet a wide range of gynaecological conditions and may well be counsellors in marital and sexual problems in addition to being drawn into the wider practise of social medicine. Where the British idea of general practice exists, the family doctor is particularly well placed to give contraceptive advice.

From whatever background they come, those who give family planning advice have an obligation to provide adequate information on the hazards of pregnancy at various stages of a woman's life as well as on the differing risks of various contraceptive techniques and on how these risks change with age. In order to give such information every family planning adviser must constantly study such subjects as risk factors applicable to particular techniques and contraceptive efficiency at differing ages. He or she must also keep abreast of knowledge about the incidence of fetal abnormality with advancing maternal age. In order to provide advice which is as unbiased as possible, the doctor or nurse should feel free from the fear of litigation in the event that a family planning procedure, after adequate explanation, gives rise to complications. Unhappily this freedom is rapidly disappearing in some western countries.

Information must be presented in a way that clients can understand. The adviser must be truly conversant not only with the local idioms and colloquial speech but also with the religious and cultural mores which are such important influences on contraceptive acceptance. Potential users must be made aware of the different risks to maternal health of various contraceptive choices as opposed to the possible failure rate or risk of pregnancy with which they are also associated. The safety of a contraceptive technique in respect to the woman using it must not be confused with its security against unwanted pregnancy. Even in the least developed parts of the world, women seeking family planning are aware that certain forms of contraception may be associated with risks to health. Indeed, because of biased media coverage of contraception, which is worldwide, most women will have an exaggerated view of the risks posed by, say, oral contraception as compared with other risks met in everyday life. It is important to try and present such risks in true perspective and certainly not to minimize them deliberately. It will be found that clients are encouraged rather than discouraged by acquaintance with the true facts, without which they are not able to make informed choices. Women in the Third World are only too well aware of the risks of being pregnant. They can hardly fail to be so.

The failure rates of different contraceptive techniques must also be presented as accurately and as fairly as possible. Here it must be remembered that in a culture where contraception has not already gained wide acceptance, user failure is likely to be far higher than in circumstances where the technique has been available and in use for a long time. When presenting comparative contraceptive failure rates, misunderstandings readily occur and merely to quote the average rates taken from textbooks may not help an individual. It is important to get across the idea that there is a ranking order of contraceptive effectiveness, with sterilization being almost totally effective, the oral contraceptive the next most effective method, IUDs not very far behind, the mechanical methods such as condoms, diaphragms and spermicides have a somewhat higher failure rate and coitus interruptus and periodic abstinence being associated with the largest number of accidental pregnancies. Even this simple ranking order may need modification in the developing world where the use-effectiveness of the Pill is commonly less than that of the IUD.

The provider's own confidence in the method being offered is of overriding importance. There is no purpose in recommending a method you yourself don't believe in. If you would not be prepared to use the oral contraceptive, or to have a vasectomy, you are unlikely to be successful in advocating these methods to others. People soon read the sincerity of the individual giving the information in something as important and personal as family planning. The person sitting opposite to you needs to know the answer to the question 'Would you use this method yourself?' In the last analysis the choice of action must always lie with the individual or couple. Only when a family planning decision is an informed one can it make its maximum contribution to maternal and child health. If counselling has been well conducted it may also lay down the foundations of a good relationship between the provider and user which may contribute to other aspects of medical care in the future.

In addition to having a 'listening ear' the physician who gives contraceptive advice must be competent in the general physical and psychological assessment of all clients, and in particular remain alert for and be capable of diagnosing unsuspected pelvic disease. For example, cancer of the ovary is a particularly lethal disease simply because it is asymptomatic until very late, so where an older woman seeks contraceptive advice there can be a unique opportunity to detect it while it is still treatable. Although most gynaecological complaints will be relatively minor and may need no more than reassurance, technical competence by all staff is essential; its absence is rapidly recognized and once this has happened, reassurance is valueless.

Whenever a family planning consultation takes place the nurse or doctor consulted should always be aware that the woman or man who mentions a minor symptom may in fact be seeking much wider reassurance. For example, a woman who complains of vaginal discharge when examination fails to reveal any such abnormality may well be asking for reassurance that she has not got venereal disease and perhaps the query arises from a suspicion of her consort's infidelity and it is at this level that she really needs to talk. Ideally the converse is also true. A specialist who has the long-term care of a woman with a chronic disease ought always to be aware of the woman's contraceptive needs and either to provide for them or to co-operate in ensuring that they are properly met. Unfortunately, this does not always happen and the woman with a chronic disease is often forced to seek the advice of a physician working in a general family planning clinic who may well lack expert knowledge of her complaint.

Interaction of medical conditions and contraceptive usage
Conditions which may be first encountered and diagnosed by the Family Planning Physician

Menstrual disorders. In young women menstrual disorders are common. Periods of amenorrhoea following emotional stress, change of occupation or travel are usually of little significance. Prolonged amenorrhoea demands the exclusion of hyper-prolactinaemia and a definitive diagnosis. In the past it was felt that women suffering from very irregular periods should not be offered oral contraception because when they came off the Pill to start a family it might be a considerable time before their menses returned. There is in fact no evidence that the menstrual irregularity is adversely affected by the Pill and such young women are not wholly suitable for other forms of contraception because their menstrual irregularities may lead to recurrent pregnancy scares. In older women who suddenly develop menstrual irregularity, the exclusion of disorders such as ovarian cysts or intrauterine pathology should precede contraceptive advice or rather should be sought for at once and barrier methods of contraception recommended as a temporary measure meanwhile.

Vulval irritation. Most cases of vulval irritation are due to a vaginal discharge (see below). Local allergic reactions or a reaction to irritating substances such as strong antiseptic detergents or deodorant sprays should be excluded. Generalized skin disorders such as lichen sclerosis or psoriasis may be found. Diabetic vulvitis, an angry red condition seen only in uncontrolled diabetics, should never be missed: super-added monilial infection may well be associated. Local vulval skin disorders, that is vulval dystrophies, may present difficult diagnostic problems but the thickened white skin of leucoplakia vulvae, particularly when associated with severe irritation and cracking of the skin calls for urgent biopsy as the condition is pre-malignant.

Various ulcerative conditions of the vulvae such as granuloma venereum, lympho-granuloma inguinale and Behcet's syndrome will normally lie beyond the competence of the family planning physician but an associated ulcer in the lip or oral cavity will strongly suggest Behcet's syndrome. Condylomata accuminata or multiple viral papillomata can be extremely irritating and individual removal or destruction is usually called for. It must always be remembered that carcinoma of the vulva, rarely encountered below the age of 45, can be associated with itching and irritation if it has developed from leucoplakia.

In none of these conditions, once the diagnosis has been made and treatment commenced, is the choice of contraceptive technique restricted.

Vaginal discharges. The vagina is a warm, moist cavity which is open to infection from the perineum and the anus. It is normally protected from such infection because it is too acid (pH 4–5) for the growth of pathogenic bacteria from the skin or bowel. This acidity is maintained by the fermentation of glycogen from the desquamated epithelial cells by Doderlein's bacillus, a normal vaginal inhabitant. Any condition which allows the introduction of more alkaline fluid by secretion, as in cervicitis, by transudation through the damaged epithelium of a cervical erosion or by irritation from a retained foreign body in the vagina, neutralizes this acidic protection so allowing infective organisms to survive and multiply. Bacterial infection of the vagina by skin pathogens is relatively rare.

Infection of this type causes a blood-stained or sero-sanguinous discharge with varying discomfort to the woman. If such discharge is present, a neglected foreign body should always be sought. After the menopause, the vaginal skin becomes atrophic and the squamous cells contain far less glycogen. Doderlein's bacillus virtually disappears and therefore much of the protective acidity is lost. Postmenopausal women are more liable to simple bacterial vaginal infections.

The most common vaginal infection is that due to the fungus *Candida albicans*. It gives rise to a scanty white and somewhat cheesy discharge with adherent white patches in the vaginal walls that are easily seen on speculum examination. Irritation is a prominent symptom. The organism can be quite difficult to demonstrate but the clinical picture is typical and obvious. Monilial infection is common in pregnancy and also in women suffering from diabetes so a specimen of urine should always be tested to exclude glycosuria. Treatment is first by anti-fungal vaginal pessaries or creams, of which there are many active varieties available. The antibiotic nystatin is generally successful and is not absorbed from either the vagina or the gastrointestinal tract, so gives rise to no systemic complications except that when given by mouth it destroys most of the normal commensal bowel bacteria and may therefore cause temporary bowel disturbances. The first treatment with nystatin is by vaginal pessaries containing 100 000 units of the antibiotic which are used twice daily for a minimum period of 21 days. In recurrent disease, reinfection from the anus is likely so in addition to a repetition of the vaginal therapy, oral nystatin tablets, each containing 500 000 units, are taken four times a day for 10 days. Recently, oral treatment of monilial infections has become feasible with the introduction of the drug ketonidazole normally supplied in 200 mg tablets. One tablet taken twice daily with food for 5 days being the normal course for vaginal infection. The efficiency of this oral treatment is still under review.

The second most common vaginal infection is that due to *Trichomonas vaginalis*, which gives rise to a slightly greenish, frothy discharge with a somewhat offensive smell. Irritation or soreness of the vulva, which may itself be inflamed, is common and so is pain at intercourse. The woman may also complain of frequency of micturition. On inspection the vaginal walls are usually red and inflamed. The diagnosis can be confirmed by mixing a drop of the discharge with warm saline and examining the unstained preparation under a microscope. *Trichomonas* is a pear-shaped organism, slightly larger than a leucocyte, and it has four flagellae, an axostyle and an undulatory membrane. It is highly motile in a fresh specimen, a feature which is diagnostic. Infection can be transmitted by intercourse and the organism often affects a sexual partner. In the male the trichomonal infection is usually asymptomatic, though a mild urethritis may occur. Treatment is by oral metronidazole (Flagyl) 200 mg three or four times a day for between five and seven days. Both partners should take the drug and the course can be repeated at a higher dosage if necessary. Metronidazole has practically no side-effects and only rarely have toxic rashes (and very rarely leucopenia) been reported. If both partners are taking the therapy, sex may be resumed when comfortable. The use of the condom cuts down the risk of infection from a male carrier of *Trichomonas*.

Diseases of the cervix. Cervical erosion is a simple and much overdiagnosed condition. The stratified squamous epithelium of the vagina changes abruptly to a columnar epithelium at, or slightly inside, the external cervical os. The junction is a zone of instability and columnar epithelium, by a process of migration or metaplasia, may be found outside the os, thereby constituting an erosion. Erosions may occur in association with cervicitis but in a simple form are usually asymptomatic and require no treatment. They tend to regress spontaneously and unless complicated by infection do not constitute a contraindication to any form of contraception.

Chronic cervicitis is common and troublesome since it may impair or destroy the normal cervical resistance to infection. Discharge is normally purulent and offensive, but pruritis is uncommon. On speculum examination, the cervix appears inflamed and enlarged Nabothian follicles may be seen. In severe cases, the endocervix will no longer be sterile and the fitting of an intrauterine device should therefore be delayed until after treatment.

If a polyp or polyps are seen at the cervix, their significance will depend upon the menstrual history. With regular menses, a simple polyp can be avulsed as an out-patient procedure without anaesthetic, but it should always be sent for histological examination. If there has been disturbed menstrual pattern or post-coital bleeding, dilatation of the cervix and diagnostic curettage are indicated. By dilating the cervix, one can ensure that the whole of the stalk of the polyp has been avulsed and curettage will exclude a hidden benign or malignant lesion.

Conditions which complicate or contraindicate pregnancy

Heart disease. In developed countries until the end of the Second World War, rheumatic heart disease was an extremely common and potentially serious complication of pregnancy but by 1970 the incidence had fallen to about 3 per 1000 women.[2] In the developing world it remains a leading cause of death among women in the fertile years. Congenital heart disease occurs in about 1 pregnant women per 1000. For women suffering from either form of heart disease the risks of pregnancy when obstetric care is good, though still increased, are less serious than in the past. In women with rheumatic heart disease, infection is potentially serious and therefore the IUD is probably not a suitable form of contraception. It has been argued that the combined pill, by increasing the risk of thrombosis and of salt and fluid retention and possibly of hypertension is contraindicated, but in fact as long as the woman is under regular and competent surveillance it would not seem logical to deprive her of the security of this form of contraception. For those patients with heart disease who are already on anticoagulants, the Pill may still be the method of choice.

Blood dyscrasias. Patients with a tendency to excessive bleeding, such as those with thrombocytopenic perpura are very suitable for combined pill contraception and possibly a Pill containing sufficient progestogen to reduce withdrawal bleeding to a minimum would be helpful. Depo-Provera is the drug of choice for women suffering from homozygous sickle-cell disease.

Hypertension. The possible relation between progestogens in the oral contraceptive and hypertension has already been discussed in Chapter 10. The Pill does not always worsen the condition, although careful monitoring is essential. The intrauterine device may be suitable for patients with hypertension.

Respiratory disorders. Women suffering from tuberculosis who are being treated with rifampicin should be warned that the antibiotic may antagonize the metabolic effects of the Pill.[16]

Diabetes mellitus. It has been suggested that the intrauterine device is unsuitable for diabetic patients because of the slightly increased risk of pelvic infection. Well-controlled diabetics are perfectly able to use the oral contraceptive although the diabetic supervision may be slightly complicated by so doing. An accidental pregnancy is more serious for diabetic women and the extra security of the Pill will generally justify any additional supervision required.

Alimentary disorders. Few alimentary disorders have any relevance to contraceptive choice. Conditions in which there is malabsorption, such as coeliac disease, ulcerative colitis, steatorrhoea or women who have had partial gastrectomy followed by intestinal hurry may well be unsuitable for Pill use because absorption is less certain. In a similar way, women taking the Pill and suffering an attack of gastroenteritis should regard the Pill as temporarily ineffective.

Diseases of the central nervous system. Epileptics taking anticonvulsants such as phenytoin may find the Pill unreliable because phenytoin potentiates its metabolic breakdown.[16] Migraine and oral contraceptive use is a controversial subject. Some women sufferers of migraine have found the condition alleviated by oral contraceptives while other women have developed the disease for the first time shortly after commencing taking the Pill. For a woman who does develop migraine when she first starts to take the Pill, it is clearly contraindicated.

Psychiatric illnesses. Some women have developed depression which has been blamed on the oral contraceptive, but other women who have suffered from severe depression have found considerable relief when on the Pill. Psychological causes for depression are likely to be of far greater importance than the Pill itself. Pyridoxin supplements have been recommended where depression is a feature. Their use remains controversial.

Women suffering from severe mental handicap of manic depressive or schizoid states, which are liable to render them temporarily incapable of looking after themselves, present particular problems of contraceptive management. The intrauterine device, where well tolerated, is probably the method of choice but injections every 90 days of depomedroxyprogesterone acetate (DMPA) or norethisterone enanthate (NET-EN) (see Chapter 10, Injectables) also provide reliable protection.

Diseases of the reproductive system. Dysfunctional uterine bleeding, when more serious reasons have been excluded, may well be treated with a high-progesterone/low-oestrogen combined oral contraceptive which will commonly regulate the cycle and reduce menstrual loss. Patient's with intramural or submucous fibroids also apparently improve with the use of the oral contraceptive and there is no evidence that fibroid growth is accelerated (see Chapter 10, Other tumours). Women suffering with endometriosis will benefit from taking the oral contraceptive cyclically, as will those suffering from primary spasmodic dysmenorrhoea: here the effects are so dramatic that if the symptoms are not improved in either of these two conditions a misdiagnosis should be considered.

Normally, premenstrual tension will be improved by the combined oral contraceptive pill and very frequently indeed it will be improved by a progestogen-only pill.

Breast disease occasionally poses problems for contraceptive counsellors. Chronic mastitis is commonly improved by the combined oral contraceptive pill and severe mastalgia by the progestogen-only pill,[10] but controversy surrounds the problem of management of the young woman who has had full treatment for carcinoma of the breast. Such a woman has not only suffered the psychological trauma inevitable with the knowledge that she has had breast cancer, but probably she has been mutilated to some degree and may well feel herself to be less sexually attractive and secure. If, at the same time, she is told that she must give up the oral contraceptive and use a less secure and aesthetically acceptable form of contraception, the threat to her sexuality is compounded, and the fear, not wholly negligible, as any gynaecologist will confirm, of an unwanted and potentially dangerous pregnancy is increased. For the woman and her family, therefore, prohibition of the Pill is by no means trivial. There is now good epidemiological evidence[14, 18, 25, 26] that the oral contraceptive is not a causative factor in the development of cancer of the breast and that women who were taking the Pill in the year preceding the diagnosis of their breast cancer are at no greater risk than women who have never taken the Pill. From epidemiological studies, as opposed to theoretical consideration of oestrogen receptors it would seem that there is no sound reason to prohibit the use of the Pill in a woman who has been treated for carcinoma of the breast. The security which the Pill can provide against accidental pregnancy is of particular importance.[6]

Family planning and preventive medicine

All who provide medical care from baby food manufacturers through druggists to nurses and doctors, have a responsibility to try and prevent avoidable disease. Nurses, midwives and doctors should always be alert for the earliest signs of incipient disease so that it may be detected before symptoms have developed so that the chance of cure is improved. This responsibility exists whether an individual asks a doctor to counter-sign a passport application, presents with an injury or disease, or is seeking contraceptive advice.

In developed countries, the provision of family planning has become particularly associated with routine preventive medicine procedures. Regular attendances for family planning consultations and supplies provide an ideal opportunity for checking blood pressure so as to detect unsuspected hypertension and the urine so as to exclude diabetes mellitus, for examining the breasts and pelvic organs for unsuspected lumps and for enquiring about a woman's general health and bodily functions, being ready to delve more deeply and examine more closely should the woman mention suggestive symptoms. Directed questions about the client's general health and well-being may suggest a possible unsuspected disease. A history of recent weight loss, a change of bowel habit, a chronic cough, a pain in the legs or chest pain on effort may all suggest the need for further investigation or referral.

Unfortunately, the ideal of combining family planning provision and preventive medicine has not always been happily achieved. Family planning organizations centrally responsible for a large number of clinics tend to enforce rigid routines which are then carried out on every visit quite irrespective of potential need. In an apprehensive individual such set-piece investigations tend to be looked upon as an obstacle course to be surmounted before family planning can be obtained. A nurse or doctor, particularly the individual's general practitioner when providing family planning advice free from the restrictions of a central organization which demands the completion of forms, can use their own knowledge and perception of the person's needs and may often provide reliable contraception at the first meeting with minimal preliminary examination. The contact this gives them can be used later to reassure and to educate towards acceptance of simple preventive medicine procedures, and, even more importantly, in basic health education. In Britain, surveys have been carried out which demonstrate that general practitioners are less likely than family planning clinics to perform various investigatory procedures and this has been widely regarded as a criticism of the general practitioners.[4] It may well be that we should regard it as evidence of their sensitivity and superior contact with the women concerned.

It is a prerequisite of good medical care that the doctor clearly understands his or her role in providing contraceptive care. Having discussed the various methods available and thereby allowed the individual or couple to make an informed choice, the doctor should have a positive idea of when and how frequently they should be seen again. Both the frequency and intensity of such follow-up will depend upon the available resources and priorities. In the West it is feasible to incorporate a large element of preventive medicine into contraceptive care, so frequent attendance with general examination including monitoring of weight, blood pressure, breast examination, cervical smear and urine testing is commonly offered. In the developing world, realistic choices must be made on the use of scarce medical resources and inappropriate screening and preventive medical procedures may deprive others in need, or drastically reduce the numbers to whom contraceptive advice can be offered. Misuse of resources does occur. In one Caribbean island, for example, it is medical policy to perform a full vaginal examination as a routine every six months. Even in developed countries, women on oral contraceptives are often seen unnecessarily frequently and for confused reasons. There are no medical reasons why a young healthy woman should be seen at all frequently once she is settled on a suitable preparation. There are no tests capable of detecting which woman is liable to develop complications, such as thrombosis, before symptoms occur. Weight gain will usually demonstrate itself quickly and be obvious at second attendance; it will certainly bring back an intelligent woman quickly if she is worried, as will abnormalities in patterns of menstruation. The Pill can be responsible for a rise in blood pressure and regular blood pressure recordings are therefore desirable. Nevertheless, after the first year on a Pill, a woman under the age of 35 does not need to be seen more than once a year. Greater flexibility in the timing of follow-up visits is necessary when an IUD is fitted, because some women will persist in its use, unwisely enduring excessively heavy periods and even becoming anaemic, rather than accepting the need to change to a different form of contraception. Early warning of such danger is obligatory and if those supervising the method are unsure that the woman would return on her own accord then routine visits are indicated.

A flexible common-sense approach to follow-up examination can enhance rather than diminish the role of the family planning worker in preventive medicine. One-third of all deaths among women aged 15 to 44 are due to cancer. More ill health will be prevented and lives saved if a clinic tries to persuade women to stop smoking rather than submitting them to expensive and controversial screening tests such as that for serum lipids. Once a doctor has advised a satisfactory method of contraception, any possible side-effects due to a woman's contraceptive method, with justice, may take second place to preventive medicine. The family planning worker may be the only professional who sees a woman with any regularity and questions about possible lumps in the breast, perhaps with a demonstration of self-examination, the taking of cervical smear and regular urine testing can be life-saving. Efforts to detect commonly-occurring diseases early are likely to be far more rewarding then screening for exceedingly rare Pill complications such as liver tumours. Advice on hygiene and on the risks of smoking and of obesity are simple but important preventive medicine measures.

Breast examination

Even in the most highly technologically developed countries the vast majority of breast cancers are detected only because the woman herself notices the lump. If possible, therefore, the breasts should be examined when giving contraceptive advice and the woman taught to palpate her own breasts, especially when she is over the age of 35. In Britain it has been found that the average size of lump which women discover is over 3 cm in diameter and by this time 50% of malignant breast tumours have developed metastases elsewhere in the body.[3]

If women can be taught a good technique of self-examination of the breasts, a larger proportion of these tumours will be first found at a stage offering a greater chance of cure. Nowadays, surgeons are becoming less radical and excision of the tumour with adjunct radiotherapy or chemotherapy is widely advocated for early breast cancer. Where this policy is known to be the local practice, women are more readily persuaded to seek and report early lesions.

Cytological screening for cancer of the cervix

Cancer of the cervix is one of the very few malignant diseases which have been shown to be preventable by early detection and eradication in their pre-malignant stages. We now possess the necessary techniques of mass cervical smear screening, preferably backed up by a colposcopic examination and directed cervical biopsy to make the diagnosis before invasive cancer has occurred. Such early diagnosis allows for local and relatively minor treatment which is almost 100% curative. If, in developed countries, we are prepared to spend sufficient money on the necessary health education, mass screening and sophisticated early treatment, not only could we virtually eliminate death from cervical cancer but few women need be submitted to major surgery or other drastic treatment for this disease.[13]

That mass cervical screening is feasible and acceptable has been conclusively shown by the pioneer British Columbia Trial where a high acceptance of screening reduced the refined death rate for cervical cancer from 11.4 per 1000 women in 1958 to 4.8 in 1974. An equally dramatic fall has occurred in the Grampian and Tayside areas of Scotland where intensive cervical screening has been successfully introduced, and this contrasts with the rest of Scotland where the refined death rate for cervical cancer has risen sharply over the same period.[12]

Some third world countries, for example Brazil, have developed cancer screening services. However, as with other programmes of preventive medicine, experience shows that initial acceptance of mass screening is primarily by the educated and privileged sections of society whereas the maximum incidence of cervical cancer is amongst the poor and underprivileged. To be successful, a cervical smear programme requires a large element of health education and propaganda from its inception. By applying a campaign of health education successfully, a high pick-up of pre-malignant cases can be achieved and the avoidance of late, expensive-to-treat cancer then makes the exercise cost-effective. A half-hearted approach providing screening facilities without widely advertising their value and acceptability can never do so.

Acceptance and usage of contraception have now spread down to the most economically and educationally under-privileged groups and those doctors and nurses who provide contraception are particularly well placed to advocate and perform cervical smear screening which is now, therefore, rightly regarded as an integral part of a family planning service in developed countries. In developing countries with limited medical resources and different health needs it is logical to introduce a contraceptive service first. Regrettably, in some countries, particularly those in Latin America, the provision of contraception was made dependent upon concomitant screening facilities and as resources are limited, neither are provided.

In Britain, the Royal College of General Practitioners has recommended that the first cervical smear should be taken within one or two years of commencing intercourse,[20] repeating it a year later to exclude a false negative and then every 3–5 years. The College specifically points out that cervical cytology screening is independent of the method of contraception used and is not a prerequisite for introducing any method. The American Cancer Society sets similar guidelines but the American College of Obstetricians and Gynecologists still recommends annual smears.[21]

Screening for sexually transmitted diseases
Since the early 1960s, there has been a considerable increase in the incidence of diagnosed sexually transmitted disease. The World Health Organization recently estimated that about 250 million people are infected annually with gonorrhoea and over 50 million with syphilis (Fig. 14.1).

Those seeking contraceptive advice are clearly sexually active and therefore potentially at risk. Doctors and nurses giving family planning advice should always be alert to detecting early venereal disease and should be aware of the difficulties and pitfalls in its diagnosis.

In all forms of sexually transmitted diseases, contact tracing is an essential part of the control. For this reason, many doctors who detect or strongly suspect venereal disease when giving contraceptive advice prefer to refer the woman or couple immediately to a specialized clinic where there will be available not only sophisticated tests but also staff experienced in tracing sexual contacts, thereby restricting the spread of the diseases. Oral contraceptives (Chapter 10), condoms (Chapter 8), spermicides (Chapter

9) and caps (Chapter 9) all appear to exert some protective effect against venereal disease while IUDs (Chapter 11) appear to be associated with a slight increase in the risk of infection.

Gonorrhoea. In men, gonorrhoea usually produces symptoms, namely purulent penile discharge and urethritis with dysuria. Prostatic massage yields a penile discharge of purulent material suitable for culture and for preparation of an air-dried slide on which haematoxylin and eosin staining will demonstrate diplococci. The incubation period is short, usually less than a week but occasionally as long as one month.[15] In women, the incubation period for gonorrhoea is longer and the symptoms, which are often trivial, are easily missed. About one-third of women have no symptoms whatsoever. In a young, sexually active woman presenting with urethritis, gonorrhoea should be excluded by culture. The para-urethral glands may be visibly inflamed and milking them downwards will produce a bead of pus at the urethra in most cases. Unfortunately there is no reliable serological test for gonorrhoea though if the disease is suspected the Gonococcal Complement Fixation Test (GCFT) may provide con-

Fig. 14.1. Incidence of gonorrhoea and syphilis and use of the Pill (England and Wales). Note that the rise in gonorrhoea preceded the introduction of the Pill.

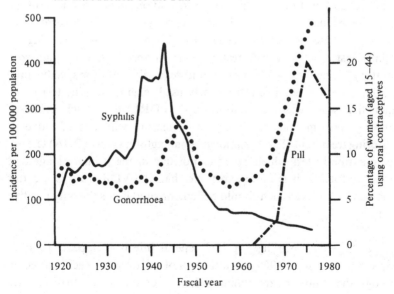

firmatory evidence; falsely negative results are common. Gonococcal salpingitis remains an important cause of infertility.

Syphilis. Although the incidence of syphilis has decreased dramatically and it is now rare in women in western society (the main reservoir of infection being homosexual males[5]) it remains an important disease worldwide.

The micro-organism *Treponema pallidum*, which causes syphilis, divides slowly, taking about 32 h for each division, so the incubation period is long: anything from 9 to 90 days. In both sexes the initial symptom is the development of a painless chancre on the penis, vulva or, very occasionally cervix. Extra-genital sites are of course common in male homosexuals but less likely to be present in clients seeking family planning advice. Untreated, the chancre will take about two months to heal. The generalized rash of secondary syphilis appears at least six weeks after infection but may be delayed for up to a year: it normally lasts for several weeks. Thus about a quarter of patients presenting with secondary syphilis still have a primary chancre. After fading of the rash, syphilis is said to be in the stage of latency, but for up to about two years from infection, muco-cutaneous relapses can occur. A history of such recurrent rashes should be taken seriously.

The diagnosis of primary syphilis entails the identification of *T. pallidum* in serum taken from the chancre or in exudate obtained by gland puncture. In practice the detection of a chancre is rare and serological testing is of far greater importance. Fortunately in the case of syphilis, reliable serological tests exist. These are of two types. Firstly, non-specific screening or standard tests (STS), which test for the presence of a standardized laboratory reagent known as reagin, and secondly, tests for specific anti-treponemal antibodies. The most widely used reagin screening test is the 'Venereal Disease Research Laboratory' (VDRL) test which is cheap, simple to perform and can be titred, a feature which is of value in monitoring treatment. The *T. pallidum* haemagglutination (TPHA) test is a specific antibody test which becomes positive in the primary stage and remains so for life; it is more expensive than the VDRL but is a better screening test,[5] a fact which should be remembered if it is the only positive finding.

Non-specific urethritis. This type of veneral infection appears to have increased rapidly since 1950 and although of mixed and largely unknown aetiology, the symptoms are similar to those of gonorrhoea with discharges and inflammation of mucous membranes, particularly in the urethra. *Chlamydia prachomatis* is one of the causative organisms. Culture facilities for the organism are not generally available except in specialized laboratories. This infection has a possible role in the aetiology of congenital abnormalities and it can also cause low-grade salpingitis and tubal occlusion.

Herpes genitalis. Herpes genitalis causes ulcerated lesions similar to herpetic lesions at other sites such as the lips. Herpes simplex virus was first isolated from a female genital infection in 1946. There are five types of virus which are known to cause genital lesions[24] although they are all broadly known as herpes type 2 as opposed to type 1 which is responsible for oral lesions. The disease became more prevalent during the 1970s and an estimated five million Americans now have genital herpes.[24] The infection is transmitted by genito–genital or oral–genital contact. In genital herpes the virus ascends to the neurons in the sacral ganglia where it can remain latent for long periods. About 80% of individuals will have recurrent infection which in some will persist throughout life and no cure is yet known. The first infection is usually the most severe and is associated with viraemia, general prodromal symptoms, itch, perineal pain, dysuria and in the case of women, dysparunia. Vesicles 1–2 mm in diameter appear on the penis or vulvae but may also occur on the buttocks, thighs or cervix. These vesicles are similar to herpetic lesions at other sites such as the lip. The inguinal glands may be enlarged and tender. The lesions usually heal in about 10 days without scarring but they may persist if secondary infection occurs. While active, the infection is painful to the sufferer but the sexual partner often is totally symptom free.

Genital herpes is thought to be a possible cause, or co-factor, of cervical neoplasia,[23] although it is still possible that genital herpes and cervical cancer are independent co-variables of a particular sexual lifestyle.[27] There is certainly sufficient evidence of a causal relation to demand careful cytological screening of all women who have suffered from this infection. Genital herpes can cause a rare but catastrophic infection of the new-born infant and Caesarean section is recommended if the conditions is demonstrably present when the woman goes into labour.

Counselling

When a couple seek contraceptive advice, they are exposing a very private part of their lives to the family planning provider. Possibly only discussions on death are more highly charged emotionally than discussion of sexual behaviour. Those who provide family planning must understand their own attitudes and responsibilities in order to help their clients. Intimate questions on sexual behaviour should be asked only where there is a specific purpose in mind. The family planning provider must avoid probing questions asked out of curiosity, or worse, the vicarious satisfaction of his or her own sexual interest. A carefully thought-out investigation of sexual behaviour can produce invaluable information but it can also, even in skilled hands, become an obstacle to the willing acceptance of family planning. Questioning every woman who seeks contraceptive advice on such subjects as frequency of coitus is an unwarranted intrusion and invites resistance. On the whole, intimate questions are more acceptable when they are asked by a doctor than by lay assistants or nurses but there can be important exceptions to this generalization.

Whoever is first faced with the individual or couple seeking contraception must try and establish rapport in order to ensure that the necessary technical information gets across, is completely understood and has met the client's needs. The family planning adviser should have a lively awareness of the numerous emotional problems of courtship, marriage and sexual behaviour which may well find expression in a couple's attitude to contraception. The time when birth control is first requested may also be the moment when help is tacitly sought for a wide range of other social and psychological problems.

Help with sexual problems may be at many different levels. A surprisingly large number of young couples in the West still harbour considerable ignorance of the wider implications of sex. Frequently, one or both may be greatly reassured to learn that whatever sexual practices they have discovered and found enjoyable are commonplace and 'normal'. In the developing world some young people, especially girls, may be literally ignorant of the relationship between intercourse and reproduction.

In the young, sexual encounters may well start on a superficial, flirtatious level and the emergence and development of sexual desire can be a sudden and frightening experience which can be helped by a simple frank discussion with an unbiased third party; the therapy is basically provided by the individual herself or himself. Newly formed or abrupt changes in sexual relationships are probably the most common cause for a sudden change in lifestyle. Here the problems may be largely social and the advice needed may be geared to an explanation of the social and legal facilities available. Finally, discussion of sexual problems may unearth more complex and deep-rooted psychological disorders which should be referred for specialist advice: the gynaecological and psychiatric couches should not be confused.

The more disturbed the client or the more difficult his or her social circumstances the greater will be the need for adequate contraceptive advice. It may be advisable to avoid probing questions in order to retain co-operation. Sometimes a medical history, or even the name or age of the sexual partner, cannot be obtained without risking loss of confidence, and it may often be necessary to sacrifice physical examination of a woman so that she feels at ease. Such a woman, as she gains confidence in her adviser, can be seen more often than usual and a developing rapport will allow long-term help to be given.

It must always be remembered that barriers to communication between social groups are greatest in the realm of sexual behaviour. Discussion and advice must be carried out in appropriate language; on the one hand, sexual intercourse may need to be described in terms of Anglo-Saxon philology and common medical terms such as 'menopause' are meaningless to some, whilst condescending chats about 'the front passage' can be equally out of place for a sophisticated woman. In the developing world these differences can be even more significant. Less than 50% of a sample of rural Mexican women identified the womb as the place 'where the baby grows' and 20% perceived the stomach and uterus to be identical. Many women believed that multiple coitus was necessary for conception. The term for intercourse 'el me user' (he uses me) illustrates a sexual or cultural attitude which is common in many societies. Contraceptives often acquire their own mythology and Mexican women frequently believe that Pills 'weaken the blood' and vasectomy was said to 'dejar de ser hombre' (stop him being a man).

In sex, as in any other activity, experience improves performance and any young couple who have a good emotional relationship will rapidly teach each other. This point can usefully be made to them and they can be reassured that so long as each always strives to please and support the other, progress is almost certain. We all encounter sexual problems from time to time but serious disturbances requiring skilled assistance are uncommon. Physical problems, however, may be a common accompaniment of early intercourse. In the woman, immediate pain or soreness on passing urine indicates little more than bruising, but if the pain on micturition occurs after a day or so's delay, this is suggestive of urinary tract infection. Daily genital hygiene for both partners is important and the old tip of passing water after intercourse can flush away stray *Escherichia coli*. Lubrication with K-Y Jelly or a similar product can relieve the trauma of early intercourse.

The problem with cystitis is that 10% of women do not respond to simple treatment. The condition tends to recur and to remain a tiresome problem over many years. Such sufferers demand specialist investigation but can be helped temporarily by the advice that rendering the urine alkaline, for example by taking a teaspoonful of bicarbonate of soda at suppertime, may ensure freedom from burning. Some of the persistent sufferers may have a poor sexual relationship and include cases of what has been called marital rape or vaginal battering.

The overall importance of good sexual adjustment can hardly be exaggerated and for those who believe that secure and acceptable contraception is fundamental to such adjustment it follows that contraceptive counselling is an important branch of preventive medicine. In this context it should be remembered that after malignancies, the most common causes of death in fertile women are accidents (including accidental poisoning) and violence (including murder). In Britain, and most certainly in the US, a woman is far more likely to be murdered than she is to die in childbirth or from abortion.[7] These sudden deaths, particularly violent deaths, are frequently associated with marital or sexual stresses and quite commonly the basic stress is related to excess fertility. If it is taken to include help with sexual problems, successful family planning may make an even greater contribution than is generally realized to the wider health of society.

Contraceptive advice for the unmarried

The provision of contraceptive advice to the married now has almost universal support but giving such help to the young and single remains controversial. Those who oppose such a service tend to forget that for the educated and knowledgeable condoms have always been available, that any public library and some churches provide literature on the ovulation method and therefore to prescribe the Pill for, say, a young unmarried student is not to do anything radically new but merely to make available a more effective method.

The average age at menarche[8] has declined in developed nations and young people are beginning sexual exploration at a correspondingly younger age. In a sample of nearly 2000 young people, Schofield found in 1965 that 30% of boys and 16% of girls aged between 17 and 19 years had experienced sexual intercourse.[22] Half of all US women are sexually active by the age of 19 years.[27] One in 10 US teenage girls become pregnant each year and 6% of these have the baby. In all, over four million teenagers are sexually active; only one million of them are married. Two-thirds of all conceptions to teenagers are unintended. In one US study one-third of very young pregnant girls aged between 13 and 15 came from families defined as living below the federal poverty line. Adolescent marriages, which so frequently result from this situation, are two to three times as likely to end in divorce and US statistics show that three out of five teenage brides are divorced within six years.[19] There are no outstanding features in the social environment: unmarried adolescents get pregnant in every type of home and background and the young woman who is unintentionally pregnant is anybody's and everybody's daughter.

The maternal death rate is up to 60% higher for young teenagers (under 15) than for women in their early twenties; low birth weight babies are twice as common and infant mortality for mothers aged 16 is 70% higher than for women aged 20–24.[19] In the US pregnancy has become the most common cause of teenage school drop-out and teenage mothers are at greatest risk of unemployment and welfare dependency. Women who begin their child-bearing below the age of 18 usually have a larger completed family size than those who successfully postpone pregnancy.[1] There is no evidence that making contraceptive advice available to the unmarried leads to prom-iscuity, but increased use (Fig. 14.2) will prevent unwanted pregnancies.

When contraceptive advice is sought by the unmarried, the experience of those providing services is that the majority have been having sexual relations for three months to one year. Many have a stable relationship and will eventually marry. National statistics support this. In New Zealand for example, where in the 1970s contraceptive policies towards the young unmarried were restrictive, there were 63 births per 1000 females aged 15–19 while in Britain, where policies had become liberal, only 44 births per 1000 occurred in the same age-group.

Since the unmarried are likely to be unready to support a child, it is important to use the most effective and acceptable method available and

Fig. 14.2. The effect of provision of contraceptive services on teenage (15–19) contraceptive practice (US 1975).

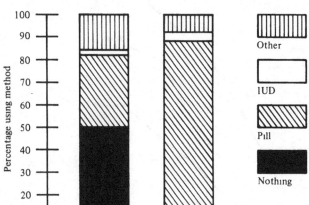

the Pill will usually be the first choice. Paradoxically, the closeness of the British general practitioner's bonds with the family may conflict with the young person's desire for privacy and confidentiality. This explains why some young people in Britain attend family planning clinics. In the US about one-quarter of those teenagers at risk of pregnancy attend private doctors, one-quarter attend clinics and half get no contraceptive advice at all.

There are marked cultural differences in patterns of teenage marriages and premarital sex. In the West premarital intercourse has become more common in the past generation (Fig. 14.3). Geographically there are great variations. In Japan in the 1970s there were 5 births per 1000 women aged 18–19 and in the US there were 58. Throughout the western hemisphere, about 60 million babies are born each year and 13 million have mothers who are still adolescents.[28]

Greater understanding and patience are needed when advising the unmarried, who will have more than their share of psychological and emotional problems. However, it is misleading to imagine as some have done, that every unmarried person who seeks contraceptive advice is in

Fig. 14.3. Cultural factors in premarital sex (black and white American women). (From Udry, J. R., Bauman, K. E. & Morris, N. M. (1975). Changes in premarital coital experience of recent decade-of-birth cohorts of urban American women. *Journal of Marriage and the Family*, **6**, 783.)

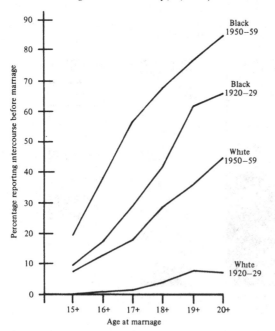

need of prolonged counselling (see this chapter, Family planning and preventive medicine). Young women in the West seem particularly frightened of contraceptive side-effects and the number discontinuing after 12 months of use of the Pill for 'fear of side-effects' rose from 16.7% in 1974 to 42.4% in 1978.[9]

Subfertility/infertility

Where a couple have been unsuccessfully attempting a pregnancy, a large variety of factors may be at work. One or the other of the pair may be truly sterile, namely suffering from some permanent and irreversible disorder which renders it impossible for them to have a child. The term sterility should only be used when the cause has been accurately diagnosed and its full implications appreciated. Subfertility is more common, and is often inaccurately referred to as infertility. It is said to exist when a couple have been having coitus regularly and reasonably frequently for one year without contraception and no pregnancy has occurred.

The precise extent of biological infecundity in any population is difficult to assess. Demographic data make no distinction between voluntary and involuntary childlessness and couples ignorant of their infertility may be counted as contraceptive users in sociological enquiries. The 1941 Indianapolis Study estimated that 9.8% of American couples interviewed were involuntarily childless and the Royal Commission on Population has suggested that 7% of English marriages are biologically infertile. Other investigators, in both countries, have arrived at broadly comparable estimates.

Infertility is widely regarded as a gynaecological problem and certainly it is usually the woman who first seeks medical advice but it is important to interview both partners. In practice, about 30–35% of all cases of infertility are due to oligo- or azoospermia, about 30–35% of cases are due to obstruction of the Fallopian tubes, 15% to disorders of ovulation (this may well be higher in westernized societies) and the remainder to mixed gynaecological or behavioural causes.

Female infertility may be either primary, where the woman has never conceived at all, or secondary, where she may have had previous full-term deliveries or abortions. If she has never conceived at all, her entire reproductive system is suspect and the investigation must include a full menstrual history and general history of all factors suggestive of endocrine disorder as well as possible causes of tubal blockage such as previous peritonitis, pelvic inflammatory disease and venereal disease, and symptoms suggestive of developing endometriosis. It is also important to enquire about the frequency of sex, and even today it is very important to make certain that the couple are in fact having true 'physiological' intercourse. In discussing these intimate questions, it is usually better that each partner be interviewed in confidence separately. Amusingly there is a definite sex bias in the reporting of frequency of intercourse, the man usually claims a higher rate than the woman. A brief physical examination falls within the ambit of any serious family planning doctor; it is particularly important in the case of the woman. Scarring may confirm details of previous operations and the nature of the scar may suggest whether or not sepsis intervened in the healing process. Hirsutism may be suggestive of endocrinal disorders as will other abnormal features of secondary sexual development. Pelvic examination may reveal anatomical problems or detect the presence of pelvic tumours, cervical abnormalities or uterine malformations. In the male, testicular atrophy may be suspected and a history of orchitis, for example, secondary to mumps infection, would be strongly suggestive. Examination of semen is a simple procedure and if a specimen can be obtained by masturbation, a drop freshly diluted with warm saline can be microscopically examined. The presence of large numbers of active motile sperm argues strongly against male infertility. A full seminal count is a more complex procedure requiring considerable expertise.

The investigation of infertility is basically a gynaecological procedure which is outside the scope of the ordinary family planning doctor. 'Anatomical' tests include a post-coital test designed to ascertain the degree of sperm invasion of the cervix by microscopical examination of cervical mucus obtained 3–8 h after intercourse. The most important group of tests are those designed to assess tubal patency. The simplest such test is the introduction of air, or preferably carbon dioxide, into the uterus followed by listening with a stethoscope on the lower abdomen for its bubbling through the tubes; a slightly more sophisticated technique uses a kymograph to measure the pressure of the gas within the uterus and thereby demonstrate its flow more accurately. The introduction of X-ray opaque dye into the uterus for a similar reason yields much greater information, particularly if the passage of the dye into and through the uterus is continuously observed by screening with an image intensifier. This test of hysterosalpingography carries a small risk of chemical or allergic reaction resulting in sterile inflammation and possible blockage of the tubes. The most modern technique is that of laparoscopy. This involves operation under general anaesthesia including examination under anaesthetic, dilatation of the cervix and curettage of the uterus combined with the introduction of carbon dioxide or nitrous oxide into the peritoneal cavity by a needle through the abdominal wall thereby creating a space into which a laparoscope or lighted telescope can be introduced to view the pelvic contents. An assistant passes watery dye up through the uterus and the laparoscopist can observe it flowing into and through the Fallopian tubes and spilling into the uterine cavity. Spasm or actual blockage of either tube can be readily seen. The ovaries are visualized and if desirable an ovarian biopsy can be taken. The technique allows the detection or exclusion of past or present pelvic inflammatory disease and endometriosis. By the use of laparoscopy, not only can the patency of the tubes be tested but also their motility and the presence or absence of adhesions around them. Hysterosalpingography remains a test of importance where an internal uterine malformation is suspected or where tubal obstruction within the uterine wall is probable.

The treatment of infertility and subfertility was greatly improved during the 1970s. Tubal blockage is exceedingly hard to correct and even when corrected the danger of ectopic pregnancy within tubes is high even though surgery in this field has been greatly improved and microsurgical techniques have established a place for themselves. The treatment of infertility due to endometriosis, nowadays a potent cause, has been rendered feasible in a small proportion of cases by newly developed drug therapy and we now also have drugs to stimulate ovaries which are failing to ovulate. Extracorporal fertilization of ova taken from the woman via the laparoscope and put directly into her uterine cavity seems to offer a simpler and soon, perhaps, a more efficient way of managing tubal blockage or endometriosis.

Psychological factors are often quoted as being important in infertility and certainly where they result in a low incidence of coitus, this may well be true. In a critical analysis of 75 papers on psychological factors affecting fertility, Noyes & Chapnic showed that over 50 different factors had been postulated and it seems that the discipline of psychiatry is not yet well established in this field and has little to contribute directly to its management.[17] On the other hand, involuntary childlessness is associated with considerable emotional trauma and stress which in turn may precipitate or disclose neurosis, sometimes with hysterical symptoms.

Large numbers of cases of infertility will, after extensive investigation, remain unexplained. Often, when conception fails to occur after one or two years has elapsed and no major or minor abnormality can be detected in either partner, the infertility is regarded as unexplained and this will be the situation in nearly half of all cases investigated. Within this group it has been shown that about 35% of couples will in fact conceive without further treatment over the next seven-year period.[11]

In some developing countries infertility is automatically 'blamed' on the woman and those who work in family planning will be playing a valuable role if they educate individuals in the fact that either partner can be 'at fault'. In some countries, in Korea for example, where there is a strong social preference for boys, even if the woman is fertile she may find herself divorced because she has a series of daughters. In defence of the woman the man should be educated that while all other genetic characteristics are provided equally by sexual partners, his sperm alone determine the sex of their children.

15

Legal and administrative aspects of family planning

In some countries the law in respect of family planning represents the prevailing social attitudes of earlier generations; in others it embodies the ideologies and aspirations of a ruling group and in yet others it is beginning to cope with the realities of existing social and economic conditions. In the majority of western countries, the law still manifestly derives from the doctrine of the mediaeval church that procreation is the primary purpose of marriage, and until well after the Second World War, the law in most European and North American countries was designed to frustrate any voluntary regulation of fertility. Most Communist states have been fundamentally pronatalist, the advocacy of family limitation on economic grounds being contrary to Marxist doctrine, although since the time of Lenin they have defended the right of women to control their own fertility. However, in China and Cuba there was a remarkable somersault during the 1970s in both politics and legal processes with regard to family planning and population. A few countries, such as Yugoslavia, Denmark, Singapore and India have used statute laws as a catalyst for social adjustment to individual needs and, where appropriate, as an expression of social policy towards limiting family size. In the US, the law has acted in a paradoxical way, alternately pushing family planning forward and burdening it with unnecessary costs. The courts have been used as arbitrators of social debate; while the British might discuss abortion or the problems surrounding contraception for teenagers in the columns of the *Times* newspaper, an American may take the same issue to the Supreme Court.

The practice of a physician, midwife, nurse and pharmacist, is legally controlled in nearly all countries. Most professional groups also have a system of internal discipline, which may well impinge upon the individual's actions with respect to the field of fertility control. The General Medical

Council in Britain can prevent a doctor working if, 'in pursuit of his profession [he] has done something with regard to it which will be reasonably regarded as disgraceful, or dishonourable by his professional brethren of good repute and competence'. Such disciplinary procedures can, for example, influence whether or not contraceptives are available to teenagers.

A patient can usually seek damages from a physician or other health personnel, or from a pharmaceutical manufacturer, if a Court of Law finds evidence of incompetence. There is no doubt that such redress is an essential and necessary part of any free society, but, over the last 20 years malpractice suits in the area of health care within the United States have become a major industry. The law in the United States is unusual in allowing attorneys both to advertise for clients and to offer deals on the basis of 'no damages, no payment'. If damages are obtained then the attorney may take a fixed, previously agreed portion which may amount to one-third or more. In Europe lawyers are not allowed to advertise and such forms of fee payment are equally debarred so that potential plaintiffs must seek a lawyer and face a possible financial loss if the court's decision goes against them. These abnormalities of the US legal scene have resulted in an enormous financial and psychological strain on those who provide health care, which, by its nature, is a vulnerable sector. For example, an American gynaecologist will pay up to US $32 000 in malpractice insurance each year while his British colleagues all pay the standard rate of £134 ($230). In many developing countries, malpractice suits are virtually unknown.

Within the United States there are three important ways in which the fear of malpractice suits influences the medical profession. Firstly, there is fear of a misdiagnosis, which in the nature of things inevitably occurs to all doctors from time to time, resulting in a malpractice suit, and in defending such a suit it may be highly desirable to record a large number of investigatory tests even if their relevance to clinical management is dubious. There is no question that the very high costs of medical care in the United States derives to a considerable extent from the routine usage of large numbers of routine tests and the frequent recourse to 'second opinions' based on medico-legal needs. Secondly, the high cost of malpractice insurance is a reflection of the cost of malpractice suits which have been successful, or settled out of court, and which can only be recovered from practitioners who eventually pass on charges to their patients. This factor applies not only to doctors but to manufacturers whose products, sold within the United States, must carry a price tag reflecting the cost of defending malpractice suits. Thirdly, as 90% of lawsuits for damages brought against drug manufacturers involve contraceptives, manufacturers are cutting down investment into contraceptive development and many promising leads, such as new developments in prostaglandins, are not being followed up as a matter of policy.

The prevalence of attorneys in the United States (1 in 411 of the population) is approximately five times that in Germany, 10 times that in France and 20 times that in Japan (1 in 9817 of the population).

Family law

Statute law defines the age of marriage. It is usually lower for women than for men. In parts of Asia, and in much of Africa, the law and social practice encourage early parenthood. The mean age of marriage for women in parts of India is 16 to 17 years. In other countries, such as Sri Lanka and Korea, the mean age of marriage has risen, becoming a major factor in the recent decline of the birth-rate. In China, changes in the marriage laws have been used to accelerate this process.[3]

The minimum legal age when a person can give valid consent to sexual intercourse in Britain is 16. Under the Sexual Offences Act (1965) it is an absolute offence to have intercourse with a girl under 13[52] irrespective of whether she consents or not. The age of 16 for giving valid consent was fixed in 1885 to protect girls from recruitment to the Victorian brothels and prior to that date had been 12. In the US there is some variation between States. In Britain the role of a doctor offering contraceptive advice to young people under the age of consent has been debated but never tested in the courts. On the one hand, such an act could be seen as aiding and abetting a crime, while on the other it could be justified as protecting the health of the individual from foreseeable adverse consequences. In 1974 the Department of Health and Social Security stated:

> . . . it is for the doctor, to decide whether to provide contraceptive advice and treatment and the Family Planning Association is advised that in doing so for a girl under the age of 16 he would not be aiding or abetting the offence of unlawful intercourse if he acted in good faith in protecting the girl against the potentially harmful effects of intercourse. He would be prudent to seek the parent's consent or tell the parents, but failure to do so would not put the doctor in jeopardy.

This statement does not have the force of the Court's decision but summarizes current British opinion. It should be noted that the law on consent is not the only statute to protect young people. The Children's and Young Persons' Acts 1963 and 1969 can be invoked when individuals under 18 are thought to be in 'moral danger'.

In other societies, such as those of pre-industrial Europe and contemporary Ireland, marriages take place at a late age as a result of social and economic pressures which are not necessarily supplemented by statute law. Conversely, in the Caribbean and parts of Africa, sexual intercourse often begins at adolescence but legal marriages are often not contracted until the parents may have had several children.

Divorce laws vary widely. For example in the 1970s the European Human Rights Commission found the Republic of Ireland as acting counter to human rights by not having any law at all on divorce. The provisions which the law makes for the protection of children also influence fertility. In the Philippines and Caribbean, for example, laws regarding child maintenance are weak and rarely enforced against the man who abandons children fathered either within or outside marriage. In other countries there are strong social pressures for blood relatives to accept responsibility for an orphaned or abandoned child, although there may be no law on adoption. In the West, adoption is an easily defined process. In the United States and UK an adopted child, on reaching the age of majority, has the legal right to discover his or her own parents. Thus adoption no longer has the anonymity of abortion or birth control, as at any time in the future a woman's child may seek her out.

Certain other aspects of reproduction are occasionally subject to legal intervention. Japan, uniquely, enforces employers to grant 'menstruation leave' in defence of a woman's 'mission of childbearing'. One or two countries, such as Papua New Guinea, have passed legislation putting feeding bottles and artificial milk formulae on medical prescription. The World Health Organization has adopted a code of practice regulating the advertising of breast milk substitutes[64] and important libel actions have surrounded the scientific debate of the consequences of promoting breast milk substitutes in the Third World.

The major issues in relation to family planning, however, revolve around the availability of contraceptives, access to the choice of voluntary sterilization and the control of abortion.

Contraceptives and the law

Contraceptive manufacture, distribution, prescription and promotion are all, from time to time, controlled by statute law, or regulations that derive from statute law.[11, 15, 38, 47, 55] Many paradoxes and archaic situations exist. Canada, for example, forbids the importation of contraceptives by post, but the Vatican City State does not! Moreover, while a state may limit access to condoms or the Pill, it cannot control the use of coitus interruptus or periodic abstinence. Groups and individuals who resist the availability of modern methods of contraception, or who wish to reverse recent liberal trends, often at the same time promote the availability of the ovulation method.

The manufacture of contraceptives is rarely prohibited. Even Ireland, Portugal and Argentina permit local production. An increasing number of countries have some type of drug regulatory authority. Unfortunately, decisions in this latter area are becoming increasingly politicized, whether in relation to Depo-Provera in the United States or the use of Section 12 of the Pharmacy Law in Japan to forbid the manufacture of steroidal contraceptives, a decision which is partly influenced by doctors who perform abortions and sometimes avoid taxes on some of the income they make. Drugs such as hormones, which are subject to the Federal Food, Drug and Cosmetic Act (Section 505), may not be exported unless approved for US use, while those such as antibiotics may be, even if adulterated or misbranded.

Patents on pharmaceutical drugs run for 17 years and may not last long enough in the modern world to enable a manufacturer to make the investment and conduct long years of testing before marketing a compound. Surgical instruments and intrauterine devices can also be patented. In an ideal world, contraceptives, like penicillin, would be best not patented, although it would be necessary to protect certain steps commercially, as with steroidal contraceptives which demand sophisticated technology and large capital investment. In the US, where the Patents Office has probably been unreasonably generous and commercial avarice unusually large, IUDs, which cost a few cents to manufacture, can cost many dollars to purchase. A provisional patent has even been granted on the use of coitus saxonicus (Chapter 5). The possibility of a patent on normal coitus, to our knowledge, has not been explored, although it would be a novel way of controlling fertility!

Price is an important factor affecting access to contraceptives, whether sold to the individual, or in bulk to a government or international agency. Some countries with overt family planning programmes, such as Thailand and India, still tax the importation of contraceptives and/or raw materials used to produce them. It should be noted that Pill and condom manufacture is a capital-intensive undertaking employing only a handful of people, several of whom require highly specialist knowledge and may be expatriates. Thus contraceptives manufactured in the Third World nearly always cost more and are often of a lower quality than those purchased in bulk from the few manufacturers already in the market place. However, the packaging of contraceptives, at least in the case of the condom, can account for up to half the cost; it is a labour-intensive undertaking and probably an appropriate first step for the transfer of the technology from developed to developing countries which must ultimately take place.

When it comes to the distribution, prescription and display of contraceptives, the trend of the last 20 years has been towards freedom of use, although as recently as 1975 Saudi Arabia banned the use of contraceptives.[41] Even when there are no absolute legal barriers to contraceptives, attention to detail is essential. Relatively minor restrictions can have a major effect on the consumer: the man who buys a tube of toothpaste because he is too shy to ask the girl in the pharmacy for a condom is a reality, as is his partner who has an unwanted pregnancy. In Britain there are no restrictions on the use or display of contraceptives providing they do not contravene the Obscene Publications Act of 1857. Contraceptive sale through vending machines is prohibited by some local authorities. Section 4(5) of the 1954 Television Act precludes the advertisement of matrimonial agencies, fortune-tellers and contraceptives.[53] In 1975 when the London Rubber Company sponsored a Formula 5000 car on the racing circuit, the BBC insisted that the name Durex (the brand name of the most popular condom in Britain) should be covered up as the offending vehicle flashed past the television cameras at over 100 m.p.h. As is often the case, this silliness brought more coverage than would otherwise have occurred and the manufacturers followed up with street hoardings of a family car, also bearing the name Durex, and the byline, *The small family car.* India takes a more straightforward attitude to advertising with slogans on public transport vehicles: *Large families miss the bus: have a first and last.*

Such limitations on promotion can have serious effects on the most vulnerable members of society. Many American states had restrictions on contraceptive promotion and distribution until the US Supreme Court's decision on *Carey* v. *Population Services* which upheld a New York decision striking down restrictions on the display of contraceptives in outlets other than pharmacies. The defence argued that contraceptives encouraged teenage sex, but the Court ruled, 'there is no evidence that teenage extramarital activity increases in proportion to the availability of contraception'. While vaginal tampons and haemorrhoid creams are widely advertised on television, brand-specific contraceptive advertisements have been prohibited either under state regulation or because of presumed hostility from programme sponsors. Interestingly, in Mexico, PROFAM uses television advertising for specific products in a way that has not yet occurred elsewhere in the Americas from Alaska to Argentina. Generic contraceptive advertising has been tested in the US, with messages such as 'Stop the stork' and those telling people to telephone a family planning clinic, but has given equivocal results.[51]

Most US state and federal legislation restricting contraceptive display and distribution can be traced back to the notorious Comstock Act of 1873 which declared contraceptives obscene and prohibited their transmission through the mails or by public carriers. It was this Act that Margaret Sanger fought against (see Chapter 1) and which she only circumvented by making physicians the key to contraceptive distribution. In 1936 the Act was partially breached. In a case known as *The United States* v. *One Package*, Justice Augustus Hand allowed 'the importation, sale or carriage by mail of things which might intelligently be employed by conscientious and competent physicians for the purpose of saving life or promoting the well being of their patients'. The Comstock Act was finally overthrown[48] in the cases of *Griswald* v. *Connecticut* (1965) and *Eisenstadt* v. *Baird* (1972).[57] Baird was arrested for distributing the spermicide Emko at a public meeting in Massachusetts. The Court ruled: 'It would be plainly unreasonable to assume that [the State] has prescribed pregnancy and birth of an unwanted child [or the physical and psychological dangers of abortion] as Punishment for fornication.' The prime legal argument against the Comstock legislation was that of the right to privacy in marriage.

Prohibitions on the distribution of contraceptives still exist in the Republic of Ireland. Under the Criminal Law Amendment Act (1935) it is unlawful 'for any person to sell or exchange, offer to advertise, or keep for sale or import into Faorstat Eireann for sale any contraceptives'. Of course, the semantic escape from such limitations is to call oral contraceptives 'cycle regulators' and tens of thousands of women use the Pill this way. The Irish Censorship Act (1929, 1946) also limits contraceptive information, although in 1973 the Irish Supreme Court upheld the individual's right to use contraceptives in the case of *Mary McGee*. It is illegal to sell a condom in Ireland but a man can belong to a charity where the subscription, purely coincidentally, is the price of a packet of condoms and which then gifts this same commodity to him! Other paradoxes exist elsewhere. For example, in Indonesia, anachronistic colonial laws still forbid the distribution of contraceptives, although the Government supports a multimillion dollar family planning programme. Even Sweden, with its tradition of sexual liberality, maintains that 'a condom vending machine must not be indicated in such a way that special attention is drawn to the fact'. This is hardly a regulation devised to please a salesman. In China, where a one-child family is encouraged, official policy is to deny contraceptives to the unmarried.

In Italy the previously restrictive section 553 of the Penal Code, which dated from Fascist times, was struck down by the Supreme Court in the 1971 *de Marchi* case. 'The problem of family planning', said the Court 'has, at the present period of history, become so important socially [that] it can no longer be considered an offence against public morals.'

The voluntary family planning movement has always tried to persuade governments to provide family planning services and lobbying by private organizations has preceded government involvement in all countries including those of eastern Europe, with the exception of China and Cuba. In Britain the Ministry of Health Memorandum 153 MCW, of 1931, permitted government clinics to give advice 'to married women for whom a further pregnancy would be detrimental to health'. The 1967 Family Planning Act removed contrived health reasons and dropped any distinction between the married and the unmarried. Contraception, voluntary sterilization and abortion are available free under the British National Health Service (NHS) and physicians and surgeons get extra item-of-service payments for certain aspects of family planning. However, fees for service to commercial and charitable institutions also survive, serving those such as working women who want and can afford a more personal, convenient service, and approximately half of all the legally-induced abortions in the country are paid for outside the NHS.

In the United States, domestic family planning services began with President Johnson's message to Congress in 1966 in which he declared: 'It is essential that all families have some access to information and services that will allow freedom to choose the number and spacing of their children within the dictates of individual conscience.' In that year, US $24 million were earmarked for family planning services.

Voluntary sterilization laws

Sterilization involves more weighty decisions than contraception and raises more complex legal issues.[36, 43, 46]

In Britain and America, although the subject was often one of uncertainty and speculation, laws forbidding sterilization never existed. For a long time in Britain, sufficient ambiguity existed in relation to vasectomy to make surgeons very wary about offering the operation because of uncertainties as to whether an aggrieved man or his wife might subsequently move a medico-legal case. Medical defence societies in England and Scotland sought counsel's opinion in 1960 and it was concluded that voluntary sterilization was not unlawful if performed on therapeutic or eugenic grounds or for any other reason, providing that full and valid consent to the operation was given. *The British Medical Journal* commented, 'whatever may be the law on sterilization, it is clearly most desirable that the Courts or Parliament should now declare it'. Unfortunately, this advice has never been taken but within the NHS special payments are made to surgeons, anaesthetists and pathologists who take part in sterilizing operations on men or women. In October 1972 a Family Planning Amendment Act was passed allowing local authorities in England

and Wales to provide voluntary vasectomy on the same basis as other contraceptive services.

In Australia there is a similar lack of legislation prohibiting sterilization, but the Attorney General of Queensland has ruled to prevent voluntary sterilization in state-funded hospitals.[6]

The law in the United States relates to sterilization in two ways. Prior to the Second World War, a number of eugenic sterilization laws were passed at State level forcing mentally defectives to be sterilized and using the operation in a punitive way. Since the Second World War, the law has been used in the opposite way to define the individual's right to free choice. Some states impose procedural requirements, such as a waiting period, and may require the operation to be done in a hospital. For example, the State of Virginia requires that 'no vasectomy shall be performed pursuant to the provision of this section prior to 30 days from the date of consent'.[56] Compulsory sterilization, whether on grounds of mental defect, criminality or some other cause, is now considered by most experts as unconstitutional in the United States.[19]

Many countries have forbidden voluntary sterilization and such laws still exist in much of Eastern Europe. Until the mid 1970s in Sweden vasectomy was illegal. Chile passed a restrictive sterilization law in 1977. As is often the case in fertility regulation, there is a wide gap between medical practice and statute law.[9] Under Article 262 of the Revised Penal Code of the Philippines, it is illegal to 'intentionally mutilate another by depriving him, either partially or totally, of some essential organ of reproduction' yet many tens of thousands of voluntary sterilizations are performed annually and the Secretary of Justice has commented that tubal ligation and vasectomy are acceptable because they 'do not involve lopping or chipping off of the organs of reproduction'. Conversely, in Brazil, the medical profession has chosen to interpret sterilization legislation in such a way that a woman seeking tubal ligation often has to submit to two or three Caesarean sections (see Chapter 12, Introduction).

Abortion laws

By the early 1980s over 70% of the world's population lived in countries with broadly liberal abortion laws while the remainder lived in countries where abortion was either totally prohibited or available only to save the life of the mother.[26,39] These latter countries include most Moslem countries,[28] the majority of the countries of Africa and Latin America and five European countries: Belgium, Ireland, Malta, Portugal and Spain.

The spirit in which the law is interpreted is often of greater importance than the law itself. For example, the Netherlands has a restrictive statute law but an extremely liberal practice with many free-standing abortion clinics openly performing large numbers of abortions on a day-stay basis for residents and visitors from less permissive neighbours, while Zambia has a liberal law, but it benefits few beyond the urban elite, who would obtain safe abortions even if they were illegal.

Russia was the first country to legalize abortion on request. On 18 November 1920, legislation was passed permitting abortion 'to be performed freely and without charge in Soviet hospitals, where conditions are assured for minimising the harm of the operation'. In 1935, as Stalin's rule tightened, abortion was forbidden. 'Our Soviet women, full-blooded citizens of the freest country of the world', wrote *Pravda*, 'have been given the bliss of motherhood. We must safeguard our family . . .'[42] The original free access to abortion was restored in 1955. Subsequently, the satellite countries of eastern Europe, with the exception of Albania, all liberalized their laws by 1960.[13, 14, 37] In recent years, certain of those countries have enacted somewhat more restrictive laws in reaction to low birth-rates.

Under British common law, abortion before quickening was not a crime prior to 1803 and abortion was legal and available throughout all the states of America at the beginning of the nineteenth century.[20, 25, 63] In England the 1861 Offences against the Person Act (Section 58) made abortion, and the intent to perform an abortion, illegal. However, the Bill was not discussed in Parliament, did not generate public debate and seems to have been more an alteration in legal drafting than any expression of mid-Victorian morality. In the US, many states adopted restrictive abortion laws in the second half of the nineteenth century. Politically, the movement was as much a manifestation of the emerging American Medical Association's desire to exclude homeopaths and chiropractors from surgical practice as it was an attempt to enforce morality, although a vocal minority led by Horatio Storer did see it that way. Storer, amongst other things, opposed the entry of women into medical practice.

Several Scandinavian countries liberalized their abortion laws before the Second World War: Iceland (1935)[18], Sweden (1938)[30] and Denmark (1939). Abortion reform in Britain was first argued between the two world wars on the grounds of the public health effects of illegal abortion. In 1938, a London gynaecologist, Alex Bourne, was acquitted of terminating a pregnancy in a 14-year-old girl who had been raped, and a precedent was set permitting therapeutic abortion.[8]

After a number of attempts, the British House of Commons amended the 1861 Offences against the Person Act in 1967.[45] An Act, which Mr David

Steel steered through Parliament, permits termination of pregnancy provided that two registered practitioners agree 'in good faith'

(a) that the continuance of the pregnancy would involve risk to the life of the pregnant woman or of injury to the physical or mental health of the pregnant woman or any existing children of her family greater than if the pregnancy were terminated; or

(b) that there is a substantial risk that if the child were born it would suffer from such physical or mental abnormalities as to be seriously handicapped.

The Act allows doctors to take into account the woman's 'actual or reasonably foreseeable environment', but insists that abortions must be performed in hospitals or registered nursing homes and that all cases must be registered. It does not apply to Northern Ireland. Several unsuccessful attempts have been made in the British Parliament to restrict the 1967 Law.

The United States had uniformly restrictive abortion laws from about 1860 and in most states abortion was permissible only to save the mother's life.[21] Even fewer hospital abortions were performed than in Britain prior to the 1967 Act. In 1962 the American Law Institute proposed that abortion should be permitted where 'pregnancy would gravely impair the physical or mental health of the mother or that the child would be born with grave physical or mental defects'.[2] This code was adopted by the State of Colorado in 1967 and 14 other states joined within the next few years. In 1970 the States of Alaska, Hawaii and New York all passed laws authorizing abortion on request and in the State of Washington a popular referendum effected the same change. In addition, numerous test cases were taken to court and finally on 22 January 1973, the Supreme Court struck down the restrictive abortion law for Texas and Georgia, making the operation available throughout the US.[58] The Supreme Court Judges reviewed existing laws with respect to the Fourteenth and Ninth Amendments and concluded 'that the right of personal privacy includes the abortion decision, but that this right is not unqualified and must be considered against important state interest in regulation'. The ruling was not based on an emotional concern for hard cases such as a woman carrying an abnormal fetus or the overburdened highly parous mother, as occurred in European arguments on abortion, but on grounds of human rights and personal freedom. With wisdom the Court decided, 'we need not resolve the difficult question of when life begins. When those trained in the respective disciplines of medicine, philosophy and theology are unable to arrive at any consensus, the judiciary, at this point in development of man's knowledge, is not in a position to speculate as to the answer.'

Following the Supreme Court ruling on abortion in 1973, Congress and State legislators passed statutes limiting access to abortion, such as those requiring that informed consent for the operation should involve a detailed description of the fetus or that spousal consent (*Planned Parenthood* v. *Danforth*, 1976) is always necessary for abortion. When these laws have been tested they have always been struck down in the State or Federal Supreme Court. The US Courts have consistently upheld an individual's right to reproductive freedom.[32] In 1979 the Supreme Court decided that a mature minor could have an abortion without 'parental consent or other parental involvement'. If the minor was not legally competent, a Court official could decide on the need to terminate a pregnancy, again without necessarily obtaining parental notification or consent. However, the Supreme Court has not overruled state or federal legislation denying tax dollars to women seeking an abortion, even when a physician determines therapeutic termination of pregnancy to be a life-saving measure (*Harris* v. *McRae* and *Williams* v. *Zbaraz*).

In the long term, the Supreme Court ruling defending a woman's right to choose a legal abortion could only be set back by the appointment of judges known to be antagonistic to abortion, by amending the US Constitution or possibly by Congressional statute. Amending the Constitution is a philosophically, legally and politically formidable process. However, by 1981, 20 amendments had been drafted, suggesting that the Constitution applies to 'unborn offspring at every state of their biological dependence', or that the fetus is a person from the 'moment' of conception.[24] The first type of amendment would logically imply a welfare state which extended protection in the way of health, food, clothing and shelter to children, adults and old people as well as to fetuses. The second type of amendment would imply the right of a child or adult to sue his or her mother for such things as smoking during pregnancy. A more threatening amendment is one that would give the states the constitutional right to pass abortion legislation and then enforce whichever state or federal law was the 'more restrictive'.[59]

Even if the philosophical problems of phrasing and a constitutional amendment which would give protection to the fetus can be overcome, an amendment still needs to be ratified by three-quarters of all the states. Amendments can be moved by Congress,[60] and there is a possibility of calling a Constitutional Convention, although such a convention has never occurred in the history of the United States and the mechanism of establishing its powers are not clearly defined: could a convention on the rights of the fetus also discuss a need for a balanced federal budget? In 1982 Senator Helms attempted to bypass the constitutional issue by proposing that 'Congress finds that the life of each human being begins at conception.'[61] However this was defeated in the Senate by a filibuster.

Freedom is always a two-way street and while US courts have defended the right of access to abortion, the Maryland Supreme Court upheld the right of a 14-year-old girl to carry her pregnancy to term when her parents attempted to force an abortion.

In 1969 the Canadian Parliament enacted a law permitting termination of pregnancy but only in hospitals, and only if a committee of at least three physicians, appointed by the hospital Board to make such decisions, recommended that abortion was necessary to safeguard the life and health of the pregnant woman. By 1978 only 30% of public general hospitals in Canada had established abortion committees, although within the private sector abortion committees had been relatively liberal. France reformed her previously restrictive abortion law in 1975 and any woman 'in distress' may seek an abortion in the first 10 weeks of pregnancy.

In the Far East, the loss of her overseas Empire resulted in serious overcrowding in post-war Japan and a high toll of death from illegal abortion. To deal with this public health problem a liberal law was passed in 1948. Many abortions go unregistered for reasons of tax evasion by those performing the operation. But, despite the non-availability of the Pill and a highly conservative attitude towards voluntary sterilization, there has been a demonstrable improvement in contraceptive practice in Japan since the mid 1950s with a corresponding decline in the number of legally-induced abortions. In 1976 the upper limit of gestation when abortion might be performed in Japan was reduced from 28 to 24 weeks.

The reform of the British law had an effect throughout the Commonwealth. In 1971 India adopted abortion legislation based on the British Abortion Law of 1967 with the additional proviso that abortion for a married woman was legal if the pregnancy was a failure of contraception, virtually allowing abortion on request for married women with children.[17,44] For the remainder of the Indian subcontinent, that is, for Pakistan, Bangladesh, Nepal and Sri Lanka, restrictive colonial laws remain.[10]

The law usually defines the person who may perform an abortion. Abortion is *de facto* and *de jure* legal in the US in the sense that the person to whom the woman normally turns for health care, namely a western-trained physician, is legally permitted to offer the operation. Abortion is *de jure* legal, but *de facto* illegal in India, where the traditional practitioners, to whom the bulk of the population turn when sick, are excluded from laws relating to termination of pregnancy and whereas less than a million legal operations occur each year, several million illegal operations continue to take place.

Menstrual therapies

The definition of when life begins has proved a stumbling block for legislators as well as for biologists and theologians. In Brazil, there is a vigorous public debate as to whether an intrauterine device should be included under abortion legislation, although to date no country has taken this step. The reverse argument, that menstrual regulation (MR, see Chapter 13, Surgical techniques) is not necessarily covered by abortion laws, has been made in some countries. In Latin America, the law requires that in order to convict an abortionist there must be proof that pregnancy has occurred, therefore MR may be a legally defensible procedure, although this has not been tested in the courts.[20] In many parts of the British Commonwealth and former Commonwealth, including Bangladesh, Pakistan, Malaysia and Sri Lanka, the law on abortion follows the text of the Indian Penal Code of 1860 and provides (Section 312) that 'whoever voluntarily causes a woman *with child* to miscarry shall . . . be punished' (emphasis added). It follows that MR cannot be found a crime. A criminal defendant is presumed innocent and the prosecution must prove all the elements of a crime, including a wrongful act (*actus reus*) and wrongful intention (*mens rea*) beyond reasonable doubt. The attempt to achieve the impossible, namely to abort a woman who cannot be proved to be 'with child' is not a crime.[7] MR is already part of the Bangladesh family planning programme, although a restrictive abortion law remains on the statute books, and is increasingly used in other countries whose law derives from the Indian Penal Code.

In England and Wales, where the 1967 Act only amends the 1861 Offences Against the Person Act which contains the words 'whether she be or not be with child', the reverse situation prevails and two doctors must be careful to form an opinion that the woman is pregnant before doing an MR.[4, 16] In April 1983 the British Attorney General ruled that use of the post-coital pill does not constitute abortion.

Consent
The user

In English law, coitus interruptus, the use of a sheath and intercourse following vasectomy have been held to constitute consummation of marriage. Informed consent for use of IUD, oral contraceptives, voluntary sterilization and abortion is a necessary ethical obligation which is being reinforced by laws and regulations in an increasing number of situations. Legal and medical disciplines have come together to establish a concept, now widely implemented, of informed consent. Briefly, this involves disclosing information to a competent person, who it is assumed understands the nature and content of the information and then makes a voluntary decision to refuse or accept the recommended medical procedure. Philosophically, the concept respects the individual and his or her freedom of choice and would seem to be especially appropriate in the area of human fertility control. Information must be given in a culturally appropriate way and include access to alternative choices: an individual who chooses sterilization because she is misinformed and unreasonably afraid of the Pill has not made an informed choice. Unhappily, particularly in the United States, the mechanism for acquiring and recording informed consent has been degraded by medico-legal concerns and the practice of 'defensive' medicine. Many consent forms are now so long and technical that they are self-defeating. Studies of their impact upon the individual supposed to give informed consent suggest that their effect is ambiguous.[23] Excessive amounts of information, the thoughtless use of medical jargon or a lack of perspective in the transmission of information relative to the other decisions that a woman must make in her domestic life can be as confusing and ethically irresponsible as a bland reassurance that all the woman needs to do is to accept an IUD or take a Pill every day and not worry about pregnancy or side-effects.

In the case of clinical trials, the volunteer should not only provide evidence of informed consent, but also understand that he or she has a right not to take part in any trial, can withdraw from a trial at any stage and should understand the risks and benefits of what is involved.[12] The US Department of Health, Education and Welfare circulated regulations governing consent for clinical research in 1974.

Problems of informed consent are even more difficult to implement in the developing world. The social distance between the physician and the patient is greater, understanding of the technical aspects of medicine is less and traditions of autonomous decision, particularly amongst women, vary. In one episode, concerning a US-financed programme of voluntary sterilization in Thailand which required US standards of informed consent, a woman refused to add her thumbprint to the appropriate form because on the only other occasion in her life when she had done this, she had been defrauded of the small amount of land that she held!

In both rich and poor countries, many, and perhaps most, individuals are looking for non-verbal clues from those who provide health care in answer to the basic question 'Doctor would you use the procedure yourself or would you offer it to your loved one?'

The physician is responsible for being well informed on the law and in the United States must be familiar with the legislation of his or her particular state. Accurate, detailed clinical records should be kept especially in the cases of sterilization and therapeutic abortion. The legal consent of the spouse or the parents in the case of a minor is not currently required for abortion or voluntary sterilization in Britain or the United States. It has been held in Britain that under the Sex Discrimination Act 'There are no forms of medical treatment or operations for which the consent of the spouse of the patient is a statutory requirement.'[54]

In Britain and the US, if the woman having an abortion is under the age of 16, the parents should be consulted whenever possible, although it remains legally proper to terminate the pregnancy even if the parents withhold consent. The US Federal Society Security Act requires that contraceptives are supplied to 'sexually active minors . . . without regard to marital status, age or parenthood . . . on a confidential basis',[31] although new regulations could override this principle. By contrast, in New Zealand, under the Contraception, Sterilization and Abortion Act, any person who directs or attempts to persuade anyone under the age of 16 to use a contraceptive, other than a parent, a registered medical practitioner or a representative of a family planning clinic approved by the Ministry of Justice, commits an offence.[27,29]

In 1982, in a major reversal of US trends in the 1970s, Secretary of Health and Human Services Schweiker set a new policy enforcing federally funded contraceptive services to notify the parents of unmarried teenagers who obtain contraceptive prescriptions.[62] This policy, like many others in the history of family planning, will hurt those teenagers who are too poor to find alternative sources and understandably will push up the fearful number of 1.2 million teenagers who conceived a pregnancy each year. So far the new 'squeal law' has been overridden by the courts.

An individual consenting to voluntary sterilization must understand that a small but measurable risk of pregnancy remains after the operation.

Medical responsibility is a two-way process and the doctor can be held liable for negligence if a woman dies, for example, as a result of failure to perform an abortion. In the context of informed choice, those who have a conscientious objection to abortion have an obligation to refer patients to those willing to provide such a service and those providing termination must also be able to deal with, or refer, problems of infertility, adoption, marriage or counselling for a single parent wishing to keep her baby.

The provider

As noted, the medical profession has its own system of rules, some of which, such as the establishment of general medical councils, stem from statute law. Most physicians try to follow a particular pattern of medical ethics and in the controversial field of contraception and abortion, their sincere convictions may come into conflict with majority practice. Only rarely will a doctor feel obliged to carry out a procedure which a society regards as criminal. More commonly, he or she, for personal or ethical reasons, may withhold advice which is legally permissible. It is interesting that, in commenting on the 1967 British Abortion Act, the Catholic bishops of England and Wales stated: 'it is not part of a doctor's duty to impose his ethical views on his patients. He should however explain to a patient seeking an abortion why he is unable to co-operate.'

When two or more doctors take care of the same individual it is essential that they communicate as freely as possible. In Britain, the Family Planning Association doctors advise an individual's general practitioner in the case of family planning advice, except in specified cases where the woman refuses permission for the prescribing doctor to communicate with her own family practitioner. When this situation arises, the physician may try to persuade the individual otherwise, but his or her first duty is always to the individual seeking advice and the possibility of withholding a prescription should not be used as a threat.

Delegation of duties

Who does what task in family planning is a major determinant of cost, and therefore of access to services, in both rich and poor countries. Clinical experience has endorsed non-physician Pill distribution and IUD insertion, but laws and regulations have not always kept pace with responsible service needs. The cost-effectiveness of family planning services turns largely on good management and the realism with which duties are delegated.[1, 33]

Non-physicians are legally allowed to prescribe Pills in 10 countries and to provide follow-up supplies in seven others.[40] IUD insertion by non-doctors is also legally permitted in 10 countries.[35] Sweden is an example of a country where midwives can prescribe oral contraceptives.[49] *De facto* oral contraceptives are available without prescription in a large part of the world, but unless the letter of the law reflects current practice, ministries of health and international agencies find it difficult to open to the poor these channels of service that the rich already use.

Fortunately, the legal doctrine of 'custom and usage' firmly establishes a medical practitioner's prerogative to delegate specified tasks, without statutory authorization. The use of checklists, written procedures and guidelines and auxiliary certification courses all reinforce this right protecting the physician and the paramedical worker.[23] Laws should be regarded as enabling rather than restrictive, but in turn, authorizations to auxiliary personnel and paramedical workers should be as specific as possible, accompanied by training and should involve appropriate supervision and adequate facilities for the referral of problem cases.

Conclusions

Many aspects of fertility regulation require a trained individual to bring his or her special skills to meet the need of the person who has chosen to limit their family. On occasions, the law can be the greatest single barrier to meeting individual needs, as occurred when Margaret Sanger attempted to provide contraceptives in the 1920s or when it still limits access to voluntary sterilization amongst the poor in Egypt and in several Latin American countries. Often, there are considerable differences between the *de jure* and the *de facto* situation.[34] The rich can usually purchase a safe abortion even when the operation is against statute law, and can nearly always secure a sterilization even if they must suffer repeated Caesarean sections or hysterectomy to achieve their goals. Elsewhere laws simply lapse. As recently as 1978 Article 416 of the Spanish Penal Code prohibited the use, sale or distribution of contraceptives, yet at least 40% of women in the fertile age-groups used some method of contraception. In yet other cases, the law is a facilitator of family planning and can be an instrument for spectacular changes, as in the US Supreme Court ruling on abortion in 1973.

Human Rights

Family planning has been proclaimed a basic human right but much remains to be done to make this right legally enforceable in the same way that the right to privacy has been enforced in the US. The 1968 Proclamation of Teheran was adopted by the International Conference on Human Rights and paragraph 16 provides that 'Parents have a basic human right to determine freely and responsibility the number and spacing of their children.' Yugoslavia has written this idea into its constitution.[50, 65] It has been argued that laws which restrict the use of contraceptives or negate the choice of voluntary sterilization are in violation of this principle. The 1982 Chinese constitution makes family planning an obligation for each citizen. In Denmark, the law *requires* a doctor attending a woman who has a term delivery or an abortion to offer contraceptive advice. In Poland a similar law requires a practitioner to give advice after termination of pregnancy. Although such statutes may be regarded as little more than an expression of good aspirations, their existence represents a civilized ideal that has not been found to cause offence to women and is in vivid contrast to the frivolous stance once common in the West, and still found throughout much of Latin America, where the physician discharges the newly delivered mother from the maternity home saying 'see you again next year'.

The basic human right to decide the number and spacing of one's children is buttressed by the application of a number of legal principles.[37] An individual has a right of *privacy and integrity* which includes fertility regulation choices and which US law providers, as noted, have extended to the field of abortion. The suppliers of family planning services can reasonably argue that in many circumstances their actions are protected by the legal principle of *necessity*. For example, anyone performing an abortion to save 'the life or health of others against imminent danger' has a reasonable legal defence. All legal systems uphold the *equal application of laws* although many aspects of contraceptive services, access to voluntary sterilization and restrictive abortion laws flaunt this principle. Finally, the basic obligation of health care personnel, and especially of physicians, is to make decisions in the best health interests of their patients. The World Health Organization has defined health 'as a state of complete physical, mental and social well-being and not merely the absence of disease or infirmity'. Many recent legal prosecutions concerning abortion in several countries (e.g. *Morgentaler*, Canada (1976); *Woolnough*, New Zealand (1976); *Roe* v. *Wade*, US (1973) and *Vuitch*, US (1971)) have been successfully defended by the application of some or all of the above basic legal principles.

In 1969 the General Assembly of the United Nations resolved that governments have a *responsibility* to provide 'knowledge and means to enable [individuals] to exercise this right' and this was interpreted by the Second International Conference on Sterilization (1973) as implying that governments are obliged not only to repeal laws against sterilization, but also to ensure that adequate surgical facilities for performing the operation exist.[43]

Tunisia has had a particularly consistent pattern of legislation dealing with the status of women, voluntary sterilization, providing for abortion (1965) where the continuation of the pregnancy would endanger the mother's health and (1973) permitting abortion on request in the first three months of pregnancy.[22] A few other countries have used the law to go one step further.

Beyond family planning

Relatively often, society perceives its fertility goals to differ from those of the individual. Many industrialized nations have given, and continue to give, tax and financial incentives for large families. In eastern Europe, particularly large financial rewards have been offered for child-bearing. Canada, France and Britain have all offered child allowances at one time or another (France currently gives a US $2500 bonus for the birth of a third child). On the whole, such incentives have not been associated with any demonstrable rise in birth-rates.

Singapore is the most frequently quoted example of a country that has passed legislation to deter couples from having children. In 1969 maternity fees were charged to high-parity women, in 1973 tax relief was limited to the first three children and, more recently, administrators have started placing the children of large families in the most inconvenient schools they can find. Although a decline in the birth-rate can be associated with each of these social policy changes, important improvements in the availability of legal abortion and voluntary sterilization took place at the same time and there is no unequivocal demonstration that such disincentives to childbearing have had a significant impact. Parents appear to be remarkably autonomous in their decisions, even if they run counter to societal ideals.

It is China that has developed the most complicated system of rewards and penalties for family size. In 1979 a one-child family campaign was announced. All who signed the one-child pledge receive a 5–8% jump in monthly income, increased living space, more food and more land for private cultivation. Those who have more than two children are unable to enroll in co-operative medical care schemes and are given adverse job assignments. By 1982 the one-child family became virtually universal in towns but was spreading less rapidly in the countryside. It is a measure of the momentum of demographic change and the predominantly young population of China that if 70% or more of all couples adopt the one-child family philosophy, the population of the country will still *grow* by over 200 million in the next 20 years, that is, adding almost as many people as now live in the US to a nation which already has approximately a thousand million people in a country of the same geographic area. The imposition of a one-child family policy is unpopular and has been accepted by the political leaders, the hospital workers and the people only because there is no viable alternative.

India has had experience with the unjust application of a law relating to population growth. In 1976 Mrs Indira Ghandi urged 'a direct assault on fertility'. A few months earlier, Maharashtra had become the first of four states to pass a compulsory sterilization law. It extended to any 'person . . . who at any time has three children, or who has more than three children on the appointed date, and such person if a male has not completed the age of 55, and if a female, has not completed the age of 45, and includes a person who having either all three male, or all three female children, has a fourth child.' These laws, however, never received the assent of the Indian President, although there is little doubt that some people were sterilized against their will during Mrs Ghandi's 'emergency rule', as local administrators, attempting to achieve the targets set for them, used police and bully squads to round up men for vasectomy. The majority of Indians, as the 1977 election defeat of Mrs Gandhi showed, rejected this coercion, and the tragedy of family planning in India has been the seeming inability of government services to make available meaningful services to all those who want them of their own free will.

Reproductive freedom

Fertility regulation, in the last analysis, is about choice. Sir Dugald Baird called family planning the 'Fifth Freedom'.[5] The freedom to determine family size, like the other great human freedom, is one which history shows individuals use responsibly. The aggregate of individual decisions concerning the means of fertility regulation can be as good as, and is often better than, society's expertise. The role of legislation should be to ensure an appropriate framework in which fertility regulation choices can be made. This should include access to accurate information, freedom to advertise and display contraceptives, the availability of the technically safest procedures, rules to ensure informed consent and mechanisms to make choices available to the socially under-privileged while at the same time avoiding coercion in all situations. Family planning may well be a human right but it is a freedom which requires continual attention if it is to flourish.

16

Conspectus

Contraception is a relatively new but increasingly important medical speciality. Until recently, birth control lacked recognition as an established entity. However, with the proven efficiency of the Pill and the IUD, both of which require a modicum of expertise to use correctly, combined with a change in the social climate whereby couples now expect real security against an unplanned pregnancy, the speciality has acquired respect and trust from other disciplines. Fertility control in its widest sense is an eclectic enterprise drawing on the theories and findings of sociology and demography. Its practitioners must always be educators and always be capable of putting into perspective the relative risks of contraceptive techniques.

Unfortunately, in the US public support for family planning is proving unstable with ambivalence about abortion and fears of the Pill and IUDs. Illogically, government support for reproductive research is uncertain and assistance to Third World family planning programmes is being challenged. In order to review where family planning stands today, and where it could go in the future, it is necessary to analyse what the providers of services have already learnt from the users, forecast possible technical developments, review the risks and benefits of contraceptive use and, finally, confront the moral issues arising from birth control practices.

Family planning as a learning process

The expansion of structured family planning services since the 1960s provides an opportunity to consider patterns of individual decision-making in the area of fertility control. Those who offer family planning choices must learn to know and to work from the knowledge and the ignorance, the aspirations and the fears, of those they try to serve. Illustrations from developing countries often provide clear-cut examples of problems which appear in a more subtle way within industrialized societies. It is interesting that studies from such places as Colombia and the Philippines demonstrate that even in traditional and developing societies people attempt to control their fertility, commonly trying to bring on a delayed menstrual period as seems to have happened throughout European history.[30, 52]

In order to use contraception, individuals must realize that it is possible for them to control or at least influence their own fertility and to have some knowledge of one or more culturally acceptable methods. Such knowledge is often lacking. A survey in Mexico showed that 29% of women did not believe it was possible to prevent a pregnancy.[55] Interestingly, the possibility of abortion was widely understood. Acceptance and use of abortion is generally the first step towards family planning since it is the first reaction to the idea that having too many children is individually and socially detrimental.

Birth planning is the outcome of a series of emotive choices. Menstruation may be seen as necessary for health but also regarded as dangerous; ambivalence towards contraception is counterbalanced by ambivalence towards childbearing. In Mexico, women refer to the practice of 'lying over', that is of suffocating a child shortly after birth and then ascribing the death to birth trauma or illness. This is regarded as morally acceptable because the infant is thought to ascend directly to heaven and become an angel. Infanticide was also one element in the demographic transition in the West.[30]

There are many individuals and couples who wish to avoid pregnancy but who fail to use a reasonable method of contraception. It is easy to label them as feckless, irrational risk-takers but it is more constructive to try, as Luker has done, to understand the decision-making involved.[33] Most of us occasionally discount future costs in favour of immediate benefits. The risk of a situation not previously encountered is especially difficult to assess. 'I didn't think I would get pregnant' says the teenager honestly stating her previous perception. By contrast, older women know they may get pregnant if they take contraceptive risks and are therefore more consistent and careful when using contraceptives, a fact already noted in discussing failure rates during various stages of family building (see Table 4.1). In all learning, practical experience is more important than pedagogic instruction. Each generation learns its social codes, particularly those concerning sex and fertility control, through its own mistakes and experience aided or impeded by information from peer groups, parents, books, films, discussions and school lavatory conversations.

Learning the remote effects of events is always more difficult than learning the effects when they are immediate. The couple who have unprotected intercourse are in the situation of the individual who smokes heavily; they may know of the long-term risk but immediate gratification overcomes their inhibitions. Pregnancy has an unpredictable relationship with intercourse; some women will get away with risk-taking for a long time and a few, who are unwittingly infertile, will get away with risk-taking all the time. A woman is likely to be more anxious about the arrival of her period after her first unprotected intercourse than after any subsequent similar exposure. Less than 1 in 20 women seeking an abortion at the British Pregnancy Advisory Service claimed that they had conceived on the first occasion on which they had ever had intercourse. A parallel with car driving may be useful. If all bad driving was inevitably associated with accidents, people would take less risks, but, like the risk of pregnancy following unprotected intercourse, careless driving usually escapes harm. Conversely, even the most careful driver is sometimes involved in an accident and unplanned pregnancies occur to the most conscientious contraceptors. We can carry the analogy further; all insurance companies know that young male drivers are worse risks than older individuals of either sex. The same mixture of lack of experience and sexual aggressiveness applies to contraceptive risk-taking.

The link between intercourse and pregnancy is unlike some other relationships in that *one* mistake can be disastrous. A fat person trying to slim may yield to the temptation of one heavy meal without irreversible destruction of their goal, but an unwanted pregnancy, when it occurs, cannot be undone by subsequent good behaviour.

The consequences of sexual risk-taking are profoundly different in the married and the unmarried. Most married couples learn the difficult process of fertility control during the time they take to build a wanted family and mistakes often appear as mistimed pregnancies, which may be relatively easy to accommodate. Nevertheless, the subjugation of women in many societies and social subgroups can still interfere with marital decision-making about family size.[24] In the case of the unmarried errors are more obvious and the costs higher. The irregularities and unpredictability of premarital coitus make birth planning more difficult and the penalties of abortion, adoption, a shot-gun marriage or bringing up the child alone are more severe.

Viewed as a learning process, the skills we acquire in the use of contraceptive technology are not qualitatively different from those of other areas of human activity. They are exceptional only in that they relate to such an intimate and important part of our lives. To pursue the driving analogy, it may be that first-generation users of contraceptives, like first-generation drivers, make more mistakes than their children and grandchildren will. Anyone who has been able to compare driving in Nigeria or Iran with that in Britain or the US will not be surprised that fertility control in these countries is also associated with more failures.

The provider and the consumer

Margaret Sanger originally brought doctors into family planning simply to make a controversial subject respectable.[18] With the rediscovery of intrauterine devices, the introduction of the Pill and the spread of abortion and sterilization, their technical skills have now become essential. Initially, doctors tended to see their role in family planning in the same way as in other aspects of medical practice, and since the main medical skills are those of diagnosis, they sought 'disease' which family planning could treat. The disease was over-fertility, particularly in the unfit, and this attitude tends to persist with regard to abortion and sterilization. Only in recent times has it come to be realized that it is better to regard family planning as a series of techniques which a doctor explains and then offers his technical skills to implement the user's choice.

Individuals seeking family planning are not 'patients' in the sense that they are sick. They are usually fit people who have made their own diagnosis; they suspect they are fertile, they know they are having sexual intercourse and they have chosen not to have a child. To some extent they have stolen the doctor's magic robes. In one sense, those who offer family planning are technicians meeting the needs of consumers and family planning demands the philosophy of marketing as well as of medicine.

Such philosophical concepts in no way diminish the place of family planning within medicine. Many aspects of medical practice have been enriched by a change in attitude which accompanied the profession's involvement in family planning during the 1960s and 1970s. In other branches of medicine the acceptability of the therapy to the user is equally important: services and therapeutic regimes are more effective when adapted to meet the needs of individuals and treatment is more acceptable when people are given information about their diseases and involved in the selection of their therapy just as they should be about contraceptive choices. At a technical level, the development and outstanding success of out-patient abortion has led to the adoption of several techniques of out-patient gynaecology and day-stay surgery not previously used.

Some health professionals find that this new role generates conflict, while others happily accept it. The attitude of doctors to sexual matters seems influenced more by their early environment than their clinical experience. Many find it hard to accept the need to explain or advertise, and even harder to appreciate that when a particular therapy or technique has been actively chosen its chance of success is thereby increased. Since Hippocrates there have been good reasons why those who practise medicine should not advertise. It would exploit human suffering to put a notice in the local newspaper claiming to be the best cancer surgeon in the city, yet when it comes to preventive medicine and family planning, promotion and advertising are important. We already recognize this by advertising clinics which will confidentially treat venereal diseases. Pain and fear will drive a sick person to medical services, whether it is a case of toothache or cancer of the rectum, but the adoption of contraception, which may well be an equally important decision, is one that a healthy couple can all too easily postpone.

In some countries, such as Denmark or India, the state promotes family planning and the obligation to use family planning is mentioned in the 1982 Chinese Constitution. In other countries, charitable organizations carry the message into the community and also provide services. An interesting hybrid system is one where the government or private institutions carry out the promotion but refer those who need services to private doctors who are then reimbursed at agreed rates for certain items of service such as IUD insertion or voluntary sterilization. The system works well in Taiwan and Korea[27] and the Marie Stopes Clinic in England has developed an interesting model, referring men seeking vasectomy to general practitioners who then contract with the charity to charge fixed fees. In Third World countries, individuals often seek help from private doctors in preference to government services which, rightly or wrongly, are commonly regarded as inferior.

The fact that family planning is a choice, rather than a remedy given in response to a medical diagnosis, means that auxiliary workers are even more important than in other branches of medicine. Nearly all the techniques involved in family planning are technically simple and rarely tax a physician's abilities. It is a disservice to an important subject to pretend otherwise. A diaphragm can be fitted and its use taught by nurses or paramedical staff. The prescription of oral contraceptives by paramedical practitioners is discussed in Chapter 10 (under Prescription). The fitting of IUDs in suitably screened women is a sufficiently simple procedure to be carried out by a nurse or midwife under appropriate supervision. Delivering a baby from the uterus involves far greater responsibility than does inserting a small plastic device into the same organ. Therapeutic abortion, especially when vacuum aspiration is used, can normally be done as an out-patient procedure. Vasectomy is a five-minute operation performed under local anaesthesia with minimal tissue exposure and is less liable to infection than the suturing of a cut finger. Most practitioners can be taught to do female sterilization by minilaparotomy. Only second-trimester abortion and certain techniques of female sterilization, such as laparoscopy, require specialist experience and well staffed back-up facilities.

The practice of family planning involves healthy people, and the individuality of disease is abolished. Every appendicectomy is a potentially difficult operation requiring adequate skill to deal with whatever abnormality or pathology may be encountered. By contrast, abortion and sterilization are repetitive operations, which in nearly every case run a routine course. These virtually identical procedures can be done quickly and in large numbers at a time, thereby being both cost-effective *and* clinically satisfactory. Success depends on practice and dedication irrespective of the operator's status in the medical hierarchy. Abortion and sterilization procedures should be concentrated so that high numbers can be performed by experienced teams rather than a few operations in a large number of different places. This also allows staff to be well rewarded for their skills while the consumer is offered cost-effective services. The end result should be a happy combination of factors providing safe, low-cost operations provided by experienced and well-paid staff.

The professional's most important function in the field of family planning is to help an individual or couple to select the most suitable method. Most aspects of family planning involve more talking than therapeutic intervention. Medical practitioners in all specialities ought to be aware of the need to advise on contraception so that unwanted pregnancies can be avoided rather than to wait until help is sought by those who are already overburdened with unintended pregnancies and desperate for help.

The quality of family planning services is a major determinant of success. In a survey of 300 women who dropped out of family planning services in Jamaica, it was found that the second most common reason for withdrawal (after complaints about the contraceptive method itself) was discouragement by the clinic routines. The times at which the clinic was open and the waiting and consequent difficulties in looking after existing children were all given as reasons why women dropped out or changed to buying their contraceptives from some more convenient source.[3]

Prejudices of the provider

It has been a repetitive theme of this book that, regrettably, the prejudices of the provider can play as great a part as the needs of consumers in determining the pattern of methods used. The provision of family planning in many countries continues to be determined by restrictive legal codes, conservative attitudes of a political elite and sometimes by inappropriate medical practice. These factors explain the wide variation in the profile of contraceptive use found in different countries and at different times within the same country. It is the attitude of providers which has determined the high use of condoms and low use of oral contraceptives in contemporary Japan and the non-use of oral contraceptives in the Indian family planning programme as against their predominant use in Malaysia. The low use of voluntary sterilization in the 1930s, 1940s and 1950s in the United States and the high use among the same population in the 1960s and 1970s was the outcome of changed medical attitudes and not demographic or cultural factors.

Medical history recounts numerous examples of uninformed prejudices delaying progress. Jenner predicted the eradication of smallpox in 1801 and in 1981 he was vindicated, but his contemporaries described vaccination as a 'discovery sent into the world by the powers of evil'. 'The law of God', cried one preacher, 'prohibits the practice: the law of man and the law of nature loudly exclaim against it.' In the case of human reproduction, convictions are often strongest where evidence is weakest. In the nineteenth century, anaesthesia in childbirth was said to be against Biblical teaching. James Young Simpson (see Chapter 13, Surgical techniques) pointed out that gynaecologists offered cold compresses to comfort women in labour, but churchmen railed against him when he offered chloroform. 'Gaining your end imperfectly' he wrote, 'according to contemporary religious views was no sin – gaining your end more fully and perfectly, is, they argue, an undiluted and unmitigated piece of evil.'[59] This is a remark which might be applied to contemporary discussions of periodic abstinence. Between the two world wars, several distinguished gynaecologists claimed that female barrier methods caused cancer. A speaker at a Congress of French Speaking Gynaecologists in 1927 cried: 'It is well known and universally admitted that the female orgasm absorbs spermatic products produced during the sexual act (and) their lack leads to both physical and psychic disorders.'[64] Marie Stopes expounded this particular theory and enthusiastically promoted the exclusive use of cervical caps, condemned IUDs and, when oral contraceptives were invented, she gave it as her sincere hope that they would never be used.[63] No doubt, similar prejudices are behind some of the statements made by contemporary medical practitioners about the side-effects of contraception, sterilization and abortion. The music hall song 'It's immoral, it's illegal or it makes you fat!' has been applied to family planning on an unforgivable number of occasions.

The optimum use of available methods

For a society to achieve low fertility two things must happen. There must be a perceived and accepted need to control family size and there must be a wide range of contraceptive methods available including the backstop of abortion to cope with the inevitable technical failures. In the industrialized world, rapid inflation and uncertainty about the future, combined with a population sufficiently educated to seek appropriate methods, has led to biological replacement and zero population growth in a few countries. Zero population growth refers to a situation in which the number of deaths and births in the country is equal; biological replacement is the situation where each couple can expect to have two progeny who themselves will reproduce in the next generation. In a society where population change has been rapid and there are many young people, it is possible to have biological replacement and a growing population at the same time. For example, Japan has biological replacement but the population continues to grow by approximately a million people a year and China has been forced to promote the 'one-child family' in an attempt to stabilize its population growth.

Despite the obvious limitations of the available methods, a society can control its fertility to within strict limits. Isolated examples of fertility decline within the developing world show that when deeply committed even very poor people can achieve a low birth-rate with current methods of contraception. In some developing countries a rapid decline in the birth-rate has occurred without unusual socio-economic development. For example, in the Indonesian island of Bali fertility fell by 35% in six years without fundamental cultural or economic changes. In the People's Republic of China the birth-rate fell from over 30 per 1000 in 1971 to approximately 17.9 per 1000 in 1979[46] but here the whole structure of the society changed dramatically.

Fertility declines most rapidly where there has been strong political leadership and where societal pressures have been mobilized to promote family planning. Nevertheless it is a fact that nowhere in the world have birth-rates fallen rapidly without users being given access to a wide choice of methods of fertility control. Unfortunately, some national family planning programmes offer only a restricted range of methods. For example, Pakistan has one of the most rapidly growing populations in Asia but the national family planning programme is limited to the provision of intrauterine devices, oral contraceptives and condoms.[50] Attitudes towards sterilization are ambivalent and, most important of all, abortion remains illegal. Whatever policies a government may set and whatever programmes international agencies may support it is in fact impossible to control human fertility with the limited choices such as now exist in Pakistan. All too often, poor, illiterate and technologically inexperienced people in developing countries are expected to control their fertility with a limited range of methods which western countries have already demonstrated to be inadequate.

Induced abortion and voluntary sterilization

Some societies, as in parts of contemporary Russia, have seen rapid declines in fertility which are almost soley due to the use of induced abortion. However, most successful countries have combined the use of abortion and contraception to lower their birth-rate. Often the abortions have been illegal, as were those which reduced the birth-rate in industrialized nations in the nineteenth and early twentieth centuries.

On the whole, the family planning community has been reluctant to accept that abortion and contraception are mutually supportive both from the point of view of the safety of the users and from that of the financing of services. Countries which have seen the most rapid decline in fertility are those such as Cuba and Tunisia which explicitly link contraception and legal abortion. Where family planning programmes have proved unusually successful, they have invariably been backed up by access to competent early abortion, even though it may have been illegal as in Taiwan, Korea and parts of Indonesia.[26] When the same services which supply contraceptives are also known to provide responsible safe abortion, family planning makes much more sense to potential users. Wherever abortion is legal, the abortion services almost invariably offer contraceptive advice, which tends to be well accepted because abortion is a good educator in contraceptive use (see Chapter 13).

Contraceptive services require a considerable investment of time and money and in a poor country they usually require heavy subsidy. Abortion services, on the other hand, can be made available at an acceptable cost in almost any part of the world. As a rule of thumb, most couples will spend a week's income to terminate an unwanted pregnancy: in Calcutta, first-trimester abortions are available for US $3–6 while in the United States they may cost $250. Abortion services generate money when run by responsible clinicians or charitable institutions. It would seem logical to use abortion profits to subsidize contraception services. Where the two are kept apart, society often feels that abortion services make unreasonable profits while those who provide exclusively contraceptive services commonly run short of money. In Britain, for example, the Family Planning Association refused to provide abortion services when the possibility arose in the late 1960s, so today it remains highly dependent on government subsidy and private philanthropy, while the Pregnancy Advisory Services, which began by meeting the need for abortion services outside the National Health Service, have successfully added contraceptive and voluntary sterilization services without soliciting outside funds.

During the 1970s, oral contraceptives and IUDs were found to present somewhat greater clinical problems than were initially foreseen, while first-trimester abortion proved to have less mortality and morbidity than even the most optimistic believed possible. Between 1972 and 1978 the risks of childbirth for an American woman were seven times as great as the risks of legal abortion. All other considerations apart, the risk to the user of controlling fertility is least when a simple method of contraception, such as the condoms, is linked with back-up legal abortion in the case of unwanted pregnancy[47,68] (Fig. 16.1).

Varying usage of the different methods of contraception
Not only does society benefit from access to a wide range of contraceptives but individuals are also likely to need different methods at different times. Fortunately, the available methods of contraception tend to complement each other. Oral contraceptives are outstandingly successful for young women to whom they offer excellent control of fertility with minimal risks. Their use is dissociated from sexual intercourse and they provide some protection against pelvic inflammatory disease. By contrast, intrauterine devices are often unsuitable for the nulliparous, are less effective than hormonal contraceptives for young women and may predispose to pelvic infection. As women get older, the risks of the Pill increase but the IUD becomes a satisfactory means of spacing pregnancies because the incidence of side-effects does not rise with age while effectiveness improves. The extremes of fertile life may require yet other patterns of contraceptive use. Where young people are experimenting with sex, the condom is useful and effective: it meets a discontinuous need and it protects against sexually transmitted diseases. It may be less useful for the older couple where sex drive may be on the wane, but here, in selected cases, vaginal barriers may be appropriate and sterilization is more likely to be acceptable.

The dramatic increase in the use of voluntary sterilization in the 1970s was perhaps the single most important event in family planning. In developed countries, most people choosing sterilization will have used a method of contraception beforehand. Often condom and coitus interruptus users will choose vasectomy, and diaphragm and Pill users tubal ligation: in other words, the same partner remains the decision-maker.[10] In developing countries, many women will have spaced their pregnancies solely by the anovulation associated with breast-feeding and therefore they may often adopt sterilization without prior use of modern contraception. Superficially, the two situations look somewhat different, but in terms of individual decision-making they deal with the same problem. Couples

Fig. 16.1. Annual number of deaths associated with control of fertility and no control per 100 000 nonsterile women, by regimen of control and by age of woman (US 1970s). (From Tietze, C., Bongaarts, J. & Schearer, B. (1976). Mortality associated with the control of fertility. *Family Planning Perspectives*, **8**, 6.)

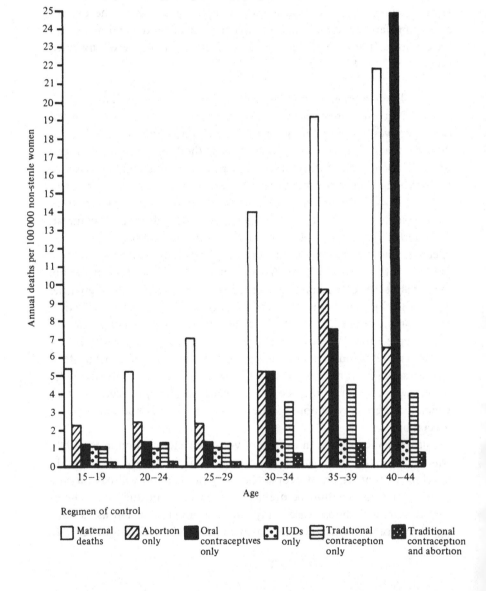

Regimen of control

☐ Maternal deaths   ▨ Abortion only   ■ Oral contraceptives only   ⬚ IUDs only   ⊟ Traditional contraception only   ⬛ Traditional contraception and abortion

often space their children reasonably, but find it much more difficult to prevent unwanted pregnancy in the long years between completing their family and menopause.

No method of fertility regulation is universally appealing. Whenever a new technique is made available, some people, who appear to have been dissatisfied with all previous options, will immediately adopt it. There will be some overlap between the new method and use of previous methods, but it is important to note that there is always a recruitment of new contraceptive users.

Future developments in fertility regulation

In real terms, the money available for contraceptive research and development reached a maximum (about US $120 million annually) worldwide in the mid 1970s, and then began to decline.[1, 19] Unfortunately the cost of developing new drugs constantly increases.[12] As a result, contraceptive research and development has slowed at the very time when the need for improved methods has become greatest[11] (Fig. 16.2). Only two new chemical entities have been accepted as contraceptive agents by the US FDA since 1968.[9] Institutions which used to conduct research have changed policies and the pharmaceutical industry has been discouraged. Governmental finance has become relatively more important. The US Government supports contraceptive research through the National Institutes of Health and the Agency for International Development and through funding universities and such institutions as the Program for Applied Research in Fertility Regulation, Family Health International (formerly the International Fertility Research Program) and the Population Council. The Government of the United Kingdom support contraceptive research in the UK through the Medical Research Council, which supports the Reproductive Biology Unit in Edinburgh and other research units, and, together with several other governments, helps to finance the Special Program of Research Development and Research Training in Human Reproduction which was initiated by the World Health Organization (WHO), Geneva, in 1972.

Possible improvements in systemic contraceptives, intrauterine devices, voluntary sterilization and the use of prostaglandins in abortion are being developed. Training is a vital factor in the successful introduction of new methods.[33]

A male Pill

Physiologically there are more sites where reproduction can be interrupted in the male than in the female but there are also more profound biological problems.[8] Men produce new sperm throughout their adult lives and there is no natural mechanism for turning off fertility in the way that pregnancy prevents further ovulation in women. The fact that new sperm cells are made continuously is both an opportunity and a threat. A number of alkylating agents, such as nitrogen mustards and triethylenemelamine inhibit sperm production. However, such drugs are too toxic for contraceptive use: metaphorically, the female contraceptive pill keeps the freezer door closed and prevents eggs being removed from the existing store while alkylating agents act like a selective weedkiller poisoning primarily sperm cells but also affecting others, and are very variable in their effectiveness. Many cytotoxic agents kill sperm. The nitrofurans reached Phase I clinical trials in the 1950s but caused unacceptable nausea. The compound bis-(dichloroacetyl)-diamine suppresses spermatogenesis without reducing hormone production from the Leydig cells and also reached

Fig. 16.2. Worldwide investment in family planning (constant US dollars 1970). (From Greep, R. O., Koblinsky, M. A. & Jaffe, Y. (1976). *Reproduction and Human Welfare: A Challenge to Research.* Cambridge, Massachusetts: MIT Press.)

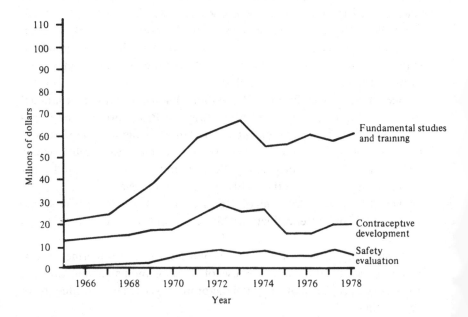

Phase I clinical trials, but severe adverse reactions occurred whenever the user drank alcohol.[23] Perhaps it could still be regarded as holding contraceptive promise for Mormons. Alpha chlorhydrin may block epididymal maturation of sperm but the therapeutic ratio is too low to permit widespread trials.

The antiandrogen cyproterone acetate[29] has been tested as a male Pill; it works by suppression of pituitary function, something which can also be achieved by giving testosterone, either by itself or with a progestogen, an effect which is analogous to that of the female oral contraceptive. Testosterone enanthate given every 10–12 days by intramuscular injection (200 mg) is an effective male contraceptive, reducing the secretion of luteinizing hormone (LH) and endogenous testosterone in exactly the same way as the female Pill inhibits the LH surge associated with ovulation and partially replaces the hormonal output from the ovary. The continuous use of testosterone enanthate is associated with periods of pituitary escape, a rise in LH levels and a temporary production of sperm leading to fertility 70–80 days later. In addition, the need for an injection every 10 days has obvious limitations. Depo-Provera and testosterone enanthate have also been used in clinical trials as a male contraceptive by Coutinho in Brazil.

Hypothalamic releasing factors present another potential route for the control of male fertility.[43, 54] Many analogues (both agonists and antagonists) of the decapeptide gonadotrophin-releasing hormone (Gn RH) have been synthesized. Phase I clinical trials have been performed using these analogues but the function of the Leydig cells (hormonal secretion) as well as sperm counts declined.

A worldwide search for plant products which will inhibit human fertility has been pursued in India, by the WHO and by individual researchers. Gossypol, or cotton seed oil, is a polyphenolic compound which when used for cooking, was observed to be associated with unintentional infertility in parts of China.[41] It may act by the inhibition of fructose utilization by the sperm. It is toxic in some animals[56] and a number of side-effects have been reported in human beings, including hypocalaemia. A Mediterranean plant with the appropriate name of the squirting cucumber (*Ecballium eleterium*) appears to have a specific effect on sperm, but has not been systematically investigated.

While a male oral Pill would be a considerable advance in family planning, given the current low levels of investment in contraceptive research and the biological complexity of interrupting male reproduction without the danger of producing abnormal sperm, it seems unlikely that such a product will be widely used in the next 10–15 years and perhaps not even before the twenty-first century.

At a more simple level, several chemical entities such as β-blockers have a direct effect on the sperm membrane leading to immobilization. Some of these may lead to improved spermicides.[45]

Sperm taken from the testes will not fertilize an egg and in most species must be exposed to the uterine environment in order to become fully capacitated. It is possible that the current oral contraceptives interfere with capacitation in the female reproductive tract. It may also prove possible to halt maturation of sperm in the male reproductive tract and the monoesters of methanesulphonic acid are effective in this way. Current work on in vitro fertilization may suggest means of preventing capacitation.

Female reproduction

Oral contraceptives imitate the suppression of ovulation during pregnancy but without the presence of a baby. Will it ever be possible to devise a hormonal contraceptive that imitates the suppression of ovulation during lactation, but without milk production? Thyroid-releasing hormone (TRH) enhances prolactin production and limited clinical trials have been conducted using the exogenous hormone to increase milk volume.

Historically, the explosion in research on hypothalamic releasing hormones during the 1970s is analogous to the work carried out on steroids and gonadotrophins between the two world wars. No doubt it will lead eventually to new developments in female contraception, just as the earlier work led on to the first oral contraceptives. Already, doses of an anti-luteinizing hormone agent as small as 50 μg on three successive days in each cycle are opening new approaches to contraception.[43, 54, 57] However, it is likely to take several years before any methods reach phase III trials and even longer before they are used on a large scale.

The choices that can be offered in family planning reflect the beliefs of society towards the acceptability and non-acceptability of various methods as expressed through religious, political, social and professional leadership, but do not necessarily reflect individual needs and may even run counter to them. In the last few years both the pharmaceutical industry and state-supported agencies have pulled back from research in the area of early abortion, yet experience shows that there is a very strong demand for a medical method of abortion in many parts of the world. It is, however, a biologically as well as a politically difficult area of research. In 1952 Theirsch conducted a clinical trial with the antimetabolite aminopterin but in his clinical series, and in subsequent illicit use of the drug, serious congenital abnormalities occurred in cases where abortion failed.

Progesterone from the corpus luteum is essential to the survival of the conceptus in the first three months of human pregnancy and a number of progesterone antagonists and inhibitors are known. Roussel-Uclaf has tested a regime of a synthetic anti-progesterone (RU-486, a 19-Norethisteroid) given for four days, either before menstruation is due or early in known pregnancy. Here we may have the makings of an effective and safe 'once-a-month' pill.

Some plant extracts, such as those from *Trichosanthsin kirilowii*, *Yuan Hua* and the Mexican 'tea' *Montana tomentosa* (zoapatle), have proven abortifacient activity and they may all act by augmenting prostaglandin synthesis.[21, 28] China is one of the few countries where research in these fields continues.

In the early 1970s, prostaglandins (PGs) were hailed as wonder drugs which might act as self-administered emmenagogues, that is by bringing on a delayed period. As with the Pill, there was a long latent interval between their discovery by von Euler in 1935 and their use in fertility regulation. When they were used, short-term side-effects and incomplete uterine evacuation proved to be problems. Species differences are important in assessing the action of PGs. PG $F_2\alpha$ and PG $E_2\alpha$ are luteolytic in rats, while in guinea-pigs and primates their main action is an oxytocin-like activity on the uterus leading to abortion.[16] There seems much less risk of a teratological effect than with compounds such as aminopterin. Naturally occurring PGs are 90% deactivated on a single passage through the lungs, but their action persists much longer if the 15-methyl group is substituted with some other group. Some second and third generation PGs are up to 30 times as effective in animals as are naturally occurring products. The substitution of halogens at various sites in the prostaglandin molecule produces substances which, unlike the natural compounds, do not require refrigerator storage.

However, while laboratory work has continued, even if at a slow rate, clinical testing has practically come to an end. The late A. Csapo began to obtain promising results with an 'impact dose' of PGs, but clinical trials have tailed off.[6] Multinational corporations have become so frightened by possible litigation and by the hostility of a vocal minority that some have made an explicit decision *not* to conduct further trials on human volunteers. Meanwhile, literally millions of women suffer the pain and dangers of traditional abortion practices. Yet today, if society wished, it might be on the verge of offering safer and perhaps even self-administered techniques for terminating very early pregnancies. One derivative of PG $F_2\alpha$, when used in a suppository, has proved successful in 49 out of 50 women with early pregnancies, up to six weeks after the last menstrual period.[72]

It has been argued earlier that unwanted pregnancies are certain to increase, particularly among the disadvantaged poor of the exploding urban shanty towns all over the Third World. Abortion is certain to reach epidemic levels. It is therefore of great importance that politicians and legislators should arrange that these abortions be performed with as little trauma to the women as possible. Vacuum aspiration is superior to sticks or knitting needles. Where legislators ignore the need and abortion remains illegal, the circumstances are ripe for exploitation. Where abortion is legal the risks are reduced from one death in every thousand criminal abortions to possibly a hundredth of this figure and in addition the openness and normality of the procedure mean that it is done with kindness and dignity; most important of all, once abortion is legalized it is automatically associated with contraception and the chances of a woman needing a repeat abortion are reduced. The essential point is that a rational attempt should be made to limit the sum total of destruction of embryonic life which inevitably occurs as people in developing societies first recognize the need to restrict their fertility. Such a programme must accept that abortion is inevitable until contraception has been made available and has had time to become absorbed culturally.

Immunological contraception

The possibility of an immunological contraceptive vaccine is an attractively simple one and has a long history. It was first explored by Landsteiner in 1899 and in 1932 Baskin took out a US patent on immunological contraception. In theory, immunological processes could interrupt human reproduction at a number of sites in both sexes.[22] Aspermatogenesis can be produced in animals by immunization techniques, but so far work has involved the use of Freud's adjuvant and this produces a painful, unacceptable local reaction.

The real need is to raise antibodies which are specific only to the selected substance and which will not react with any other essential metabolites. There are molecular differences between placental gonadotrophins and pituitary gonadotrophins and these have been exploited by Talwar[66] and others in trying to vaccinate women against circulating gonadotrophins, without damaging other aspects of the pituitary control of the sexual cycle.[62] Some progress has been made in this field but the vaccine, like that against cholera, is relatively short lived and as its effect wears off, the woman may conceive but then abort at increasingly late stages of pregnancy. We do not yet know if this unacceptable drawback can be overcome.[62] A more promising line might be to try to raise antibodies against the zona pellucida which appears to contain a number of unique proteins.[15] One of the obvious difficulties is getting sufficient antigen on which to experiment but perhaps a new generation of bioengineering techniques will overcome this problem. Once again research into fertilization may yield new possibilities for contraception.

Channels of distribution

The search for a totally effective, fully reversible contraceptive without side-effects is likely to be a long one. However, steps which require minimal investment can be taken to broaden the availability of current and potential methods. A contraceptive need not necessarily be bought by the sex for which it is physiologically appropriate. In Japan about one-fifth of condom sales are by women to women. In Bangladesh, most oral contraceptives are purchased over the counter by husbands to give to their wives and condoms are often purchased by servants for the head of the household. A comparison of continuation rates for oral contraceptives when provided directly to women and when given indirectly through their husbands has already been discussed (Chapter 10, Oral contraceptives: Preparations; Fig. 10.4).

Public and private channels of family planning service complement each other in several ways. The private world includes the physician in private practice but also encompasses the pharmacist and even the barber selling condoms. The private channel is older, often extensive and cost-effective, but sometimes the most needy are excluded by economic circumstances from access to private services. Selected subsidy to private channels of distribution has proved an acceptable and economic way of widening contraceptive use.

Reproductive mortality and morbidity

Human reproduction and its control are associated with three separate types of mortality. Firstly, there are the deaths which are directly related to reproduction. Less obvious, but of greater numerical significance among western women, is the way in which the age of childbearing influences disease patterns later in life: especially important is the relation between early childbearing and the *reduced* risk of breast cancer. Thirdly, there are the well-documented risks associated with contraceptive use.[47, 68]

Pregnancy and childbirth

Women carry most but not all of the risks of contraception. The risk to the fetus and infant is closely correlated with its mother's pattern of childbearing and such items as the interval since the last delivery.[34] As contraceptives become more sophisticated, some risks, beginning with vasectomy, will begin to be shared by men. Coitus itself, like most good things in life, also carries a measurable chance of death, and a not insignificant number of cardiovascular accidents and coronary thromboses occur to men and women during sexual intercourse.

The greatly reduced risk of pregnancy and labour to both mother and child has been one of the undisputed triumphs of western medicine in the last half century. In the developing world pregnancy broadly carries the same risks that our great-grandmothers faced. The difference in such risks between countries and areas, or even between racial groups within a country, is the best measure we have of medical care. The maternal mortality rate is the number of women dying annually from complications of pregnancy, childbirth or puerperium per 1000 live births and still-births. It is a prime index of the general health of a community. Whether the background level of maternal mortality is high or low, rising age and parity are highly correlated with increased risk of death and, within every age-group, there is a higher risk with the first pregnancy than with a second or third, while beyond this the risk increases again with each increasing parity until it reaches and exceeds the level prevailing for first maternities.

Perinatal mortality includes both still-births and infant deaths occurring within 1 week of delivery. It is expressed in terms of the number of deaths per 1000 live births. The perinatal mortality closely parallels the maternal mortality rate, being high for first births and low for second and third births, but rising steeply thereafter with increasing parity. The disproportionately heavy mortality suffered by women of high parity and low economic status has been revealed in a large number of studies.

The infant mortality rate is the number of deaths during the first year of life per 1000 live births. It clearly reveals the persistence of those factors which have been seen to affect survival even at the intrauterine stage. A poor economic and social environment, which is statistically correlated with an increase in perinatal deaths, tends to exacerbate the already reduced life chances of the younger infants in a large family.

Over the past generation, maternal mortality has declined precipitously in most developed countries. In England and Wales in 1950 there were 281 deaths due to the abortion or other complications of pregnancy and childbirth while in 1975 only 19 such deaths occurred.[70] In Europe, North America and Australasia it is probably approaching an irreducible minimum. Under-registration of deaths remains a problem[53] but it is clear that the most important factor contributing to the decline is improved maternal health and nutrition; part of that decline has been due to improvements in obstetric services but part has also been due to the spread of contraception and to a very significant reduction in the number of high-risk pregnancies amongst older women of high parity. In some developing countries, such as Sri Lanka, maternal mortality is also falling, showing that even an over-stretched and poorly financed medical service can do a great deal to avoid death in childbirth. Most of the world's deaths which are due to childbirth and abortion now occur in those countries where untrained traditional birth attendants still practise.

It is estimated that between 1980 and the year 2000, 3000 million babies will be born and in 2000 million of these deliveries, no trained person will be present. Deaths amongst this group cannot be less than one in a thousand and may be two or three times this level. It is likely that in Bangladesh 20 000 women die each year as a result of childbirth or abortion. In the world as a whole, 2–4 million women will probably die this way before the end of the century. If this carnage occurred in one place, there would be an upsurge of humanitarian concern, but because the women die one at a time, the magnitude of the problem is not recognized.

The provision of family planning, often as the first element of primary health care that can be made available, can do a great deal to reduce this wastage.[31, 67] A third of all pregnancies in the world at the present moment are not wanted and most of these are in older women of higher parity who are at greatest risk of death and injury in childbirth. The infant of the older woman is also at greatest risk and in Cairo, for example, a woman over 35 years of age having her fourth or higher delivery is more than three times as likely to suffer perinatal loss as a woman aged 19–34 having her first baby.[2]

Not only do many women die because they lack skilled care in pregnancy and childbirth but very large numbers suffer avoidable injuries. Severe tearing of the vulva and vagina is common and following long, obstructed labour the tissues separating the vagina from the bladder or from the rectum are destroyed leaving permanent connection between these organs with loss of urinary or rectal continence. Because of lack of skill, even more fetal or infant lives are lost than those of mothers and finally an unknown but large number of those infants who survive unsupervised pregnancy and birth suffer avoidable disabilities, particularly spasticity and mental retardation.

The contrast in the outcome of pregnancy is one of the most marked differences between rich and poor countries. The health policies which should follow from this tragic division are simple to understand and to implement. Wherever women are beyond the attention of trained midwives backed up by the possibility of referral to an obstetrician, then the availability of oral contraceptives without prescription and access to as many family planning options as possible, including legal abortion and the choice of voluntary sterilization, are steps that need to be taken if mortality is to decline.

Postponement of childbearing

While emphasis has rightly been put upon the health benefits of fertility control, it must also be recognized that there are some disease penalties for postponing childbearing. There is a strong correlation between late childbearing and developing cancer of the breast in later life and, as noted in Chapter 10 (under Cancer of the breast), in the West cancer of the breast has reached epidemic proportions. Fibroids, endometriosis and ovarian cancer are all more common in nulliparous women and in women who have their first child late in life.

It seems therefore, that events early in the fertile life have a considerable influence on pathologies which develop in middle age and later. The modern world too easily forgets that long intervals of menstruation are a product of civilizea living. Over the past 100 years, the average age of the menarche has declined, that of the menopause may have risen and the first delivery occurs later, with fewer pregnancies and less and shorter breast-feeding, so that women are exposed to more ovulatory cycles. Perhaps menstruation is more dangerous than we think.

The response of many women that the Pill is 'unnatural' is superficial. Hormonal contraceptives suppress ovulation and flatten levels of hormone output and this may explain the accumulating evidence that the Pill has a protective effect against ovarian and endometrial cancer and against benign breast disease. It would be over-simple to suggest that today's steroidal contraceptives meet the twin goals of contraception and ensuring a healthy body at the menopause in a fully satisfactory way, but it is reasonable to suggest that they may prove the first, halting step in this direction. Certainly, physicians and medical scientists might be wise to set the goal of developing methods of contraception which are not only simple, reversible and have a minimum of harmful effects but which also forestall the pathologies associated with late childbearing and non-pregnancy. It is possible that in 100, or even 500 years' time, women may still be using a systemically active method of contraception, at least for some part of their reproductive lives, both to prevent pregnancy and to mimic those changes in the life-long pattern of reproduction associated with protection against breast cancer and other forms of reproductive pathology which occur when pregnancy is delayed or never takes place at all. To delay childbearing by the use of a condom or periodic abstinence may eventually prove more unnatural than using hormonal contraceptives.

It is a fact of life that men still use their reproductive systems as did their stone-age ancestors and in much the same way as evolution programmed it. Men are not faced with the complex, interlocking and difficult to predict pathologies which face women in the modern world.

It would be useful to have fundamentally new methods of fertility regulation, such as immunization, but hormonal methods may remain important for the very reason that they bring about widespread changes in the woman's physiology. No doubt the current generation of Pills and injectables is open to significant improvement and it cannot be denied that these contraceptives have totally unwanted and potentially lethal effects, but it is still possible that if and when the final equation of risks and benefits is written, then benefits may outweigh risks, all considerations of pregnancy prevention apart.

Risks and benefits of contraceptive use

All methods of fertility regulation have real or suspected hazards. Those of the Pill and the IUD are well documented. Abortion and sterilization carry the risks of surgery and even in the case of vasectomy there has been debate about possible long-term immunological hazards. It has been suggested that the use of spermicides and periodic abstinence may give rise to congenital abnormalities. One study of ovarian cancer even suggested the asbestos particles originating from the powder used on condoms may be the cause.[39] In short, only coitus interruptus has never been associated with speculation, however remote, about lethal consequences.

There has been a lack of perspective from the medical profession, decision-makers and the media in assessing and in reporting the possible risks of contraceptive use. When it was pointed out to one Indian family planning leader that widespread distribution of oral contraceptives would prevent many more deaths resulting from childbirth than it could possibly cause through side-effects, she countered 'Ah, but deaths in childbirth are *natural* deaths[!]' Human judgement must be exercised by anyone working in the field of family planning and those risks which are agreed to exist need to be put into a realistic perspective. As a first step, it seems reasonable to balance the risks of contraceptive use against non-use. There have been remarkable improvements in obstetrics and the chance of death in childbirth in the developed world is now exceptionally low. In Britain and America, a woman is more likely to be murdered than to die in childbirth. Nevertheless, the dangers of death due to pregnancy are still greater than the dangers associated with any method of contraception with the single exception of the older woman on the Pill. Only for the woman of 35 who smokes are the immediate risks of the Pill greater than that of becoming pregnant and dying in childbirth.[68] In the developing world, the health benefits of contraceptive use are correspondingly greater.[47] In countries where abortion is illegal, every method of contraception, however distributed and to whatever age-group, is in the health interests of women.

Sexual activity is a powerful driving force for all healthy, mature people and contraceptives should not be judged by the same criteria as bronchodilators and laxatives. Rather they must be set against the background of their social consequences, and the chance of death resulting from contraceptive use may be reasonably compared with some other risks which are taken daily. There are a large number of recreational activities that are far more dangerous than taking the Pill. In the US there are 5000 boating and swimming fatalities a year and there is a greater likelihood of a death in the family if father buys an outboard motorboat than if mother uses oral contraceptives. In America one person a day falls out of a boat while fishing and drowns and two people a week die in their baths. Between 1970 and 1978, 118 young men died playing American football at school.[36] Sitting at home is no protection against rare adverse events and 6500 people a year (2.9 per 100 000 of the population) die from household fires in the US, while accidental poisoning caused 3374 deaths (1.6 per 100 000 of the population) in 1977.[37] In England and Wales there were 674 accidental poisonings in 1974. Car accidents are the leading cause of death to US infants and children (8 per 100 000) but only 7% wear seat belts or ride in protective rear seats. One useful way of describing risks is to suppose that all causes of death could be removed so that we live forever except for the risk under consideration. Some examples of how long we would live are given in Table 16.1.

It is curious that the US Congress votes more than $200 million a year for the control of drugs and yet seems unable to pass any laws restricting the use of firearms. Between 1963 and 1973, 46 121 Americans were killed fighting in Vietnam and 84 646 were killed at home in the US with hand guns. A male born into a big US city has a 1 in 33 chance of being murdered[35] while a US Serviceman during the Second World War had a 1 in 50 chance of being killed. In the United States, a citizen is more likely to be killed by the *accidental* use of firearms than by the deliberate use of contraceptives.

Almost without exception, the consequences of contraception are beneficial and contribute significantly to the health and well-being of the community. One of the effects of the modernization of contraceptive practice appears to have been a greater feeling of security among sexual partners and an increase in coital frequency. Between 1965 and 1970 mean coital frequency among women in the US who were married and living with their husbands increased by almost a quarter and this could be partly accounted for by the increased use of such highly effective methods of contraception as the Pill and vasectomy.

In contrast, many societies permit drugs and other practices which are either of questionable value or are demonstrably harmful.[14] The ill effects of alcohol and tobacco, which are tolerated solely because they provide comfort and pleasure, are outstanding causes of mortality and morbidity, but they are inadequately regulated by civil law or by social custom and fall outside the sphere of medical prescription. Thirty thousand deaths from lung cancer occur yearly in Britain and the majority can fairly be attributed to smoking. By the end of the century more British men will have died from smoking-induced cancer than from two world wars. Moreover, the correlation that exists between heart disease and smoking probably accounts for even more deaths than that between smoking and lung cancer. The American Heart Association estimates that over 300 000 deaths annually in the US are due to smoking-induced lung and cardiovascular diseases. Cigarettes have now become the most common cause of death in the West. The risk to the woman who smokes seems every bit as large as that to a man[13] and if a pregnant woman smokes, the next generation is also affected: for every 10 cigarettes smoked in pregnancy, her new-born infant will be 0.1 g under-weight. In real terms, the risk of the Pill is equivalent to smoking one cigarette a day. It would indeed be in the health

Table 16.1. *How long would a person live if they had only one risk of death? (US and UK data)*

Risk	Life expectancy (years)
Smoking 40 cigarettes per day	100
Riding a motorcycle 10 h per week	300
Drinking a bottle of wine per day	1 300
Driving a car 10 h per week	3 500
Power boating once a month	6 000
Having a baby every year	10 000
Playing football twice a week	25 000
Staying home for 200 h per year watching television (man aged 16–68)	50 000
Using oral contraceptives (non-smoker)[a]	63 000
Travelling by train 100 h per year	200 000
Using an IUD	200 000
Being struck by lightning	10 000 000
Being hit by a falling aeroplane	50 000 000

[a] The calculation only considers cardiovascular risks and omits the benefits of the Pill, such as reduced ovarian cancer. The risks of other steroidal contraceptives, such as injectable Depo-Provera are omitted. To date, no human deaths have been associated with these drugs and, as of the present, they would have to be associated with a separate category of 'immortality' in the above Table!
Sources: Modified, with additions, from R. Rochat and R. Hatcher.

interest of society to put cigarettes on prescription and oral contraceptives in vending machines.

Setting policies

While there should be no attempt to trivialize the proven side-effects of various contraceptive measures, it is equally important to build a realistic perspective on which the user, the health worker, politicans and legislators can make sound decisions. Manifestly, such a rational perspective exists in neither developed nor developing countries. Society does not always put money and effort where it will bring the biggest return. The US spends an estimated $5 000 000 to avoid a death from accidental exposure to radiation in a nuclear power plant[25] but has thousands of unguarded railway crossings which are responsible for a thousand deaths a year.[38]

Few studies have been conducted on the public perception of risks and benefits, but Lichtenstein and her colleagues have tested the ability of subjects to judge the frequency of various lethal events.[32] A group of well-informed US citizens was asked to make comparisons such as 'Is tuberculosis more or less likely than drowning?' There was a consistent tendency to overestimate small risks of death while underestimating common ones, which was especially marked in the case of well-publicized causes of death. For example, Lichtenstein's test subjects rated tornados as a more frequent cause of death than asthma, although in reality they present only one-twentieth of the risk and deaths due to botulism were rated 100 times as common as they really are. Contraceptive risks are obvious candidates for public overestimation because they are rare, dramatic, well publicized and have the added attraction of being related to sex.

The medical profession is not immune to its own fashions or to public pressure. While disease prevalence should not determine priorities in health, neither should it be irrelevant. The total elimination of cancer would add on average only 2 years 6 months to the expectation of life of a western child at birth.[71] This is not to submerge millions of individual tragedies in an average and undermine advances that have been made and need to be made, but it is to emphasize the huge success of preventive medicine, of which family planning is one element, in the western world.

Third World policy makers often set unjustifiably conservative policies on Pill distribution and other aspects of family planning while turning a blind eye to common causes of death. In Kenya each year there is one fatal traffic accident and 10 injuries for every mile of paved road. In the same country, parliamentarians have asked for Depo-Provera (where no associated human death has been proven or suspected) to be banned, partly as a result of stimuli from US-based groups. Nearly half of all the prescriptions written in the Nairobi teaching hospitals are for three or more drugs and one must wonder how much iatrogenic disease follows such practices.

No systematic effort has been made by Third World leaders to warn about the dangers of smoking. The consumption of cigarettes is growing rapidly in developing countries and smoking-related deaths can be expected to rise rapidly in the next 10–20 years.[65,71] The WHO's Director General has called smoking 'Probably the largest single preventable cause of ill health in the world'. Tobacco is not controlled by the FDA and American cigarettes are exported aggressively and without a health warning. Politicians, such as Representative L. H. Fountain (whose Congressional hearings did much to confuse public knowledge about oral contraceptives in the 1960s) and Senator Helms (one of the leaders of the Right to Life movement in America) both staunchly defend government subsidies to the US tobacco industry.

Ethical implications

In the contemporary world moral issues are often more important than social or technical issues in limiting universal access to the full range of contraceptive measures.

Biological issues

Insight into the reproductive behaviour of our nearest relative, the great ape, highlights several important aspects of our own sexuality. Although genetically similar (man and chimpanzees have 97% of their DNA in common) the great apes and man show a variety of mating patterns and a wide range of copulatory frequencies. In the orang-utan, gorilla and chimpanzee, the female only accepts the male for a few days around the time of ovulation and for much of her life she is either pregnant or lactating. The adult male gorilla and orang-utan may only mate once a year or less and the weight of their testes is only 0.017% (in the gorilla) of their total body weight, the external genitalia being relatively very small. However, there are marked differences in body size and build in gorillas, reflecting competition between the males, each of whom strives to have a harem of females. The chimpanzee, by contrast, lives in promiscuous bands and an adult male chimpanzee may mate literally one thousand times as frequently as his cousin the male gorilla. The chimpanzee testes weigh 0.269% of the total body weight.[58]

Unlike the other apes the human female shows no variation in sexual behaviour associated with ovulation, and mating can take place at any time during the menstrual cycle or during pregnancy and lactational amenorrhoea. Human testes are not as large in relation to body weight as they are in the chimpanzee, but their size does allow for mating three or four times a week without any reduction in the number of sperm in the ejaculate. The penis is uniquely large in *Homo sapiens* and the attractiveness of the female is signalled partly by the unique development of the breasts which occurs at puberty, whereas in all other primates it occurs with the first birth. As Charles Darwin[7] correctly understood, reproductive behaviour is determined by, and in turn helps to shape, further evolution. To the biologist, the artificial control of fertility in the modern world merely attempts to restore a pattern of reproduction that prevailed before civilized living produced a number of artificial changes in the way in which women used their reproductive system.

Early in its fetal development the human ovary contains approximately six million oocytes, each genetically unique. Most degenerate before puberty. A few commence development each cycle, but of these all but one (or occasionally two) degenerate and even if a woman has six babies she would still only express one part in a million of her genetic potential. A man produces 50–300 million sperm every day, again each sperm is genetically unique. Thus over a fertile lifetime one man produces an equivalent genetic diversity as has been expressed by all the human beings that have ever been born even though, as an individual, he would clearly be limited by race and many other inherited characteristics. The loss of gametes and early embryos involved in the formation of the next generation appears to be part of Nature's richness and diversity. There is no discomfort to the biologist if millions of sperm are caught in a condom or if the necessary, natural healing processes of miscarriages are replicated in artificial situations.

Religious issues

All the world's major religions endorse the idea of responsible parenthood, although several have reservations on one or other methods of fertility regulation. Islam makes a number of positive statements about family planning. The Prophet Mohammed endorsed the use of *al-azl* or coitus interruptus for socio-economic reasons and for the health of the woman. The Koran recommends at least two years' breast-feeding after delivery.[42] The Buddhist scriptures contain the phrase 'Too many children make you poor'.

Christianity has found it most difficult to accept the need to regulate fertility for several reasons. The teaching of an imminent second coming by Christ's disciples diverted the attention of the first Christians from a concern with procreation and the Early Fathers of the Church, taking their cue from the Stoics, added to the problems of Christian teachings on reproduction by drawing their conclusions about *natural law* from the wrong animals. They assumed that if the dog or goat mated once for each pregnancy then man should do the same. For much of the history of Christendom, sexual intercourse was regarded as a regrettable necessity for reproducing the human race; at best a remedy for concupiscence.[44] It was something that should be engaged in as infrequently as possible, with the minimum of pleasure and only when procreation was possible. The Protestants were the first to step away from this idea although theirs was hardly a giant leap forward for humanity. In 1908 the Lambeth Conference of Anglican bishops had regarded 'with alarm the growing practice of artificial restriction of the family'. In 1930 the same Conference accepted contraception in cases where abstinence was impossible and in 1931 the Federal Council of Churches in the US approved a 'careful and restrained' use of contraception. Only in 1958 did the English bishops truly endorse family planning. The Central Conference of Rabbis in America followed the same evolution as the Anglicans. The Catholic Church is still in the midst of a similar revolution, and like most prolonged revolutions it is leaving many casualties behind.[49, 61]

Pope John XXIII's second Vatican Council (1962–65) (Vatican II) placed the purpose of marriage (i.e. human sexuality, or the love which sexual intercourse expresses) on an equal plane with the procreative aspect.[40] In contradistinction to mediaeval attitudes, sexual intercourse for non-procreative purposes is accepted and the use of human reason to avoid pregnancy, as expressed in different patterns of periodic abstinence (see Chapter 7) is now totally acceptable and the Church regards intercourse to express love during intervals of natural infertility, lactation, pregnancy and after the menopause as licit. A sample of Catholic priests in New York State found that 30% of the younger priests even questioned aspects of the Church's teaching on abortion. Catholic moralists, however, remain divided as to whether there is any fundamental difference between periodic abstinence and, say, the use of a condom. Some maintain that the two acts are an equivalent use of human reason designed to achieve a common goal, while others maintain that intercourse without the interference of an appliance or hormones remains an ideal. Within the discipline of moral theology failing to achieve an ideal may be technically evil, but the use of so-called artificial methods of contraception can remain a best choice in a number of situations, given the limitations of the human condition. In short, with some hesitancy and some nuancing of the situation, many Roman Catholic moral theologians from Rome to Lima now accept the use of contraceptive methods. During the last few days of Vatican II, a second evolution in Catholic thinking took place with the first explicit statements in the history of the Catholic Church on religious toleration and ecumenism: a long-standing teaching was totally reversed. If and when such a formal change on contraception will take place is uncertain, although the precedents are several and genuine.

Unhappily, there have been a number of idiosyncratic papal teachings which apparently run counter to this broad evolution in thought and practice. On 29 July 1968 Pope Paul VI, rejecting the majority advice of his own Commission on birth control, explicitly condemned modern methods of contraception in his encyclical *Humanae vitae*. The encyclical gave rise to a great deal of intellectual and emotional pain but did not halt the process set in motion by Vatican II and during the 1970s the majority of Catholics, encompassing laity, priests and theologians, not only exposed the ideal of responsible parenthood but also ceased their intellectual and political opposition to the availability of family planning services. Whereas in the years 1950–51 80% of Catholic women either used no method of contraception or used exclusively the rhythm method early in marriage, by 1971–75 only 9.5% of women at a similar stage of family building avoided modern methods of contraception (Fig. 16.3).

Despite this massive shift of conscience in members of the Church, Pope John Paul II has continued to condemn artificial contraception in many of his personal teachings and has astonished many contemporary theologians by harking back to the early teaching of the Church concerning the resurrection of the body, which, as late as 1982 he claims would still be male or female and, while united in marriage, sex and procreation would have no part in the life eternal.[69]

Such lack of perspicacity helps to link the church leadership to a vocal minority of Catholics who seem to be bent on reversing the dictum of Vatican II; the Right to Life movement has a significant, although by no means exclusive, input from Catholic laity and some priests. It has built a simplistic and emotional symbolism around certain perceived aspects of abortion and the so-called 'abortion mentality' and has linked up with other groups such as the World Organization Ovulation Method Billings (WOOMB) to attack all other methods of contraception and Mothers Organized for Morality (MOMS) to attack the availability of family planning services.

Technological issues

Technical changes and advances undoubtedly raise ethical problems. Modern medicine has altered human reproduction in four important areas:

(a) It is possible to control conception.
(b) Childbirth has become a highly technical event with fetal monitoring and the possibility of Caesarean section.
(c) Traditional patterns of breast-feeding have been greatly abbreviated or eliminated.
(d) The gametes and early zygote can be manipulated in artificial insemination and extra-corporal fertilization.

Unfortunately, much ethical analysis of the issues has been piecemeal and, until recently, has concentrated on intercourse almost to the point of obsession. Either all these changes demand equal concern or none of them should be considered. If artificial methods of contraception are con-

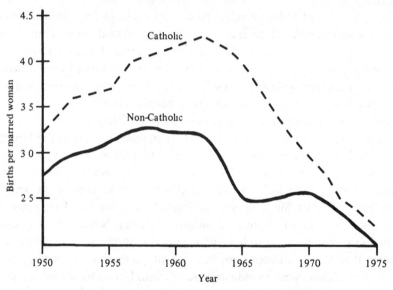

Fig. 16.3. Catholic and non-Catholic family size and contraceptive usage 1950–75 (US). (Source: Westoff, C. F. & Jones E. F. (1979). The end of the Catholic family. *Demography*, **16**, 215.)

Catholic 1965
58.5% Using contraception
21.8% Pill
31 8% Rhythm
3.8% Sterilized

Non-Catholic
70.0% Using contraception
30 7% Pill
4 2% Rhythm
10.6% Sterilized

Catholic 1975
76.4% Using contraception
34.2% Pill
5.9% Rhythm
26.0% Sterilized

Non-Catholic
79.9% Using contraception
34.3% Pill
1.7% Rhythm
33 1% Sterilized

demned, why isn't artificial feeding of an infant? If adoption of a child for the whole of infancy, childhood and adolescence has become legally accepted, should not transplanting a fertilized egg from a donor to a recipient woman for nine months become similarly acceptable?

New techniques sometimes produce more fear than they need to. If a method of sex selection is perfected it would most likely be used on a wide scale in a country like Korea, where a marked preference for sons still exists.[73] If widely adopted it could change the sex ratio in the next generation, but this would automatically introduce a self-correcting mechanism once the number of women began to fall, because their social value would then rise, eventually bringing sex equality.

Do contraceptives cause immorality?

For many people the key question about contraception is not the morality of individual methods but the possible adverse societal consequences of controlling fertility. Nearly all societies have well defined moral codes limiting intercourse to specified sexual partnerships. Illegitimate pregnancy is frequently strongly condemned and even today in some parts of the world, such as the Lebanon, the unmarried woman who becomes pregnant will become a social outcast and may even be killed by her own family. In such societies many people believe that great social problems may follow the making of contraception freely available. Even in Britain, family practitioners who have been qualified for 20 years or longer strongly believe the possession of contraceptive information is often an incitement to promiscuity.[17] Modern methods of contraception change many of the rules which society found necessary to impose on sexual conduct in the past. Since the Second World War, there have been marked and sometimes rapid changes in patterns of sexual behaviour, although different parts of the world have gone in different directions. There is no doubt that the prevalence and duration of premarital intercourse has increased in many western industrialized nations but such changes are also part of broad historical rhythms which extend back over several centuries.[30, 60]

While sexual behaviour has become more liberal in the West at a time of increasing contraceptive availability, the reverse has occurred in the People's Republic of China where a thousand million people have undergone one of the most dramatic changes in sexual behaviour in human history, moving from a society with a dual standard of morals for men and women including widespread prostitution and sexual exploitation, to one where late marriage is associated with a high degree of chastity, extramarital intercourse is unusual and where there is an almost Victorian concern with masturbation. This change has taken place over three decades during which the use of contraceptives, voluntary sterilization and legal abortion has grown to such an extent that today the pattern of use of modern methods of contraception, in, say, California and China is remarkably similar even though they have moved in opposite directions in patterns of sexual behaviour.

There is a great deal of other evidence that the availability or non-availability of the means to control fertility and patterns of sexual behaviour are unrelated. The abortion law in the Republic of Singapore is almost a Xerox copy of the 1967 British Act, yet in Britain in 1979, 61.1% of women having legal abortions were unmarried whereas in Singapore in the same year it was 24.3%. In other words, access to the means of fertility control does not of itself determine patterns of sexual behaviour, which are more dependent on cultural factors, work opportunities, the affluence of young people and the degree of parental authority. Conversely, Great Britain and New Zealand have a common cultural tradition but in Britain contraception is available to the unmarried and abortion is legal whereas in New Zealand abortion is illegal and contraception difficult for the unmarried to obtain. There are more illegitimate pregnancies in New Zealand than there are in Great Britain and again it would seem that access to the means of fertility control is not a major determinant of sexual morals but merely of the social outcome.

Considered from the viewpoint of the individual, contraception enhances a sexual responsibility. Is the woman who refuses premarital intercourse for the simple reason that she is afraid of pregnancy more or less moral than her contemporary who refrains from intercourse even though she has the power to control her own fertility? 'Ignorance', wrote a nineteenth-century judge upholding the publication of Annie Besant's works (see Chapter 1) 'is no more the mother of chastity than true religion.'[5]

Looking for a consensus

When the world is changing rapidly, as it is now, individuals cast around for simple explanations of complex events, particularly at times of economic difficulty and national disillusionment. Adolf Hitler came to power at a time of devastating inflation and national humiliation. The abortion rate in Germany was exceptionally high and family planning clinics were beginning to function. One of the first acts after the Nazi seizure of power was to ban the advertisement and display of contraceptives and to close down all birth control clinics. Before the Nazi Socialist Party marched into Czechoslovakia, it marched into the bedrooms of its own citizens; abortions were termed 'acts of sabotage against Germany's future' and the courts imposed 6- to 15-years jail terms on convicted abortionists.[20]

At the moment there is widespread fear about economic instability and the United States is still recovering from defeat in South East Asia. In the United States legislation is once more being drafted to overturn the free access to contraception, sterilization and abortion which was so painfully won during the 1960s and 1970s. Abortion has become an issue uniting an otherwise diverse series of groups and the record of US politicians is being judged on the single issue of whether they are for or against abortion. In Europe, by contrast, the temperature of the abortion debate has fallen with the passage of time. 1980 was the first year since the change in the British abortion law that a Private Member's Bill was not launched in an attempt to modify or reverse it. 1981 saw a nationwide referendum in Italy overwhelmingly support the continuation of a liberal abortion law, despite the active and personal participation of the Pope.

Will the deep division of opinion that still exists concerning the moral aspects of family planning, especially in relation to abortion, ever be bridged?

Fortunately, the problem is not without precedent: basically it is one of religious toleration. Those with differing opinions on the ethics of fertility regulation do not differ on the basic facts about population, human reproduction or human sexuality. They do, however, make different assertions over the moral interpretation of these facts, just as different religions hold different assertions about the theological interpretation of temporal life. There is no Biblical basis for any rejection of reproductive freedom[51] and in the end human problems must be resolved by human means, with toleration of sincerely held but opposing ideals.[4]

To ask biologists to define when human life begins, as the US Congress did in 1981, is as philosophically unreasonable as to ask an astronomer to look for the Pearly Gates with a telescope. It should be no more surprising to find an abortion clinic in a city where a substantial number of people believe abortion to be wrong than it is to find a church, a mosque and a synagogue in the same city, all of which express profoundly different spiritual interpretations of the observable world in which we live.

A basic human freedom

The ability to control one's own fertility gives to each individual a major degree of freedom and choice, greater than is provided by any other aspect of health care. Effective contraception not only allows choice to the individual but also provides many positive factors in community health.

Unplanned pregnancies are most common in young women and in older women who already have what they had hoped was their completed family. Pregnancy and childbirth are particularly dangerous to the very young and to older women who have borne many children. Avoidance of unwanted pregnancy is therefore an important aspect of maternal health. Equally important is the fact that children unwantedly conceived have a higher neonatal and infant mortality. Planning and spacing of pregnancies is beneficial to mother, child and family and so to the community.

Despite the obvious need for research into fertility regulation and into its organization to make current technology more widely available, progress is limited by parsimonious investment and even available methods are often misunderstood by physicians as well as by potential users.

In order to progress, family planning, involving as it does complex interactions with so many aspects of private and public life and its adequate but still clumsy technology, needs to be approached with realism and pragmatism. However, as with anything else connected with sex, it arouses strong emotional reactions and prejudices in legislators and doctors as well as in the public at large and rigid absolutist attitudes obstruct rational assessment.

Contraceptive practice is most likely to assume its rightful role in the world if its advantages are carefully defined and its colourful but destructively controversial history is understood. The availability of fertility regulation is still too often limited by community attitudes which uphold the status quo in relation to reproductive and sexual behaviour, blocking access to contraception and sterilization and commonly proving intolerant of abortion. Such attitudes have already wasted important decades. With the current explosion in the world's population there is no historical reason to believe that we can avoid the return of famine, war and pestilence to restore the imbalance between births and deaths, yet we spend over US $100 *per capita* per year for every man, woman and child on the planet for military purposes but only 25 cents per person per year on family planning.

Family planning is an essentially democratic enterprise. The freedom to determine family size, like the other great human freedoms, is one used responsibly by individuals. The aggregate of individual decisions concerning fertility regulation can be as good as, and sometimes better than, society's expertise.

Democracy and demography have the same linguistic root and for many people the right of access to contraception may be even more important than the right of access to the ballot box.

References

1 The history of contraception

1 Allbutt, A. H. (1886). *The Wife's Handbook: How a Woman Should Order Herself During Pregnancy . . . With Hints . . . on Other Matters of Importance, Necessary to be Known by Married Women.* London.
2 Baker, J. R. (1935) *The Chemical Control of Contraception.* London: Chapman and Hall.
3 Baker J. R. (1962). Personal communication.
4 Brown H. & Leech, M. (1920). *Anthony Comstock Roundsman of the Lord.* London.
5 Carleton, H. M & Phelps, H. J. (1933). Birth control Studies III. Experimental Observations on the Grafenberg Ring Contraceptive Methods. *Journal of Obstetrics and Gynaecology of the British Empire,* **40**, 81.
6 Charles, E. (1932) *The Practice of Birth Control.* London.
7 Comstock, A. (1880). *Frauds Exposed, How the People Are Deceived and Robbed, and Youth Corrupted.* New York: Patterson Smith.
8 Contraceptive Handbill (1823) Form B. *To the Married of Both Sexes in Genteel Life.* Place Collection, **61**, pt 11. British Museum, London.
9 Cronin, A. J. (1937). *The Citadel.* London: Gollancz.
10 Darwin, C. (1871). *The Descent of Man.* London.
11 Douglas, E. T. (1969) *Margaret Sanger· Pioneer of the Future* New York. Holt, Rinehart and Winston.
12 Fryer, P. (1965). *The Birth Controllers.* London. Secker and Warburg.
13 Hall, R. *Marie Stopes.* London· Virago
14 Harrison, R (1900) General Practitioners and family planning in Sheffield. *Lancet,* **1,** 1275
15 Florence, L. S. (1930). *Birth Control on Trial.* London.
16 Houghton, V. (1962). The International Planned Parenthood Federation (IPPF). *Eugenics Review,* **53**, 149 and 201
17 Jaffe, F. S., Dryfoos, J. G. & Corey, N. (1973). Organised family planning programs in the U.S 1968–1972. *Family Planning Perspectives,* **5**, 73.
18 Knowlton, C. (1937). *Fruits of Philosophy or Private Companion of Adult People,* ed. N. E. Himes. Mount Vernon, New York.
19 Ladurie, E. Le Roy. (1979). *Montaillou The Promised Land of Error.* New York· Vintage Books.
20 Committee of the Malthusian League (1913) *Hygienic Methods of Family Limitation.* London.

21 Memorandum to the Ministry of Health, June 1957
22 Murphy, F. X. (1981). Catholic perspectives on population issues. *Population Bulletin*, **36**, 1.
23 National Birth Rate Commission (1927). *Medical Aspects of Contraception*.
24 Owen, R. D. (1831). *Moral Physiology or, a Brief and Plain Treatise on the Population Question*, 3rd edn. New York.
25 Potts M. (1982). History of Contraception. In *Gynecology and Obstetrics*, vol. 6, ed. J. J. Sciarra, G. I. Zatuchni & M. J. Daly, ch. 8, p. 1 Philadelphia, Pennsylvania. Harper and Row.
26 *Practitioner*, July 1923.
27 Quaife G. R (1979). *Wanton Wenches and Wayward Wives Peasants and Illicit Sex in Early Seventeenth Century England* London· Croom Helm
28 Russell, B. & Russell P. (1937). *The Amberley Papers*. London. Allen and Unwin
29 Sigerist, H. (1950). *History of Medicine*, Vol 1. New York Oxford University Press.
30 Simms, M. (1977). Birth Control in the 20s. *World Medicine*, April, P. 67
31 Society for the Provision of Birth Control Clinics (SPBCC) Annual Report (1927–28). London.
32 Stopes, M. C. (1918). *Wise Parenthood A Sequel to 'Married Love'. A Book for Married People*. London· Putnam and Co
33 Stopes, M. C. (1918). *Married Love. A New Contribution to the Solution of Sex Difficulties*. London. Putnam and Co.
34 Suitters, B. (1973). *Be Brave and Angry Chronicles of the International Planned Parenthood Federation* (IPPF) London: IPPF.
35 Temkin, O (1956). *Soranus' Gynaecology*. Baltimore, Maryland.
36 Queen Victoria. Letter to the King of the Belgians, 5 January 1841. In *The Letters of Queen Victoria, A Selection from Her Majesty's Correspondence between the years 1837 and 1861*, Vol. 1, ed. A. C Benson and Viscount Esher, p. 321. London: John Murray (1907).
37 Ward, A M. (1969). Family Planning clinics in Sheffield. *Journal of Biosocial Science*, **1**, 207.
38 Watson, F. (1950). *Dawson of Penn*. London.

2 Patterns of family planning

1 Banks, J. A. (1954). *Prosperity and Parenthood*. London· Routledge and Kegan Paul.
2 Caldwell, J. & Caldwell, P. (1977). The role of marital sexual abstinence in determining fertility. a study of the Yoruba in Nigeria. *Population Studies*, **31**, 193
3 Chandrasekhar, S. (1981). *'A Dirty Filthy Book'*. Berkeley, California: University of California Press
4 Christopher, E. (1980). *Sexuality and Birth Control in Social and Community Work*. London. Temple Smith
5 David, H. P. (1970). *Family Planning and Abortion in the Socialist Countries of Central and Eastern Europe*. New York Population Council
6 Davies, H J. (1971). *Intrauterine Devices for Contraception*. Baltimore, Maryland. Williams and Wilkins
7 Dawson D. A., Meng, D. J. & Ridley, J C (1980). Fertility control in the United States before the contraceptive revolution. *Family Planning Perspectives*, **12**, 76
8 Eaton, J. W. & Mayer, A. J. (1953). A social biology of very high fertility

among the Hutterites· The demography of a unique population. *Human Biology*, **25**, 206.

9 Fluhmann, C. F. (1956) *The Management of Menstrual Disorders.* Philadelphia, Pennsylvania and Jordan· W. B. Saunders.

10 Friedman, R., Siew-Ean Khoo & Bondan Supraptilak (1981). Use of modern contraception in Indonesia. a challenge to the conventional wisdom. *International Family Planning Perspectives*, **7**,3

11 Frisch, R. E. (1974). A method of prediction of age of menarche from height and weight at ages 9 through 13 years. *Pediatrics*, **53**, 384.

12 Frisch R. E., Wyshak G. & Vincent, L. (1980). Delayed menarche and amenorrhea in ballet dancers. *New England Journal of Medicine*, **303**, 17.

13 Frommer, D. J. (1964). Changing age of the menopause. *British Medical Journal*, ii, 349.

14 Glass, D. V. & Eversley, D E. C. (1965). *Population in History*. London: Edward Arnold.

15 Howell, N. (1971). *Demography of the Dobe !Kung*. New York· Academic Press

16 Innes, J. W. (1938). *Class Fertility Trends in England and Wales 1876–1934*. Princeton, New Jersey Princeton University Press.

17 Lesthaeghe, R. J. (1977). *The Decline of Belgian Fertility. 1890–1970*. Princeton, New Jersey· Princeton University Press

18 Lewis-Faning, E. (Ed.) (1949). *Family Limitation and its Influence on Human Fertility in the Past Fifty Years*. London: Her Majesty's Stationery Office (HMSO)

19 Manvell, R (1976). *The Trial of Annie Besant and Charles Bradlaugh*. New York. Hayden Press

20 McLaren, A. (1978). *Birth Control in Nineteenth Century England* London: Croom Helm.

21 Mohr, J. C. (1978). *Abortion in America*. Oxford Oxford University Press.

22 Parish, T. M. (1935). A thousand cases of abortion. *Journal of Obstetrics and Gynaecology of the British Empire*, **42**, 1107.

23 Parkes, A. S. (1976) *Patterns of Sexuality and Reproduction*. Oxford: Oxford University Press.

24 Peel, J (1962). Contraception and the medical profession. *Population Studies*, **18**, 133

25 Peel, J. (1966). The Hull Survey. I. The survey couples. *Journal of Biosocial Science*, **2**,1.

26 Potts, M. & Bhiwandiwala, P. (Eds) (1979). *Birth Control: an International Assessment*. Lancaster, England MTP Press

27 Potts, M., Diggory, P. & Peel, J. (1977). *Abortion*. Cambridge: Cambridge University Press

28 Potts M. & Selman, P. (1979). *Society and Fertility* Plymouth, England: Macdonald and Evans.

29 Rainwater, L. (1960) *And the Poor Get Children*. Chicago: Quadrangle Books.

30 Rowntree, G. & Pierce, R. M (1961). Birth Control in Britain. Part 1. *Population Studies*, **15**,3. Part 2. *Population Studies*, **15**,121.

31 *Royal Commission on Population (1949) Report* London: HMSO.

32 Taylor, C., Neuman, J. & Kelly, N. (1976). The child survival survival hypothesis. *Population Studies*, **30**, 263.

33 van de Walle, E. & Knodel, J. (1980). Europe's fertility transition· New evidence and lessons for today's developing world. *Population Bulletin*, **34**, 1.

34 Webb, S. (1906). *The Declining Birth Rate*. London: Fabian Society.

35 Whelpton, P. K. & Kiser, C. V. (1946). *Social and Psychological Factors Affecting Fertility*, 5 vols. New York: Millbank Memorial Fund.

36 Wrigley, E. A. (1969). *Population and History*. London. Weidenfeld and Nicolson.
37 Yaukay, A. (1961). *Fertility Differences in a Modernising Country*. Princeton, New Jersey: Princeton University Press

3 The population explosion

1 Altman, D. & Piotrow, P. T. (1978). Community based commercial contraceptive distribution *Population Reports*, Series J, 19.
2 The Fourth Conference of the Asian Parasite Control Organization (1977). Tokyo *Proceedings of the Asian Parasite Control Organisation.*
3 Barney, F. A. (1980). *Global 2000 Report to the President of the US*. New York· Pergamon Press.
4 Council on Environmental Quality (1981). *Global Future Time to Act.* Washington, D.C.· US Department of State.
5 International Fertility Research Program (1981). *Surgical Family Planning Methods. the Role of the Private Physician*. Research Triangle Park, North Carolina: International Fertility Research Program (IFRP).
6 Pi-chao Chen (1981). *Rural Health and Birth Planning in China*. Research Triangle Park, North Carolina: IFRP.
7 Potts, M (1982). Contraceptive needs of the developing world. In *Reproduction in Mammals*, ed. C. R. Austin & R. V Short, Book 5. Cambridge: Cambridge University Press.
8 Potts, M. & Bhiwandiwala, P. (1979). *Birth Control an International Assessment*. Lancaster, England: MTP Press
9 Potts, M. & Selman, P. (1979). *Society and Fertility*. Plymouth, England: McDonald and Evans.
10 Simon, J. L. (1977). *The Economics of Population Growth*. Princeton, New Jersey: Princeton University Press.
11 Simon, J. L. (1981). *The Ultimate Resource* Princeton, New Jersey: Princeton University Press.
12 Viravaidya, M. & Potts, M. (1979) Involving the community. Thailand. In *Birth Control. an International Assessment*, ed. M. Potts & P. Bhiwandiwala. Lancaster, England: MTP Press.

4 The safety and effectiveness of contraceptive methods

1 Atkinson, C , Schearer, S. B., Harkavy, O. & Lincoln, R. (1980). Prospects for improved contraception. *Family Planning Perspectives*, 12, 173.
2 British Standards Institute (1966). BS 4028.
3 British Standards Institute (1979). BS 3074.
4 Butts, H. A. (1972). Legal requirements for condoms under the Federal Food, Drug and Cosmetic Act. In *The Condom. Increasing Utilization in the United States*, ed. M. H. Redford, G. W Duncan & D. J. Prager, p. 202. San Francisco: San Francisco Press.
5 Center for Disease Control, Atlanta, Georgia (1980). Morbidity and Mortality. *Weekly Reports*, 29, (20) 229.
6 Committee on the Safety of Medicines (1972). *Carcinogenicity tests of Oral Contraceptives*. London· Her Majesty's Stationery Office (HMSO).
7 Corfman, P. & Siegel, D. (1968). Epidemiological problems associated with studies of the safety of oral contraceptives. *Journal of the American Medical Association*, 203, 148

8   Diggory, P. (1981) The long-term effects upon the child of perinatal events. In *Changing Patterns of Childbearing and Child Rearing*, ed. R. Chester, P. Diggory & M B. Sutherland, p. 23. London and New York: Academic Press.
9   Djerassi, C. (1970). Birth Control after 1984. *Science*, **169**, 941.
10 Djerassi, C. (1979). *The Politics of Contraception*. New York W. W. Morton.
11 Eckstein P., Jackson, M. C N & Millman, N. (1969) Comparison of vaginal tolerance tests of spermicidal preparations in rabbits and monkeys. *Journal of Reproduction and Fertility*, **20**, 85.
12 Engel, L., Strauchen, J. A., Chiazze, L. & Heid, M. (1980). Accuracy of death certification in an autopsied population with specific attention to malignant neoplasms and vascular disease. *American Journal of Epidemiology*, **111**. 99.
13 Greep, R. O , Koblinsky, M. A. & Jaffe, F. S. (1976) *Reproduction and Human Welfare A challenge to Research*. Cambridge, Massachusetts: MIT Press.
14 Hahn, D. W., Homm, R. E. & McKenzie, B. E. (1979). Evaluation of new vaginal contraceptives In *Vaginal Contraceptives New Developments*, ed. G. I. Zatuchni, A. J. Sobrero, J. J. Speidel & J. J Sciarra, p 234. Hagerstown, Maryland· Harper and Row.
15 Hardy, M. R. (1972). Condom Testing In *The Condom Increasing Utilization in the United States*, ed. M. H Redford, G. W. Duncan & D. J. Prager, p. 210. San Francisco: San Francisco Press.
16 Henry, L. (1961). Some data on natural fertility. *Eugenics Quarterly*, **8**, 81.
17 Hiyoshi, Y., Omae, T. & Takeshita, C. (1977). Malignant neoplasm found by autopsy in Hisayama, Japan, during the first ten years of a community study. *Journal of the National Cancer Institute*, **59**, 13.
18 Hulka, J. F. (1969). A mathematical study of contraceptive efficiency and unplanned pregnancy. *American Journal of Obstetrics and Gynecology*, **104**, 443.
19 Inman, W. H. (1970) The study of adverse reactions to drugs. *Procedures of the Royal Society of Medicine*, **63**, 1302.
20 International Fertility Research Program (1981). *Reproductive Age Mortality Surveillance (RAMOS)*. Research Triangle Park, North Carolina: International Fertility Research Program (IFRP).
21 *IPPF Medical Handbook* (1964) ed. R. Kleinman, 2nd edn. London: International Planned Parenthood Federation (IPPF).
22 James, G., Patton, R. E & Meslin, A S. (1955). Accuracy of cause of death statements on death certificates *Public Health Reports*, **70**, 39.
23 Jain, A. & Savin, I. (1977). Life table analysis of IUDs · problems and recommendations. *Studies in Family Planning*, **8**, 26.
24 Masters, W. M., Kolodny, R. C. & Johnson-Masters, V. E. (1979) *In Vivo* testing of intravaginal contraceptives. In *Vaginal Contraceptives· New Developments*, ed. G I. Zatuchni, A. J. Sobrero, J. J. Speidel & J. J. Sciarra, p. 256. Hagerstown, Maryland Harper and Row
25 Measman, M. A. & Lipworth, L. (1956) Accuracy of certification of cause of death. *Studies on Medical and Population Subjects No. 20* London HMSO.
26 Pearl, R. (1932) Contraception in 2000 women. *Human Biology*, **4**, 363.
27 Potter, R. G. & Sagi, P. C. (1962). Some procedures for estimating the sampling fluctuations in contraceptive failure rate. In *Research in Family Planning*, ed C. V Kiser, p 389. Princeton, New Jersey, Princeton University Press.
28 Potts, M. (1979). Perspectus on fertility control. *International Journal of Gynaecology and Obstetrics*, **6**, 449
29 Potts, M. & Paxman, J. (1983). *Contraceptive Testing and Distribution*. In press.

30 Quinn, J.J. (1979). Condoms' manufacturing and use. In *Vaginal Contraceptives: New Developments*, ed. G.I. Zatuchni, A.J. Sobrero, J.J. Speidel & J.J. Sciarra Hagerstown, Maryland: Harper and Row.

31 Ravenholt, R & Frederiksen, H. (1968). Numerator analysis of fertility patterns. *Public Health Reports*, **83**, 449.

32 Ross, W S. (1977). *The Life/Death Ratio*. New York: Readers Digest Press.

33 Sander, F.U. & Cramer, S.O. (1941). A practical method for testing the spermicidal action of chemical contraceptives. *Human Fertility*, **6**, 134.

34 Short, R V. & Baird, O.T (Eds.) (1976). *Contraceptives of the Future*. London: The Royal Society.

35 Stopes, M. (1925). *The First Five Thousand*. London. Putnam and Co

36 Tietze, C. & Lewit, S. (1968). Satisfactory validation of contraceptive methods: use-effectiveness and extended use-effectiveness. *Demography*, **5**, 931.

37 US Federal Register (1980) 45(241) 82016–92049.

38 Weikel, J H. & Nelson, L.W. (1977). Problems in evaluating chronic toxicity of contraceptive steroids in dogs. *Journal of Toxicology and Environmental Health*, **3**, 167.

39 Westoff, C.F., Potter, R.G. & Sagi, P.C. (1963). *The Third Child*. Princeton, New Jersey: Princeton University Press.

40 WHO (1978). *Steroidal Contraception and the Risk of Neoplasia*. Technical Report Series 619 Geneva: WHO.

5 Traditional methods

1 Bernard R. & Potts, M. (1978). Seasonality of birth in Baroda, India. *Journal of Biosocial Science*, **10**, 409

2 Cartwright, A. (1970). *Parents and Family Planning Services*. London: Routledge and Kegan Paul.

3 Deys, C M. & Potts, M. (1972). Condoms and things. In *Schering Workshop on Contraception The Masculine Gender* Advances in the Biosciences, Vol. 10, p. 287. Oxford: Pergamon Press.

4 Florence, L S. (1956). *Progress Report on Birth Control*. London.

5 Freedman, R., Whelpton, P.K. & Campbell, A.A. (1959). *Family Planning, Sterility and Population Growth*. New York: McGraw Hill.

6 Gopalaswami, R.A. (1962). Family Planning: outlook for government action in India. In *Conference on Research in Family Planning, New York, Oct. 1960*, ed. C. V. Kiser, p. 67. Princeton, New Jersey: Princeton University Press.

7 Haendly, P. (1925). Eine neve methode (endgültigen oder auch temporaren) der sterilisterung der frau (bildung einer doppelten scheide durch quere kolporrhaphia). *Zentrablat für Gynakologie*, **49**, 2404.

8 Henry, L. (1956). *Anciennes Familles Genevoises. Etudes demographiques. XVIe–XXe siecle*. Institut National d'Etudes Demographiques, Travaux et documents, no 26 Paris: Presses Universitaires de France.

9 Hollingsworth, T. H. (1957). A demographic study of the British ducal families. *Population Studies*, **11**, 4

10 Kinsey, A C., Pomeroy, W B., Martin, C E. & Gebhard, P H (1953). *Sexual Behaviour in the Human Female* Philadelphia, Pennsylvania: W. B. Saunders.

11 Lewis-Faning, E. (Ed.) (1949). *Family Limitation and its Influence on Human Fertility during the Past Fifty Years* London: Her Majesty's Stationery Office (HMSO).

12 Himes, N. (1963). *Medical History of Contraception*. New York: Gamut Press.

13 Noonan, J.T (1965). *Contraception A History of its Treatment by the Catholic Theologians and Canonists*. Cambridge, Massachusetts Harvard University Press.

14   Omran, A. R. (1972). A resume of Islam's position on family planning and abortion In *Induced Abortion a Hazard to Public Health?* Ed. I R. Nazer, P 348. Beirut· International Planned Parenthood Federation (IPPF).

15   Phadke, A. M & Marathe, S. P. (1966). Scotal suspenders and male infertility. *Indian Practitioner*, p. 739.

16   Pi-chao Chen (1981). *Rural Health and Birth Planning in China*. Research Triangle Park, North Carolina· International Fertility Research Program (IFRP).

17   Potts, M. (1967) Abortion in Eastern Europe. *Eugenic's Review*, **60**, 232

18   Potts, M (1972). Coitus interruptus In *Clinical Proceedings of the First International Planned Parenthood Federation S.E. Asia and Oceania Regional Medical and Scientific Congress*, p. 241 Sydney, Australia: Australian and New Zealand Journal of Obstetrics and Gynaecology.

19   Robinson, D. & Rock, J. (1967). Intrascrotal hyperthermia induced by scrotal insulation: effect on spermatogenesis. *Obstetrics and Gynaecology*, **29**, 217

20   Sinha, J N. (1955). *All India Conference on Family Planning, Lucknow, 2 Jan. 1955*. Bombay· Family Planning Association of India.

21   Stone, A. & Himes, N E. (1938). *Practical guide to Birth Control Methods*. New York. Viking Press.

22   Stycos, J. M. & Back, K. W. (1955) *The Family and Population Control*. Chapel Hill, North Carolina: University of North Carolina.

23   Westoff, C. F. (1953). In *Social and Psychological Factors affecting Fertility*, ed. P. K. Whelpton & C. V. Kiser, Vol. 3. New York: Millbank Memorial Fund.

24   Wislocki, E. (1933). Locations of testes and body temperature. *Quarterly Review of Biology*, **8**, 385 and 748.

25   Wrigley, E. A. (1969) *Population and History*. London· Weidenfeld and Nicolson.

6   Contraception and lactation

1   Campodonico, I., Guerrero, B. & Landa, L. (1981). Effect of a low-dose oral contraceptive (150 mcg levonorgestrel and 30 mcg ethinyloestradiol) on lactation. *Clinical Therapeutics*, **1**, 454.

2   Cronin, T. J (1968) Influence of lactation upon ovulation *Lancet*, ii, 422.

3   Cunningham, A. S. (1979). Morbidity in breast-fed and artificially fed infants. *Journal of Pediatrics*, **95**, 685.

4   Delvoye, P., Delogne-Desnoeck, J. & Robin, C. (1980). Hyperprolactinaemia during prolonged lactation, evidence for anovulatory cycles and inadequate corpus lutem. *Clinical Endocrinology*, **13**, 243.

5   Dusitsin, N., Chompootaweep, S. & Tankeyoon, M. (1977). The effect of postpartum tubal ligation on breast-feeding. VI Asian Congress of Obstetrics and Gynaecology. Bangkok, Thailand.

6   Guiloff. E., Ibarra-Polo, A., Zanartu, J., Toscanini, C., Mischler, T. W. & Gomez-Rogers, C. (1974). Effects of contraception on lactation. *American Journal of Obstetrics and Gynecology*, **118**, 42

7   Hoffman, S. L , Chowdhury, A. K. M. A. & Sykes, Z. M. (1980). Lactation and fertility in rural Bangladesh. *Population Studies*, **34**, 337.

8   Howie, P. W.. McNeilly, A. S., Houston, M. J., Cook, A. & Boyle, H. (1981). Effect of supplementary food on suckling patterns and ovarian activity during lactation. *British Medical Journal*, **283**, 757.

9   Jain, A. K & Bongaarts, J. (1981). Breast-feeding: patterns, correlates, and fertility effects. *Studies in Family Planning*, **12**, 79.

10   Janowitz, B , Lewis, J. H., Parnell, A , Hefnau, F., Younis, M. N. & Setout, C A. (1981). Breast feeding and child survival in Egypt *Journal of Biosocial Science*, **13**, 287

11   Jelliffe, D B & Jelliffe, E. F. P. (1978). *Human Milk in the Modern World.* Oxford Oxford University Press.

12   Jordan, B. (1978). *Birth in Four Cultures.* Montreal. Edan Press.

13   Kaern T (1967) Effect of an oral contraceptive immediately postpartum on inhibition of lactation *British Medical Journal*, iii, 644

14   Kamal, I., Hefnawi, F , Ghoneim, M., Talaat, M., Younis, N., Tagui, A. & Abdalla, M. (1969) Clinical biochemical and experimental studies on lactation. II Clinical effects of gestagens on lactation *American Journal of Obstetrics and Gynecology*, **105**, 324

15   Klaus, M. H. & Diaz-Rossello, J (1980). Breast feeding 1980. *Pediatrics in Review*, **1**, 289.

16   Knodel, J. & Debavalya, N (1980). Breast-feeding in Thailand Trends and differentials, 1969–79. *Studies in Family Planning*, **11**, 355

17   Knodel, J. & van de Walle, E (1967). Breast-feeding, fertility and infant mortality· an analysis of some early German data. *Population Studies*, **21**, 109.

18   Konner, M. & Worthman, C. (1980). Nursing frequency, gonadal function and birth spacing among !Kung hunter–gatherers. *Science*, **207**, 788.

19   Lean, T H (1967). Optimum insertion time for IUD after delivery. In *Proceedings of the 8th International Conference of IPPF*. Santiago· International Planned Parenthood Federation.

20   McCann, M F & Laskin, L. S (1981) Breast-feeding, fertility and family planning. *Population Reports*, series J, 527.

21   McNeilly, A. S. (1979) Effects of lactation on fertility. *British Medical Bulletin*, **35**, 151.

22   Montagu, A. (1979). Breast-feeding and its relationship to morphological, behavioural and psychocultural development. In *Breast-feeding and Food Policy in a Hungry World*, ed. D. Raphael, p. 189 New York. Academic Press.

23   Nilsson, S. & Nygren, K. G. (1980). Debate on the use of hormonal contraceptives during lactation. *Research in Reproduction*, **12**, 1.

24   Potter, R G., Kobrin, F. E. & Langsten, R. L. (1979). Evaluating acceptance strategies for timing of postpartum contraception. *Studies in Family Planning*, **10**, 151.

25   Potts, M. & Whitehorn, E (1980). Contraception and the lactating woman. In *Research Frontiers on Fertility Regulation*, ed. G. I Zatuchni, M. H. Labbock & J J. Sciarra, p. 117 Hagerstown, Maryland· Harper and Row

26   Rogers, B. (1978). Feeding in infancy and later ability and attainment: a longitudinal study. *Developmental Medicine and Child Neurology*, **20**, 421.

27   Short, R. V. (1979) Lactation – the central control of reproduction. In *Breast-feeding and the Mother. Ciba Foundation Symposium*, **45**, 179.

28   Sosa, R., Kennell, J. H., Klaus, M. & Urrutia, J J (1979). The effect of early mother–infant contact in breast-feeding, infection and growth In *Breast-feeding and the Mother. Ciba Foundation Symposium*, **45**, 179.

29   Tietze, C. (1966). Contraception with intra-uterine devices. 1959–1966. *American Journal of Obstetrics and Gynecology*, **96**, 1043.

30   Tyson, J. E., Perez, A & Zanartu, J. (1976). Human lactational response to oral thyrotropin releasing hormone *Journal of Clinical Endocrinology and Metabolism*, **43**, 760.

31   Tyson, J. E. (1977). Neuroendocrine control of lactational infertility. In *Fertility Regulation During Human Lactation*, ed. A. S. Parkes, A. M. Thomson, M. Potts & M. A. Herbertson. (*Journal–Biosocial Science Supplement*, **4**, 23.)

32   Walker, W A. & Isselbacher, K.J. (1977) Intestinal antibodies. *Physiology in Medicine*, **297**, 767.
32   Whitehead, R G. & Prentice, A. M. (1981). Food supplements and breast milk output. *Lancet*, i, 667.
34   Wing, J.P. (1977) Human versus cow's milk in infant nutrition and health *Current Problems in Pediatrics*, **8**, 1.

7   Periodic abstinence

1   Berger, G.J. (1980). Medical risks associated with 'natural' family planning. *Advances in Planned Parenthood*, **15**, 1.
2   Billings, E.L , Brown, J. B., Billings, J.J & Burger, H.G. (1972). Symptoms and hormonal changes accompanying ovulation *Lancet*, i, 282
3   Billings, J.J. (1970). *The Ovulation Method*. Melbourne, Australia Advocate Press.
4   Blandau, R.J. (Ed.) (1975). *Aging Gametes Their Biology and Pathology*. Proceedings of the International Symposium on Aging Gametes, Seattle, Washington, 13–16 June 1973 Basel: S. Karger.
5   Bomsel-Helmreich, O. (1976). The aging of gametes, heteroploidy, and embryonic death. *International Journal of Gynaecology and Obstetrics*. **14**, 98.
6   de Bethune, A.J. (1963). Child spacing. the mathematical probabilities. *Science*, **142**, 1629.
7   Dorairaj, K. (1981) *Fertility Control in India Natural Family Planning as an Alternative Strategy*. New Delhi, India: Indian Social Institute.
8   Ferin, J., Thomas, K. & Johnson, E. D. B. (1973). Ovulation detection. In *Human Reproduction Conception and Contraception*, ed. E. S. E. Hafez & T. N. Evans, p. 260. Hagerstown, Maryland: Harper and Row.
9   Freedman, R , Whelpton, P. K. & Campbell, A. A. (1959). *Family Planning, Sterility and Population Growth*. New York· McGraw Hill.
10   German, J (1968) Mongolism, delayed fertilization and human sexual behaviour. *Nature*, **217**, 516.
11   Grady, W. R , Hirsch, M B., Keen, N & Vaughn, B (1970–76). Differentials in contraceptive use failure among married women aged 15–44 years: United States Washington, DC, duplicated paper
12   Guerrero, V. & Rojas, D I. (1975) Spontaneous abortion and aging of human ova and spermatozoa. *New England Journal of Medicine*, **293**, 573.
13   Guerrero, R (1978). The Aging of gametes. the known and the unknown *Linacre Quarterly*, **45**, 345.
14   Guy, F & Guy, M. (1973). The Mauritius program. In *Proceedings of a Research Conference on Natural Family Planning*, ed. W. A. Uricchio & M. K. Williams, p. 239. Washington, DC Human Life Foundation.
15   Hartman, C. G (1962). *Science and the Safe Period a Compendium of Human Reproduction* Baltimore, Maryland: Williams and Wilkins
16   Himes, H E. (1963) *Medical History of Contraception* New York Gamut Press
17   Iffy, L. & Wingate, M B (1970). Risks of rhythm method of birth control *Journal of Reproductive Medicine*, **5**, 11.
18   Iffy, L. (1979). Myths and facts about the etiology of ectopic pregnancy. In *New Techniques and Concepts in Maternal and Fetal Medicine*, ed. H. A. Kaminetzky & L. Iffy, p 78. New York von Nostrand Reinhold.
19   Jaramillo-Gomez, M. & Londono, J. B. (1968). Rhythm: a hazardous contraceptive method *Demography*, **5**, 433.

20 Jongbloet, P. H (1971). *Mental and Physical Handicaps in Connection with Overripeness Ovopathy.* Leiden, The Netherlands H E Stenfert Kroese N. V.

21 Jongbloet, P. H. (1970) The intriguing phenomenon of gamethopathy and its disastrous effects on human progeny *Maandschrift voor Kindergeneesk*, **37**, 261.

22 Jongbloet, P. H (1975). The effects of preovulatory overripeness of human eggs on development seasonality of birth In *Aging Gametes Their Biology and Pathology* ed R J Blandau, p. 300. International Sympsosium on Aging Gametes, Seattle, Washington. Basel S Karger.

23 Jongbloet, P H & Van Erkelens-Zwets, J H J (1978). Rhythm methods: are there risks to the progeny? In *Risks, Benefits and Controversies in Fertility Control*, ed. J J. Sciarra, G. I. Zatuchni & J J Speidel, p. 520. Hagerstown, Maryland Harper and Row.

24 Kippley, J. & Kippley, S (1975). *The Art of Natural Family Planning.* Cincinnati, Ohio: Couple to Couple League

25 Klaus, H. (1982) Natural family planning a review *Obstetrical and Gynaecological Survey*, **37**, 128.

26 Klaus, J., Goebel, J. M , Muraski, B , Egizio, M. T., Weitzel, D , Taylor, R. S , Flagan, M. U , Flagan, E. K , Flagan, K & Hobday, K (1979). Use effectiveness and client satisfaction in six centres teaching the Billings Ovulation Method. *Contraception*, **19**, 613.

27 Knaus, H. (1929). Die periodische Frucht-und Unfruchtbarkeit des Weibes. (Periodic fertility and infertility in women) *Zentralblatt für Gynakologie*, **53**, 2193.

28 Lasken, L. (1981) Periodic abstinence: How well do new approaches work? *Population Reports*, Series **I**, 1.

29 Latz, L. J (1934). *The Rhythm of Sterility and Fertility in Women.* 4th edn. Latz Foundation. Chicago

30 Uricchio, W A & Williams, M K (Eds) (1973). *Proceedings of a Research Conference on Natural Family Planning* Washington, DC. Human Life Foundation.

31 Marshall, J. (1968). A field trial of the basal-body-temperature method of regulating births *Lancet*, ii, 8.

32 Marshall, J (1976). Cervical mucus and basal-body-temperature method of regulating births field trial *Lancet*, ii, 282

33 Marshall, J. (1968) Congenital defects and the age of spermatozoa. *International Journal of Fertility*, **13**, 110.

34 Mastroianni, L. (1974). Rhythm Systematized chance taking *Family Planning Perspectives*, **6**, 209.

35 Medina, J. E , Cinfuentes, A. & Delgado, C (1980). Acceptance of natural family planning methods in Colombia. Presented at International Federation for Family Life Promotion Second International Congress, Navan, Ireland. 24 Sept –1 Oct. 1980

36 Naggan, L. & MacMahon, B. (1967) Ethnic differences in the prevalence of anencephaly and spina bifida in Boston, Massachusetts. *New England Journal of Medicine*, **277**, 119.

37 Noonan, J. T. (1965). *Contraception a History of its Treatment by the Catholic Theologians and Canonists* Cambridge, Massachusetts· Harvard University Press.

38 Oechsli, F. W. (1976). Studies of the consequences of contraceptive failure. final report. University of California (duplicated paper)

39 Ogino, K. Ovulationstermin und Konzeptionstermin. (Ovulation day and conception day) *Zentralblatt für Gynakologie*, **54**, 464

40   Poltawska, W. (1980). The effect of the contraceptive attitude on marriage. *International Review of Natural Family Planning*, **4**, 187

41   Rowntree, G & Pierce, R. (1961). Birth Control in Britain Part 1 *Population Studies*, **15**, 3. Birth control in Britain Part 2. *Population Studies*, **15**, 121.

42   Seguy, J & Simmonet, J (1933). Recherche de signes directs d'ovulation chez la femme. (Research on direct signs of ovulation in women) *Gynecologie et Obstetrique*, **28**, 756.

43   Short, R V (1977) The discovery of the ovaries In *The Ovary*, Vol 1, ed. S. Zuckerman. San Francisco. Academic Press.

44   Squire, W (1868). *Puerperal temperatures Transactions of the Obstetrical Society, London*, **9**, 129

45   Thibault, C (1970). Normal and abnormal fertilization in mammals *Advances in the Biosciences*, **6**, 63

46   Tietze, C , Poliakoff, S.R. & Rock, J. (1951). The clinical effectiveness of the rhythm method of contraception. *Fertility and Sterility*, **2**, 440.

47   Treloar, A. A. (1972). Variations in the human menstrual cycle. *Proceedings of a Research Conference on Natural Family Planning*, ed. W. A. Urichio & M. K. Williams, p. 32 Washington, DC The Human Life Foundation.

48   Udry, J. R. (1968) Coital frequency, delayed fertilization and outcome of pregnancy. *Nature*, **219**, 618.

49   Van de Velde, T H. (1905). *Uber den Zusammenhang Zwischen Ovarialfunction, Wellenbewegung und Menstrualblutung und uber die Entstehung des sogenannten Mittelschmerzes.* (On the relationship between ovarian function, periodicity and menstrual flow, and on the origins of the so-called Mittelschmerz) Haarlem, The Netherlands. F Bohn.

50   Vickers, A. E. (1969) Delayed fertilization and chromosomal abnormalities in mouse embryos. *Journal of Reproduction and Fertility*, **20**, 69.

51   Welch, J P. (1968) Down's syndrome and human behaviour *Nature*, **219**, 506.

52   World Health Organization (1981) A prospective multicenter trial of the ovulation method of natural family planning. 1. The teaching phase. *Fertility and Sterility*, **36**, 152.

8   The condom

1   Ajax, L. (1972) How to market a nonmedical contraceptive: a case study from Sweden. In *The Condom Increasing Utilization in the United States*, ed. M. H. Redford, G W Duncan & D. Prager, p 50. San Francisco: San Francisco Press.

2   Altman, D & Piotrow, P (1980). Social marketing does it work. *Population Reports*, Series **J**, 21.

3   Arnold, C. (1973). A condom distribution program for adolescent males. In *Readings in Family Planning A challenge to Health Professionals*, ed. D. McCallister. St Louis, Missouri: C. V. Mosby.

4   Barlow, D. (1977) The condom and gonorrhoea. *Lancet*, **ii**, 811.

5   Bauman, K. E. & Udry, J R. (1972). Contraception in an urban Negro sample. *Journal of Marriage and the Family*, **34**, 115.

6   Bernstein, E L (1940). Who was Condom? *Human Fertility*, **5**, 172.

7   Black, T. R. L. & Harvey, P. D. (1976). A report on a contraceptive social marketing experiment in rural Kenya. *Studies in Family Planning*, **7**, 101.

8   Boswell, J. (1950) *Boswell's London Journal, 1762–1763*. London· Yale Edition.

9   Coleman, S. (1981) The cultural context of condom use in Japan. *Studies in Family Planning*, **12**, 28.

10 Deys, C M. & Potts, D M. (1972). Condoms and things. *Advances in the Biosciences*, **10**, 287.

11 Debhanom Muangman (1978) *Report on measurement of Thai male genital sizes and recommendation for appropriate condom usage.* Mahidal University, Bangkok: Faculty of Public Health

12 Dingwall, E. J (1953) Early contraceptive sheaths. *British Medical Journal*, I, 40

13 Eugenic Protection Law (of Japan) (1949). Article III, para. 4.

14 Finkel, M L. & Finkel, D. J. (1975) Sexual and contraceptive attitudes and behaviour of male adolescents. *Family Planning Perspectives*, **7**, 256.

15 Fisher, M (1963). A local authority contraceptive clinic: a survey of its effectiveness *Medical Officer*, **110**, 175–80.

16 Gjorjov, A. N. (1976) *Barrier Contraception and Breast Cancer.* Basel, Switzerland: S. Karger.

17 Glass, R , Vessey, M & Wiggins, P. (1974). Use-effectiveness of the condom in a selected family planning clinic population in the United Kingdom. *Contraception*, **10**, 591.

18 Harvey, P D. (1972). Condoms in America. In *The Condom, Increasing Utilization in the United States*, ed. M. H. Redford, G. W Duncan & D. J. Prager. San Francisco. San Francisco Press.

19 Himes, N. (1963). *Medical History of Contraception.* New York Gamut.

20 Kane, F J., Lachenbruch P. A , Lokey, L., Chafetz N., Auman, R., Pocuis, L. & Lipton, M. A. (1971). Motivational factors affecting contraceptive use. *American Journal of Gynecology and Obstetrics*, **110**, 1050.

21 Koyama, I & Oato, N. (1972). Condom use in Japan. In *The Condom. Increasing Utilization in the United States*, ed M. H Redford, G. W. Duncan & D J Prager San Francisco: San Francisco Press

22 Lack, S G. (1975) Innovative approach to male family planning. a success story American Public Health Association meeting, Chicago (duplicated paper)

23 Levin, H (1968) Commercial distribution of contraceptives in developing countries: past, present and future *Demography*, **5**, 941

24 Louis, T & Ciszewski, R (1979) Social marketing – Sri Lanka and Bangladesh In *Birth Control An International Assessment*, ed M. Potts & P. Bhiwandiwala Lancaster, England MTP Press

25 Rattner, H (1925). Dermatitis of the penis from rubber *Journal of the American Medical Association*, **105**, 1189.

26 Rowntree, G & Pierce, R. M (1961). Birth control in Britain, Part 1. *Population Studies*, **15**, 3. Birth control in Britain, Part II. *Population Studies*, **15**, 121

27 Lamont, J M (1972) Fish with rubber bands Scottish Fisheries Bulletin. June, p. 17. In *The Condom Increasing Utilization in the United States*, ed. M. H. Redford, G W. Duncan & D. J. Prager. San Francisco: San Francisco Press.

28 Peberdy, M (1965). Domiciliary family planning In *Biosocial Aspects of Social Problems*, ed. J E. Meade & A S. Parkes. New York. Plenum.

29 Peel, J. (1972) The Hull family survey II. Family planning in the first five years of marriage. *Journal of Biosocial Science*, **4**, 333.

30 Potts, M & McDavitt, J. (1975). A spermicidally lubricated condom *Contraception*, **11**, 701.

31   Potts, M (1973) The glorious Japanese condom *World Medicine*, 7 March, p 27.

32   Quinn, J J. (1979) Condoms: manufacturing perspectives and use In *Vaginal Contraceptives, New Developments*, ed. G. I. Zatuchni, A. J. Sobrero, J. J Speidel & J. J. Sciarra, p. 66. Maryland Harper and Row.

33   *The Machine* (1744). London.

34   Tietze, C (1970) Relative effectiveness In *Manual of Family Planning and Contraceptive Practice*, ed M. S. Calderone, p. 268. Baltimore, Maryland Williams and Wilkins

35   US Department of Health and Human Sciences (1980). Contraceptive efficacy among married women aged 15–44 United States. National Center for Health Statistics *Vital and Health Statistics*, Series **23**, no 5

36   Voge, C I B (1933) *The Chemistry and Physics of Contraception*. London: Cape.

37   Westoff, C. F., Potter, R G , Sagi, P C. & Mischler, E. G. (1961). *Family Growth in Metropolitan America*, p. 38. Princeton, New Jersey· Princeton University Press

38   Westoff, C. F., Herrera, L F. & Whelpton, P. K. (1953). Social and psychological factors affecting fertility *Milbank Memorial Fund Quarterly*, **31**, 291

39   Whelpton, P. K., Campbell, A A. & Patterson, J. E. (1966) *Fertility and Family Planning in the United States* Princeton, New Jersey: Princeton University Press.

9 Vaginal contraceptives: chemical and barrier

1   Arnuwatra Limsuwan, Somboon Vachrotai, Surakaiti Achananuparp & Manaswi Unhanantha (1978). A Clinical trial of a vaginal preparation regimen for the prophylaxis of gonorrhea. *Journal of the Medical Association of Thailand*, **62**, 435

2   Austin, C. R. & Short, R. V (Eds.) (1982). *Reproduction in Mannals, vol 1. Germ Cells and Fertilization*. Cambridge: Cambridge University Press.

3   Begum, S. F , Liao, W C., McCann, M F & Ahmad, N. (1980) A clinical trial of Neo Sampoon vaginal contraceptive tablet *Contraception*, **22**, 573

4   Berger, G. S , Keith, L. & Moss, W (1975). Prevalence of gonorrhoea among women using various methods of contraception *British Journal of Venereal Diseases*, **51**, 307

5   Casanova, J. (1725–1798) *The Memoirs of Jacques Casanova de Seingalt*. London Navarre Edition, 1922.

6   Coleman, S J. (1979) Spermicides – simplicity and safety are major assets. *Population Reports*, Series **H**, 79.

7   Cole, C H., Lacher, T G , Bailey, J C & Fairclough, D L (1980). Vaginal chemoprophylaxis in the reduction of reinfection in women with gonorrhoea. *British Journal of Venereal Diseases*, **56**, 314.

8   Cutler, J C & Singh, B (1982) Demonstration of a spirocheticidal effect by chemical contraceptives in *Treponema pallidum. Bulletin of the Pan American Health Organization*, **16**, 59

9   Edelman, D. A & Thompson, S (1982) Vaginal contraception – an update. *Contraceptive Delivery Systems*, **3**, 75

10   FDA Panel (1980) Vaginal contraception and other vaginal drug products for over-the-counter human use. *Federal Register*, **45**, no 241, p 82016

11   Finch, B. E (1963). Balls, feathers and caps. In *Contraception Through the Ages*, ed B E Finch & H. Green, p 38 Springfield, Illinois: Charles C Thomas

12   Hardy, N R. & Wood, C (1972). Vaginal contraception. In *New Concepts in Contraception*, ed. M Potts & C Wood, p 103. Lancaster, England. Medical and Technical Publishing (now MTP Press)

13   Harris, R. W. C., Brinton, L. A., Cowdell, R M., Skegy, D. C G, Smith, P. G., Vessey, M. P. & Doll, Sir Richard (1980). Characteristics of women with dysplasia or carcinoma in situ of the cervix uteri. *British Journal of Cancer*, **42**, 359.

14   Jick, H., Walker, A M , Rothman, K J , Hunter, J. R., Holmes, L B., Watkins, R. N., D'Ewart, D. C , Danford, A. & Madeen, S. (1981) Vaginal spermicides and congenital disorders *Journal of the American Medical Association*, **245**, 1329

15   Kelaghan, J., Rubin, G. L , Ory, H W & Layde, P. M. (1982) Barrier method contraceptives and pelvic inflammatory disease. *Journal of the American Medical Association*, **248**, 184

16   Keown, K. K. (1977) Historical perspectives on intravaginal contraceptive sponges *Contraception*, **16**, 1.

17   Keith, L., Berger, G. S. & Jackson, M. A (1981). Vaginal contraceptive methods *Current Problems in Obstetrics and Gynecology*, **4**, 1.

18   LaFitte, F. (1963). *Family Planning in the Sixties*. Birmingham, England: British Pregnancy Advisory Service

19   Lee, T. Y., Utidjian, H M D , Singh, B., Carpenter, U. & Cutler, J. C. (1972). The potential impact of chemical prophylaxis on the incidence of gonorrhoea *British Journal of Venereal Diseases*, **48**, 376.

20   Lee, R. U., Dillon, W. P. & Bachler, E (1982). Barrier contraceptives and toxic shock syndrome. *Lancet*, 1, 221.

21   Mann, T (1964). *Biochemistry of Semen and the Male Reproductive Tract*. London· Methuen

22   Melamed, M R., Koss, L G , Flehinger, B J , Kelisky, R P & Dubrow, H. (1969). Prevalence rates of uterine cervical carcinoma in situ for women using the diaphragm or contraceptive oral steroids. *British Medical Journal*, iii, 195.

23   Mensinga, D. M (1882). *Fakultative Sterilate*. Leipzig

24   Newson, J. & Newson, E (1963). *Patterns of Infant Care in an Urban Community* Harmondsworth, Middlesex· Penguin Books Ltd.

25   Peel, J (1963) The manufacture and retailing of contraceptives in England. *Population Studies*, **17**, 113

26   Pierce, R. M. & Rowntree, (1961). Birth control in Britain, Part 2. *Population Studies*, **15**, 121.

27   Potts, M. (1979) The importance of vaginal contraception. In *Vaginal Contraceptives New Developments*, ed G. I. Zatuchni, A. J. Sobrero, J. J. Speidel & J J Sciarra, P 347. Hagerstown, Maryland Harper and Row.

28   Pratt, W F., Grady, W R , Menken, J A. & Trussel, J (1979). An overview of experience with vaginal contraceptives in the United States In *Vaginal Contraceptives New Developments*, ed. G. I Zatuchni, A J. Sobrero, J J. Speidel & J J Sciarra, p 82. Hagerstown, Maryland Harper and Row

29   Raabe, N. & Frankman, O (1975) C-Film as a contraceptive. *British Medical Journal*, iv, 286

30   Rendon, A I , Covarrubias, J , McCarney, K E , Marion-Landais, G. & Luna de Villar, J (1980) A controlled, comparative study of phenylmercuric acetate, nonoxynol-9 and placebo vaginal suppositories as prophylactic agents against gonorrhea *Current Therapeutic Research*, **27**, 780

31   Rock, J , Barker, R. H. & Bacon, W B (1947) Vaginal absorption of
     penicillin. *Science*, **105**, 13

32   Schell, W. B. & Wolff, H H (1981) Ultrastructure of human spermatozoa in
     the presence of the spermicide nonoxynol-9 and a vaginal contraceptive
     containing nonoxynol-9 *Andrologia*, **13**, 42.

33   Shelton, J. D. & Higgins, J E (1981) Contraception and toxic-shock
     syndrome. a reanalysis. *Contraception*, **24**, 631

34   Sobrero, A (1979) Spermicidal agents: effectiveness, use and testing. In
     Vaginal Contraceptives New Developments, ed. G. I. Zatuchni., A J. Sobrero,
     J J. Speidel & J J Sciarra Hagerstown, Maryland Harper and Row.

35   Stim, E M (1980) The nonspermicide fit-free diaphragm method· a new
     contraceptive method *Advances in Planned Parenthood*, **15**, 88

36   Stopes, M. (1961). *Birth Control Today*, 12th edn. London. Hogarth Press.

37   Tatum, H. J. & Connell, E. B. (1981). Barrier contraception: a comprehensive
     review. *Fertility and Sterility*, **38**, 1

38   Terris, M. & Dalmann, M C. (1960) Carcinoma of the cervix· an
     epidemiologic study. *Journal of the American Medical Association*, **174**, 1847

39   Tietze, C., Lehfeldt, H. & Liebman, H G (1953) The effectiveness of cervical
     caps, a contraceptive method *American Journal of Obstetrics and Gynecology*,
     66, 904.

40   Tietze, C. & Lewitt, S (1967). Comparison of 3 contraceptive methods.
     diaphragm with jelly or cream, vaginal foam and jelly/cream alone *Journal of
     Sex Research*, **3**, 295.

41   Vessey, M. P. & Wiggins, P. (1974). Use-effectiveness of the diaphragm in a
     selected family planning clinic population in the United Kingdom.
     Contraception, **9**, 15.

42   Vessey, M P., Doll, R., Peto, R , Johnson, B & Wiggins, P. (1976). A long-
     term follow-up study of women using different methods of contraception – an
     interim report. *Journal of Biosocial Science*, **8**, 373.

43   Wortman, J (1976). The diaphragm and other intravaginal barriers *Population
     Reports*, Series **H**, 57

44   Wilde, F A (1838). Das weibliche Gebar-Unvermogen· Eine medicinisch-
     juridische Abhandlung Zum Gebrauch fur practische Geburtshelfer, Aerzte,
     und Juristen.

45   Zaneveld, L J. D. (1976). Sperm enzyme inhibitors as antifertility agents. In
     Human Semen and Fertility Regulation in Men, ed. E S E. Hafez, p. 570. St
     Louis, Missouri. C. V. Mosby

10   Steroidal contraceptives

1   Ablin, J., Vittek, J. & Gordon, G G (1973) On the mechanism of the
     antiandrogenic effect of medroxyprogesterone acetate. *Endocrinology*, **93**, 417

2   Adadevoh, B K. & Dade, O. A. (1977). Contraception and
     hemoglobinopathies in Ibadan, Nigeria. an evaluation of the effect on
     anaemia. *Tropical Geography and Medicine*, **29**, 77.

3   Adams, D. B., Gold, A. R. & Burt, A. D. (1978). Rise in female sexual activity
     at ovulation blocked by oral contraceptives. *New England Journal of Medicine*,
     229, 1145.

4   Adams, P. W., Godsland, I , Melrose, J., Niththyananthan, R., Oakley, N. W.,
     Seed, M. & Wynn, V. (1980). The influence of oral contraceptive formulation
     on carbohydrate and lipid metabolism. *Journal of Pharmacotherapy*, **3**, 54.

5 Albright, F (1945). Disorders of the female gonads. In *Internal Medicine its Theory and Practice*, ed J. M. Musser, p. 959 Philadelphia, Pennsylvania Lea and Febiger

6 Ambrus, J L., Gillette, M , Nolan, C , Jung, O , Regallo-Spavento, S., Spavento, P., Novick, A , Suchetzbky, C & Ambrus, C M. (1981) Estrogens and endometrial cancer. *Journal of Medicine Clinical, Experimental and Theoretical*, **12**, 81

7 Anonymous (1981) OCs have minimal effect on gallbladder disease *Contraceptive Technology Update*, ii, 105.

8 Antunes, C M F , Stolley, P D , Rosenshein, N. B., Davis, J C., Tonascia, J A., Brown, C , Burnett, L , Rutledge, A , Pokempner, M & Garcia, R (1979). Endometrial cancer and oestrogen use. *New England Journal of Medicine*, **300**, 9

9 Applesweig, N (1973) The development of systemic contraceptives. In *Response to Contraception*, ed. M. Roland Philadelphia, Pennsylvania: W B. Saunders.

10 Armed Forces Institute of Pathology, Hepatic Branch and Center for Disease Control, Bureau of Epidemiology, Family Planning Evaluation Division (1977) Increased risk of hepatocellular adenoma in women with long term use of oral contraceptives. *Morbidity and Mortality Weekly Report*, **26**, 293.

11 Bacon, J F & Shenfield, G. M. (1980) Pregnancy attributed to interaction between tetracycline and oral contraceptives *British Medical Journal*, **280**, 293.

12 Bain, C W W., Rosner, B , Speizer, F. E , Belanger, C. & Hennekens, C M (1981). Early age at first birth and decreased risk of breast cancer. *American Journal of Epidemiology*, **114**, 705.

13 Bancroft, J. (1980). Human sexual behaviour. In *Reproduction in Mammals*, vol. 8, Human Sexuality, ed C. R Austin & R V. Short Cambridge Cambridge University Press

14 Bancroft, J , Davidson, D W , Warner, P. & Tyrer, C (1980) Androgens and sexual behaviour in women using oral contraceptives *Clinical Endocrinology*, **12**, 327.

15 Bartlemez, G. W., Corner, G W. & Hartman, C G. (1951). Cycle changes in the endometrium of the rhesus monkey (*Macaca mulatta*) *Contribution to Embryology, Carnegie Institute*, **34**, 99.

16 Barnes, R. W., Krapf, T , Hoak, J C. (1978). Erroneous clincial diagnosis of leg vein thrombosis in women on oral contraceptives *Obstetrics and Gynecology*, **51**, 556

17 Beard, J. (1897) *The Span of Gestation and the Cause of Birth*. Jena, Germany.

18 Beck, L R , Pope, V Z., Cowsar, D R , Lewis, D H. & Tice, T R (1980) Evaluation of a new three month injectable contraceptive microsphere system in primates (baboon) *Contraceptive Delivery Systems*, **1**, 79

19 Beck, L R , Ramos, R A , Flowers, C E., Lopez, G Z., Lewis, D. H. & Cowsar, D. R (1981). Clinical evaluation of injectable biodegradable contraceptive system. *American Journal of Obstetrics and Gynecology*, **140**, 799.

20 Belsey, M. A , Russell, Y & Kinnear, K. (1979). Cardiovascular disease and oral contraceptives: a reappraisal of vital statistics data. *International Family Planning Perspectives*, **5**, 2.

21 Benagiano, G (1977) Long-acting systemic contraceptives. In *Regulation of Human Fertility*, ed E. Diczfalusy, p 323 Proceedings of a World Health Organization Symposium. Copenhagen: Scriptor.

22 Benagiano, G. (1977) Multinational clinical evaluation of two long-acting injectable steroids norethisterone enanthate and medroxyprogesterone acetate *Contraception*, **15**, 513.

23   Benagiano, G & Fraser, I. S. (1981). The Depo-Provera debate commentary on the article 'Depo-Provera a critical analysis' *Contraception*, **24**, 493.

24   Benagiano, G & Goldzeiher, J W. (1979). Effects of contraception on progeny *Reviews in Perinatal Medicine*, iii, 115.

25   Bennion, L. J , Ginsberg, R. L., Garnick, M. B. & Bennett, P H. (1976). Effects of oral contraceptives on the gall bladder bile of normal women *New England Journal of Medicine*, **294**, 189

26   Beral, V & Colwell, L. (1980). Randomised trial of high doses of stilboestrol and ethisterone in pregnancy long-term follow-up of mothers *British Medical Journal*, **281**, 1098.

27   Beral, V , Ramcharan, S. & Faris, R (1977). Malignant melanoma and oral contraceptive use among women in California. *British Journal of Cancer*, **36**, 804

28   Berger, G. S., Edelman, D. A. & Talwar, P P (1979) The probability of side effects with Orval, Norinyl 450 and Norlestrin. *Contraception*, **20**, 447

29   Bergsjjo, P , Langeren, M. & Aas, T (1974). Tubal pregnancies and women using progestogen-only contraceptives. *Acts Obstetrica et Gynecologica Scandinavica*, **53**, 377

30   Berkowitz, R S., Goldstern, D P , Marean, A. R. & Bernstein, M. (1981) Oral contraceptives and postmolar trophoblast disease. *Obstetrics and Gynecology*, **58**, 474.

31   Bishun, N. P. (1976). Chromosomes and oral contraceptives. *Proceedings of The Royal Society of Medicine*, **69**, 353.

32   Black, M. M , Barday, T M C , Cutler, S. J., Mankey, B. F. & Asire, A. J. (1972). Association of atypical characteristics of benign breast lesions with subsequent risk of breast cancer. *Cancer*, **29**, 338.

33   Boston Collaborative Drug Surveillance Programme (1973) Oral contraceptives and venous thromboembolic disease, surgically confirmed gall bladder disease, and breast tumour *Lancet*, i, 1399

34   Bottiger, L. E., Boman, G , Ekland, G & Westerholm, B. (1980). Oral contraceptives and thromboembolic disease effects of lowering oestrogen content. *Lancet* i, 1097

35   Boyce, J C., Lu, T., Nelson, J. H & Furchter, R. G (1977). Oral contraceptives and cervical cancer. *American Journal of Obstetrics and Gynecology*, **128**, 761.

36   Bracken, M. B. (1979). Oral contraception and twinning an epidemiological study *American Journal of Obstetrics and Gynecology*, **133**, 432

37   Bracken, M B , Holford, T. R , White, C. & Kelsey, T. L. (1978). Role of oral contraception in congenital malformations of offspring *International Journal of Epidemiology*, **7**, 309.

38   Bracken, M. B. & Holford, T R (1981) Exposure to prescribed drugs in pregnancy and association with congenital malformations. *Obstetrics and Gynecology*, **58**, 336

39   Bradley, D. P., Wingerd, J., Petitti, D B , Krauss, R M & Ramcharan, S. (1978) Serum high-density-lipoprotein cholesterol in women using oral contraceptives, oestrogens and progestins. *New England Journal of Medicine*, **299**, 17.

40   Brain, M. G , Harris, J. J. & Winsor, W (1971). Hypertension, oral contraceptive agents and conjugated oestrogen. *Journal of Internal Medicine*, **74**, 13.

41   Breckenridge, A M , Back, D J & Orme, M (1979) Interactions between oral contraceptives and other drugs. *Pharmacology and Therapeutics*, **7**, 617.

42   Briggs, M. H. & Briggs, M (1979) Plasma lipoprotein changes during oral contraception *Current Medical Research Opinion*, **6**, 249

43   Briggs, M H. & Briggs, M A (1980). A randomized study of metabolic effects of four oral contraceptive preparations containing levonorgestrel plus ethinyloestradiol in different regimens In *The Development of a New Triphasic Oral Contraceptive*, ed. R. B Greenblatt, p 79, Lancaster, England MTP Press

44   *British Medical Journal* (Editorial) (1976) Amenorrhoea after oral contraception, ii, 660.

45   *British Medical Journal* (Editorial) (1980) Drug interaction with oral contraceptive steroids. **281**, 93

46   *British Medical Journal* (Editorial) (1973) Hair loss and oral contraception ii, 499

47   *British Medical Journal* (Editorial) (1978). Small-bowel ischaemia and the contraceptive pill, i, 4.

48   *British Medical Journal* (Editorial) (1972) The pill and porphyria ii, 603

49   Brooks, G G. (1974) Anaphylactic shock with medroxyprogesterone acetate A case report. *Journal of Louisiana State Medical Society*, **125**, 397.

50   Buell, P (1973). Changing incidence of breast cancer in Japanese-American women *Journal of the National Cancer Institute*, **51**, 1479

51   Bye, P G T & Elstein, M (1973) Clinical assessment of a low-estrogen combined oral contraceptive *British Medical Journal*, ii, 389.

52   Candy, J & Abell, M R (1968) Progestogen-induced adenomatous hyperplasia of the uterine cervix *Journal of the American Medical Association*, **203**, 85

53   Carr, D M. (1967). Chromosomes after oral contraceptives. *Lancet*, ii, 830.

54   Cartwright, A (1970) *Patients and Family Planning Services*. London Routledge and Kegan Paul

55   Casagrande, J T., Pike, M. C , Ross, R K., Louie, E. W., Rey, S & Henderson, B E (1979). Increased ovulation and ovarian cancer. *Lancet*, ii, 170

56   Chez, R A (1978) Proceedings of the Symposium 'Progesterone, progestins and fetal development' *Fertility and Sterility*, **30**, 16

57   Choudhury, R R , Chompootaweep, S & Dusitsin, N. (1977) The release of prolactin by medroxyprogesterone acetate in human subjects *British Journal of Pharmacology*, **59**, 433

58   Christiansen, R E (1980) The relationship between maternal smoking and the incidence of congenital anomalies. *American Journal of Epidemiology*, **112**, 684.

59   Christopher, E (1980). *Sexuality and Birth Control in Social and Community Work* London Temple Smith

60   Chumnijarakij, T & Poshyachinda, V (1975). Postoperative thrombosis in Tahi women *Lancet*, i, 1357

61   Cohen, C J , Deppe, G & Bruckner, H. W. (1977) Treatment of advanced adenocarcinoma of the endometrium with melphalan, 5 fluorouracil and medroxyprogesterone acetate A preliminary study *Obstetrics and Gynecology*, **50**, 145

62   Collaborative Group for the Study of Stroke in Young Women (1973) Oral contraception and increased risk of cerebral ischemia or thrombosis *New England Journal of Medicine*, **288**, 871

63   Collette, M J A., Linthorst, G & Waard, F (1978) Cervical carcinoma and the pill. *Lancet*, i, 441

64   Committee on the Safety of Medicines (1972) *Carcinogenicity of Oral Contraceptives*, p 23 London Her Majesty's Stationery Office (HMSO)
65   Coulam, C B , Annegers, J F , Abboud, C F , Laws, E R & Kurland, L. T (1979) Pituitary adenoma and oral contraceptives *Fertility and Sterility*, **31**, 25
66   Coutinho, E , Diaz, S , Croxatto, M B , Nielsen, N C , Sandez, F A , Segal, S & Nash, M (1978). Contraception with long-acting subdermal implants. I. An effective and acceptable modality in international clinical trials II. Measured and perceived effects in international clinical trials. *Contraception*, **18**, 315
67   Coutinho, E. M & De Souza, J C. (1966) Conception control by monthly injections of medroxyprogesterone suspension and a long-acting oestrogen. *Journal of Reproductive Fertility*, **15**, 209
68   Crawford, F E (1981) The effect of cigarette smoking on plasma concentrates of oral contraceptive steroids *British Journal of Clinical Pharmacology*, **11**, 638
69   Crawford, J. S (1973). Respiratory distress syndrome. *Lancet*, i, 858.
70   Currie, J N & Billings, J. J (1980). Strokes and contraceptive medication *The Medical Journal of Australia*, January 25, p. 58.
71   Czeizel, A (1980) Are contraceptive pills teratogenic? *Acta Morphologica Academiae Scientiarum Hungaricae*, **28**, 177
72   Dabancens, A , Prado, R , Larraguibel, R. & Zanartu, J. (1974). Intraepithelial cervical neoplasm in women using intrauterine devices and long acting injectable progestogens as contraceptives *American Journal of Obstetrics and Gynecology*, **119**, 1052
73   Dahlberg, K (1982) Some effects of depo-medroxyprogesterone acetate (DMPA) observations in the nursing infant and long-term use *International Journal of Gynaecology and Obstetrics*, **20**, 43
74   Dalton, K (1964) *The Premenstrual Syndrome*. London William Heineman
75   Dam, R R , Huerta, H A., Valenzuela, F L., de Mier, M A., de Monarrez G C , Cisneros, E O , Macias, M Z. & Perkin, G W. (1979). Use and acceptance of the 'paper pill' A novel approach to contraception. *Contraception*, **19**, 273
76   Dao, T L , Morreal, C , Nerroto, T (1973) Urinary estrogen excretion in men with breast cancer *New England Journal of Medicine*, **289**, 138
77   de Ceulaer, K , Gruber, C , Heyes, R & Serjeant, G. R. (1982) Medroxyprogesterone acetate and homozygous sickle cell disease *Lancet*, ii, 229
78   de Jager, E (1982) A new progestogen for oral contraception *Contraceptive Delivery Systems*, **3**, 11
79   Demacker, P N. M , Schade, R. W B., Stalenhoef, A F. H. & Stuyt, P. M. J. (1982). Influence of contraceptive pill and menstrual cycle on serum lipids and high-density lipoprotein cholesterol concentrations *British Medical Journal*, **284**, 1213.
80   Dhal, K., Kumar, N , Rastogi, G K. & Devi, P. K (1977). Short term effects of norethisterone enanthate and medroxyprogesterone acetate on glucose, insulin, growth hormone and lipids. *Fertility and Sterility*, **28**, 156.
81   Djerassi, C. (1973). Steroidal contraceptives in the People's Republic of China. *New England Journal of Medicine*, **289**, 533.
82   Djerassi, C. (1976) Manufacture of steroidal contraceptives technical versus political aspects. *Proceedings of the Royal Society*, B, **195**, 175
83   Donde, V. M & Virkav, K. D (1975). Biochemical studies with once-a-month contraceptive pill containing quinestrol and quinestanol acetate. *Contraception*, **11**, 681.

84 Drill, V A (1966). *Oral Contraceptives* Toronto McGraw Hill.
85 Dubrow, H., Melamed, M. R , Flehinger, B J., Kelisky, R P & Koss, L. J (1969). A study of the factors affecting a choice of contraceptive. *Obstetrical and Gynecological Survey*, **24**, 1012.
86 Edmondson, H. A , Henderson, B. E & Benton, B (1976) Liver-cell adenomas and oral contraceptives. *New England Journal of Medicine*, **294**, 1064.
87 Edmondson, M A , Reynolds, T B , Anderson, B & Benton, B. (1977). Regression of liver cell adenoma associated with oral contraceptives. *Annals of Internal Medicine*, **86**, 180
88 Esquirel, A & Laufe, L E (1968) Conception control by a single monthly injection. *Obstetrics and Gynecology*, **31**, 636.
89 Evans, D A , Hennekens, C H , Miao, L , Laughlin, L W , Chapman, W. G , Rosner, B., Taylor, J. O. & Kass, E. H. (1978). Oral contraceptive use and bacilluria in a community based study. *New England Journal of Medicine*, **299**, 536
90 Evrard, J. R , Buxton, B M. & Erikson, D (1976). Amenorrhea following oral contraception *American Journal of Obstetrics and Gynecology*, **124**, 88
91 Fasal, E & Paffenbarger, R. S. (1975) Oral contraceptives as related to cancer and benign lesions of the breast. *Journal of the National Cancer Institute*, **55**, 767.
92 Faundes, A , Hardy, E., Reyes, Q., Pastene, L. & Portes-Carrasco, R. (1981). Acceptability of the contraceptive vaginal ring by rural and urban populations in two Latin American countries. *Contraception*, **24**, 393.
93 Ferenczy, A (1978). How progestogens effect endometrial hyperplasia and neoplasia. *Contemporary Obstetrics and Gynecology*, **11**, 137.
94 Fisch, I R , Freedman, S M. & Myatt, A. V (1972). Oral contraceptives, pregnancy and blood pressure *Journal of the American Medical Association*, **222**, 1507.
95 Foster, H W. (1981). Contraceptives in sickle cell disease. *Southern Medical Journal*, **76**, 543.
96 Frank, D W , Kirton, K T. & Murchison, T. E. (1979). Mammary tumours and serum hormones in the bitch treated with medroxyprogesterone acetate or progesterone for four years. *Fertility and Sterility*, **31**, 340.
97 Fraser, I S. & Weisberg, E (1981). A comprehensive review of injectable contraception with special emphasis on depo medroxyprogesterone acetate *The Medical Journal of Australia*, i, 3.
98 Frederiksen, H. & Ravenholt, R. T (1970). Thromboembolism, oral contraceptives and cigarettes. *Public Health Reports*, **85**, 197.
99 Fries, H. & Nillius, S. T. (1973). Dieting, anorexia nervosa and amenorrhoea after oral contraceptive treatment. *Acta Psychiatrica Scandinavica*, **49**, 669.
100 Fuertes de la Haba, A (1973). Changing patterns in cervical cytology among oral and nonoral contraceptive users *Journal of Reproductive Medicine*, **10**, 3.
101 Gambrell, D., Massey, F. M.; Castaneda, T. A. & Buddie, A. W. (1979). Breast cancer and oral contraceptive therapy in premenopausal women. *Journal of Reproductive Medicine*, **23**, 265.
102 Garcia, C. R., Goldzieher, J. W. & Massey, J. B. (1973). Oral Contraceptives. In *Human Reproduction Conception and Contraception*, ed. E. S. E. Hafez & T. N. Evans, p. 335. Hagerstown, Maryland: Harper and Row.
103 Gellman, V. (1964). *Manitoba Medical Review*, **44**, 104
104 Giosis, M. & Cavalli, P. (1963). The effect on the female foetus of prolonged treatment with 6-methyl-17 hydroxyprogesterone acetate (MPA) during pregnancy. *Panminerva Medica*, **5**, 107
105 Goldzieher, J W. (1973). The evaluation of clinical and therapeutic

information. In *Human Reproduction Conception and Contraception*, ed.
E S E Hafez & T N Evans, p 607 Hagerstown, Maryland Harper and
Row.

106 Goldzieher, J. W , Moses, L E , Averkin, E., Sched, C. & Taber, B. Z. (1971).
A placebo-controlled double-blind crossover investigation on the side effects
attributed to oral contraceptives. *Fertility and Sterility*, **22**, 609.

107 Goldzieher, J. W. (1978) Research on the safety of oral contraceptives in
developing countries. Duplicated report of Southwest Foundation for Research
and Education, San Antonio, Texas.

108 Graf, K. J. & El Etreby, M F (1979) Endocrinology of reproduction in the
female beagle dog and its significance in mammary gland tumour genesis. *Acta
Endocrinology*, **222**, Supplement 1.

109 Grant, A. (1973). Postpill anovulation. *International Journal of Fertility*, **18**, 44.

110 Green, G. R & Sartwell, P E. (1972). Oral contraceptive use in patients with
thromboembolism following surgery, trauma or infection *American Journal of
Public Health*, **62**, 680

111 Greenberg, G (1975). Hormonal pregnancy tests and congenital
malformations *British Medical Journal*, ii, 191.

112 Greenspan, A. R., Hatcher, R A , Moore, M , Rosenberg, M. J & Ory, H. W.
(1980) The association of depo-medroxyprogesterone acetate and breast
cancer. *Contraception*, **21**, 563

113 Grounds, M (1974). Anovulants thrombosis and other associated changes.
Medical Journal of Australia, ii, 440.

114 Guiloff, E., Berman, E., Montiglio, A , Osorio, R. & Lloyd, C. (1970). Clinical
study of a once-a-month oral contraceptive quinestrol–quinestanol. *Fertility
and Sterility*, **21**, 110

115 Haberlandt, L (1921) Uber hormonale Sterilisierung des Weiblichen
Tierkorpers. *Munch Med Woschenschr*, **68**, 1577

116 Haberlandt, L. (1931) *Die hormonale Sterilisierung des Weiblichen* Organismus
Thesis, Jena, Germany Fischer.

117 Harlap, S. & Davies, A. M. (1978) *The Pill and Births the Jerusalem Study.
Final Report*, 219 pp US Department of Health, Education and Welfare
Bethesda, Maryland. National Institute of Child Health and Development
(NICHD), Center for Population Research.

118 Harlap, S , Davies, A M. & Baras, M (1981) Complications of pregnancy
and labor in former oral contraceptive users. *Contraception*, **24**, 1.

119 Haspels, A A (1976). Interception: post-coital estrogens in 3016 women.
Contraception, **14**, 375.

120 Hassain, A. A. (1981) Nasal absorption of natural contraceptive steroids in
rats – progesterone absorption. *Journal of Pharmacological Science*, **20**, 466

121 Heinonen, O P , Slone, D , Monson, R R., Hook, E. B. & Shapiro, S (1977).
Cardiovascular birth defects and antenatal exposure to the female sex
hormones *New England Journal of Medicine*, **296**, 67

122 Herbst, A A (1974) Clear cell adenocarcinoma of the vagina and cervix in
girls analysis of 170 registry cases *American Journal of Obstetrics and
Gynecology*, **119**, 713

123 Hines, D C & Goldzieher, J W (1969). Clinical investigation a guide to its
evaluation. *American Journal of Obstetrics and Gynecology*, **105**, 450.

124 Hoppe, G (1977) A new hormonal combination as a treatment for women
with signs of virilisation like acne, seborrhea and hirsutism VII *Asian
Congress of Obstetrics and Gynecology, Bangkok*, p 268

125 Hoover, R., Gray, L A , Cole, P. & MacMahon, B (1976) Menopausal
estrogens and breast cancer *New England Journal of Medicine*, **295**, 401.

126 Horwitz, R. I., Horwitz, S. M., Feinstein, A. R & Robboy, S J. (1981).
     Necropsy diagnosis of endometrial cancer and detection bias in case-control
     studies. *Lancet*, ii, 66.
127 Hoyle, M., Kennedy, A., Prior, A. L. & Thomas, G. E. (1977). Small bowel
     ischaemia and infarction in young women taking contraceptives and
     progestational agents. *British Journal of Surgery*, **64**, 533.
128 Huber, D. M., Kahn, A. R. & Brown, K. (1980). Oral and injectable
     contraceptives· effects on breast milk and child growth in Bangladesh. In
     Research Frontiers in Fertility Regulation, ed G. I. Zatuchni, p 127
     Hagerstown, Maryland Harper and Row
129 Huber, S. C , Huber, D A., Khan, A R., Chakraborty, J., Chowdhury, A. Y.,
     Rahman, M & Chowdhury, A I (1980) Oral contraceptives and family health
     in Bangladesh. *International Journal of Gynaecology and Obstetrics*, **18**, 268.
130 Hull, M. G. R., Savage, P. E., Bromham, D. R., Jackson, J. A. M. & Jacobs,
     H S. (1981) Normal fertility in women with post-pill amenorrhea *Lancet*, i,
     1329.
131 Ing, R., Ho, J. M. C. & Petrakis, M. L (1977) Unilateral breast-feeding and
     breast cancer. *Lancet*, ii, 124.
132 Inman, W. H. W. (1979). Oral contraceptives and fatal subarachnoid
     haemorrhage. *British Medical Journal*, ii, 1468.
133 Inman, W. H. W., Vessey, M. P., Westerholm, B. & Engelund, A. (1970).
     Thromboembolic disease and steroidal content of oral contraceptives. *British
     Medical Journal*, ii, 203.
134 International Fertility Research Program (1980). RAMOS (Reproductive Age
     Mortality Surveillance) Research Triangle Park, North Carolina: IFRP
135 Irey, N. S , Manion, W. C. & Taylor, H. B. (1970). Vascular lesions in women
     taking oral contraceptives *Archives of Pathology*, **89**, 1.
136 Jain, A. (1976). Cigarette smoking, use of oral contraceptives and myocardial
     infarction. *American Journal of Obstetrics and Gynecology*, **126**, 301.
137 Janerich, D T , Dugan, J M , Standfast, S. J. & Strite, L. (1977). Congenital
     heart disease and prenatal exposure to exogenous sex hormones. *British
     Medical Journal*, i, 1058.
138 Jeffcoate, T. N. A., Miller, J , Ross, R F. & Tindall, V R. (1968). Puerperal
     thromboembolism in relation to the inhibition of lactation by oestrogen
     therapy. *British Medical Journal*, iv, 19
139 Jennett, W B & Cross, J N. (1967). Influence of pregnancy and oral
     contraception on the incidence of stroke in women of child-bearing age
     Lancet, i. 1019.
140 Jick, H., Walker, A. M , Watkins, R. N., D'Ewart, D., Hunter, J R., Danford,
     A , Madsen, S , Dinan, B J & Rothman, K. J. (1980). Oral contraceptives and
     breast cancer *American Journal of Epidemiology*, **112**, 577
141 Jones, E. F., Beniger, J. R. & Westoff, C F. (1980). Pill and IUD
     discontinuation in the United States, 1970–1975. the influence of the media.
     Family Planning Perspectives, **12**, 293
142 Jordan, W. M. (1961) Pulmonary embolism *Lancet*, ii, 1146.
143 Joshi, J. U., Joshi, U. M , Sankolli, G M. & Saxena, B N. (1980). A study of
     interaction of a low-dose combination oral contraceptive with anti-tubercular
     drugs *Contraception*, **21**, 617.
144 Karim, M., Ammar, A & El Mahgoug, S. 1971). Injected progestogen and
     lactation *British Medical Journal*, i, 200.
145 Kass, H (1960) Hormones and host resistance to infection *Bacteriological
     Review*, **24**, 177
146 Kaufman, D W , Shapiro, D., Slone, C , Rosenberg, L , Miettinen, O. S ,

Stolley, P. D., Knapp, R. C , Leavitt, T., Watrang, W. G , Rosemchein, M B., Lewis, J. L , Schottenfelt, D & Ingel, R. L (1980). Decreased risk of endometrial cancer among oral contraceptive users. *New England Journal of Medicine*, **303**, 1045.

147   Kay, C. R. (1980) The happiness pill? *Journal of the Royal College of General Practitioners*, **30**, 8

148   Kay, C R., Smith, A & Richards, B. (1969) Smoking habits of oral contraceptives users. *Lancet*, ii, 228.

149   Kelsey, J L., Molford, T. R., White, C , Mayer, E. S., Kitly, S. E. & Acheson, R. M (1978). Oral contraceptives and breast disease an epidemiologic study *American Journal of Epidemiology*, **10**, 236

150   Kent, D. R (1981). Oral contraceptives and hepatic vein thrombosis *Journal of Reproductive Medicine*, **26**, 21.

151   Kent, D. R., Nissen, E D. & Nissen, S. E. (1977). Liver tumours and oral contraceptives. *International Journal of Obstetrics and Gynaecology*, **15**, 137

152   Khoo, S. K. & Correy, J F (1981) Contraception and the "high risk" woman. *The Medical Journal of Australia*, i, 61.

153   Kistner, R. W. (1959) Histological effects of progestogens on hyperplasia and carcinoma in situ of the endometrium. *Cancer*, **12**, 1106.

154   Klarsen, D. J., Rapp, E F. & Hirte, W. E (1976) Response to medroxyprogesterone acetate as a secondary hormone therapy for metastatic breast cancer in postmenopausal women. *Cancer Treatment Report*, **60**, 25.

155   Kleinman, R. L. (Ed.) (1974). *Family Planning Handbook for Doctors*. London: International Planned Parenthood Federation (IPPF).

156   Klinger, H. P., Glasser, M & Kava, H. W. (1976). Contraceptives and the conceptus. 1. Chromosome abnormalities of the fetus and neonate related to maternal contraceptive history. *Obstetrics and Gynecology*, **48**, 40.

157   Koetsawang, S (1977). Injected long-acting medroxyprogesterone acetate· Effect on human lactation and concentrations in milk. *Journal of the Medical Association of Thailand*, **60**, 57

158   Koetsawang, S (1980). Management of abnormal bleeding with steroidal contraceptives. In *Steroidal Contraception and Mechanisms of Endometrial Bleeding*, ed. E Diczfalusy, I. S. Fraser & F T G Webb, p. 50. Geneva: World Health Organization.

159   Lachnit-Fixson, U. (1980). Clinical investigation with a new triphasic oral. In *The Development of a New Triphasic Oral Contraceptive*, ed. R. B. Greenblatt, p 99. Lancaster, England· MTP Press

160   Laragh, J H., Sealey, J. E. Lidingham, J. G. G. & Newton, M. A. (1967). Oral contraceptives, renin, aldosterone and high blood pressure *Journal of the American Medical Association*, **201**, 918.

161   Lawson, D. H., Davidson, J. F. & Jick, H. (1977). Oral contraceptive use and venous thromboembolism absence of an effect of smoking. *British Medical Journal*, ii, 729

162   Lawson, D. H., Jick, H , Hunter, J. & Madsen, S (1981) Exogenous estrogens and breast cancer. *American Journal of Epidemiology*, **114**, 710.

163   Lednicer, D. (Ed.) (1970). *Contraception The Chemistry of Fertility Control*. New York· Marcel Dekker.

164   Leiman, G. (1972). Depo medroxyprogesterone acetate as a contraceptive agent–Effect on weight and blood pressure. *American Journal of Obstetrics and Gynecology*, **114**, 97.

165   Liang, A. P., Greenspan, A., Layde, P. M., Shelton, J D., Hatcher, R. A., Potts, M. & Michelson, M. J. (1983). The risk of breast, uterine corpus and ovarian cancer in women using depo-medroxyprogesterone acetate. *Journal of the American Medical Association*, **249**, 2909

166 Lindhe, J. & Bjorn, A L (1967) Influence of hormonal contraception on the gingiva of women Journal of Periodontal Research, **2**, 1
167 Lingeman, C H (1974) Etiology of cancer of the human ovary a review. *Journal of the National Cancer Institue*, **53**, 1603
168 Linos, A , Worthington, J. W., O'Fallon, W. M. & Kurland, L. T. (1978). Rheumatoid arthritis and oral contraceptives. *Lancet*, i, 871.
169 Litt, B. D (1975). Statistical review of carcinoma in situ reported among contraceptive users of Depo-Provera Memorandum of 17 June 1974, to United States Food and Drug Administration hearing on Depo-Provera 7 May 1975.
170 Loudon, N. B , Foxwell, M., Potts, D. M , Guild, A. L & Short, R. V (1977) Acceptability of an oral contraceptive that reduces the frequence of menstruation: the tri-cycle pill regimen. *British Medical Journal*, ii, 487
171 MacCorquodale, D W., Thayer, S. A. & Doisy, D. A. (1936). *Journal of Biological Chemistry*, **115**, 435
172 MacMahon, B , Cole, P., Brown, J B , Aoki, K , Lin, T M., Morgan, R W & Woo N.-C (1971) Oestrogen profiles of Asian and North American women. *Lancet*, ii, 900.
173 MacMahon, B , Cole, P & Brown, J (1973). Etiology of human breast cancer. a review *Journal of the National Cancer Institute*, **50**, 21.
174 MacMahon, B., Cole, P., Lin, T M., Lowe, C R , Merra, A P , Ravnihar, B , Salker, E. J., Valarras, V. G & Yusa, S (1970). Age at first birth and breast cancer risk. *Bulletin of the World Health Organization*, **43**, 209
175 Maine, D. (1978). Depo the debate continues. *Family Planning Perspectives*, **10**, 362.
176 Mann, J I. & Inman, W. H. W. (1975). Oral contraceptives and death from myocardial infarction. *British Medical Journal*, ii, 245
177 Mann, J. I., Doll, R , Thorogood, M., Vessey, M. P. & Water, W. E. (1976). Risk factors for myocardial infarction among young women. *British Journal of Preventive and Social Medicine*, **30**, 94
178 Mann, J I , Inman, W H. W. & Thorogood, M (1976). Oral contraceptive use in older women and fatal myocardial infarction. *British Medical Journal*, ii, 445.
179 Mann, J. I., Thorogood, M., Waters, W. E & Powell, C. (1975). Oral contraceptives and myocardial infarction in young women a further report. *British Medical Journal*, iii, 631
180 Mann, J. I., Vessey, M. P , Thorogood, M. & Doll, Sir Richard (1975) Myocardial infarction in young women with special reference to oral contraceptive practice. *British Medical Journal*, ii, 241.
181 March, C. M., Mishell, D. R. & Klitzky, O. (1979). Galactorrhea and pituitary tumors in postpill and non-postpill secondary amenorrhea. *American Journal of Obstetrics and Gynecology*, **134**, 65.
182 Markush, R E & Seigel, D G (1969) Oral contraceptives and mortality trends from thromboembolism in the United States *American Journal of Public Health*, **59**, 418
183 Matthews, P M., Millis, R R. & Haywood, J. L (1981). Breast cancer in women who have taken contraceptive steroids *British Medical Journal*, **282**, 774
184 McDaniel, E. B. & Pardthaisong, T (1973) Depo medroxyprogesterone acetate as a contraceptive agent. Return of fertility after discontinuation of use *Contraception*, **8**, 407
185 McDaniel, E B. & Potts, M (1979). Depo medroxyprogesterone acetate and endometrial carcinoma. *International Journal of Gynaecology and Obstetrics*, **17**, 297

186   McLeod, S. C. (1979). Endocrine effects of oral contraceptives. *International Journal of Gynaecology and Obstetrics*,16, 518.

187   Meade, T. W., Greenberg, G. & Thompson, S. G. (1980). Progestogens and cardiovascular reaction associated with oral contraceptives and a comparison of the safety of 50µg and 30µg oestrogen preparation. *British Medical Journal*, 280, 1157.

188   Medawar, P. B. & Hunt, R. (1978). Vulnerability of methylcholanthrene-J-induced tumours to immunity caused by syngeneric foetal cells. *Nature*, 271, 164

189   Medical Journal of Australia Leading Article (1979). Hounding the pill. ii, 206.

190   Melamed, M R., Koss, L. G., Flehinger, B. J., Kelisky, R. P. & Dubrow, H. (1969). Prevalence rates of uterine cervical carcinoma in situ for women using the diaphragm or contraceptive oral steroids. *British Medical Journal*, iii, 195.

191   Michael, R. P. & Kereme, E. B. (1968). Pheromones in the communication of sexual status in primates. *Nature*, 218, 746.

192   Millar, J H. D. (1961). The influence of pregnancy on disseminated sclerosis. *Proceedings of the Royal Society of Medicine*, 54, 4

193   Miller, P. (1981). Personal communication.

194   Min, F. H. (1981). Studies on long-acting oral contraceptives. In *Symposium on Recent Advances in Fertility Regulation*, ed C. C. Fen, D. Griffin & A. Wollman. Geneva: Atar SA.

195   Minkin, S. (1980). Depo-Provera; A critical analysis. *Women and Health*, 5, 49. New York Haworth Press

196   Mishell, D. R., Thornicroft, I. H., Nakamura, R. M., Nagata, Y. & Stone, S. G. (1973) Serum estradiol in women ingesting combination oral contraceptives. *American Journal of Obstetrics and Gynecology*, 114, 923.

197   Mishell, D R. (1976) Long-acting contraceptive formulations In *Regulation of Human Fertility*, ed. K S. Moghissi & T. N. Evans. Detroit, Michigan: Wayne State University Press

198   Mishell, D R. (1982). Noncontraceptive health benefits of oral steroidal contraceptives. *American Journal of Obstetrics and Gynecology*, 142, 809

199   Morris, N. M. & Udry, J. R. (1971). Sexual frequency and contraceptive pills. *Social Biology*, 18, 40.

200   Morrison, A S., Jick, H. & Ory, H. W. (1977). Oral contraceptives and hepatitis. A report from the Boston Collaborative Drug Surveillance Program. *Lancet*, i, 1142.

201   Muramatsu, M. (1974). Personal communication

202   Murphy, J. E. (1968) The influence of oral contraceptives on surgical attendances in general practice. *Clinical Trials Journal*, 5, 141

203   Nash, H (1975) Depo-Provera. A review. *Contraception*, 12, 377.

204   Nash, H , Robertson, D. M. & Jackanicz, T. M. (1978). Release of contraceptive steroids from sustained release dosage forms and resulting plasma levels *Contraception*, 18, 395

205   Nilsson, L. & Solvell L. (1967) Clinical Studies on Oral Contraceptives – a randomized, double-blind, crossover study of four different preparations (Anovlar, Lyndiol, Ovulen and Voledan). *Acta Obstetrica et Gynecologica Scandinavica*, 46 (Supplement 8), 1.

206   Nora, J. J & Nora, A M (1979). Cumulative evidence implicating exogenous progestogen/estrogen in birth defects. *New Techniques and Concepts in Fetal Medicine*, ed. H. A. Kaminetzky, L. Iffy & J. A. Apuzzio, p 19 London Van Nostrand Reinhold.

207   Notelovitz, M. (1981). Low-dose oral contraceptive usage and coagulation. *American Journal of Obstetrics and Gynecology*, 141, 71

208 Nudemberg, F., Kothari, M., Karam, K & Taymov, M (1973) Effects of the 'pill-a-month' on the hypothalamic-pituitary-ovarian axis *Fertility and Sterility*, **24**, 135

209 Ortiz, A , Hiroi, M & Stanczyk, F Z. (1977) Serum medroxyprogesterone acetate concentrations and ovarian function following intramuscular injection of depo medroxyprogesterone acetate *Journal of Clinical Endocrinology and Metabolism*, **44**, 32

210 Ory, H , Naib, Z , Conger, S. B., Hatcher, R A. & Tyler, C W (1976) Contraceptive choice and prevalence of cervical dysplasia and carcinoma in situ *American Journal of Obstetrics and Gynecology*, **124**, 573.

211 Ory, H W. (1974). The negative association between surgically confirmed functional ovarian cysts and use of oral contraceptives *Journal of the American Medical Association*, **228**, 68

212 Ory, H. W (1979). The health effects of fertility control In *Contraception Science, Technology and Application*, p 110 Proceedings of a Symposium Washington DC National Academy of Sciences.

213 Ory, H. W (1982) The noncontraceptive health benefits from oral contraceptive use *Family Planning Perspectives*, **14**, 182.

214 Ory, H W , Conger, S. B , Naib, Z., Tyler, C. W. & Hatcher, R. A. (1977). Preliminary analysis of oral contraceptive use and risk of developing premalignant lesions of the uterine cervix. In *Pharmacology of Steroid Contraceptive Drugs*, ed S. Garattini & H W Berendes, p 211. New York Raven Press.

215 Ory, H. W , Cole, P , MacMahon, B., Hoover, R (1976). Oral contraceptives and assessment *Family Planning Perspectives*, **12**, 278

216 Ory, M , Cole, P , MacMahon, B., Hoover, R (1976) Oral contraceptives and reduced risk of benign breast disease *New England Journal of Medicine*, **294**, 419

217 Paffenberger, R. S., Faral, E , Simmons, M E. & Kampert, J B (1977) Cancer risk as related to the use of oral contraceptives during the fertile years *Cancer*, **39**, 1887

218 Paffenberger, R. S , Kampert, J. B., Chance, H. G (1979) Oral contraceptives and breast cancer risk. In *The Regulation of Fertility Evaluation and Perspectives*, p 93 Paris Institut National de la Recherche Medicale.

219 Petitti, D. B & Wingerd, J (1978) Use of oral contraception, cigarette smoking and the risk of subarachnoid haemorrhage. *Lancet*, ii, 234

220 Pike, M C Henderson, B E , Casagrande, J T , Rosario, I & Gray, G. E. (1981) Oral contraceptive use and early abortion as risk factors for breast cancer in young women. *British Journal of Cancer*, **43**, 72.

221 Pincus, G., Garcia, C. R., Rock, J., Paniagua, M., Pendleton, A , Larrague, F , Nicholas, R , Bomo, R. & Pean, U (1959) Effectiveness of an oral contraceptive *Science*, **130**, 1981.

222 Pincus, G (1965) *The Control of Fertility* New York Academic Press.

223 Pinotti, J A , Mancusi, M H , Lima, J P R & Lane, E (1973). Alterations in the mammary glandular epithelium following the use of oral contraceptives In *Fertility and Sterility Proceedings of the Seventh World Congress*, ed. T Hasegawa, M Hayashi, F. J. G Ebling & I. W. Henderson, p. 865 Amsterdam, The Netherlands· Excerpta Medica.

224 Poller, L (1978) Oral contraceptives, blood clotting and thrombosis *British Medical Bulletin*, **34**, 151

225 *Population Reports* (1974) Oral contraceptives–50 million users. Series **A**. 1.

226 *Population Reports* (1975). Advantages of orals outweigh disadvantages Series **A** 29

227   *Population Reports* (1975) Minipill – a limited alternative for certain women. Series A, 53
228   *Population Reports* (1975) Injectables and implants Series K, 1
229   *Population Reports* (1977) Debate on oral contraceptives and neoplasia continues· answers remain elusive. Series A, 69.
230   *Population Reports* (1979). OCs – Update on usage, safety and side effects. Series A, 136
231   Porter, J , Jones, W (1981) Postcoital contraception *Medical Journal of Australia*, 1, 85
232   Potts, M , Feldblum, P. J., Chi, I-c , Liao, W & Fuertes-de La Haba, A (1982) The Puerto Rico oral contraceptive study an evaluation of the methodology and results of a feasibility study *British Journal of Family Planning*, 7, 99.
233   Pramik, M J (Ed) (1978) *Norethindrone the first three decades* Palo Alto, California Syntex
234   Pritchard, J A & Pritchard, S A (1977) Blood pressure response to estrogen–progestin oral contraceptive after pregnancy-induced hypertension. *American Journal of Obstetrics and Gynecology*, 129, 733
235   Pye, R J., Meyrick, G , Pye, M. J. & Burton, J. C. (1977). Effect of oral contraception on sebum excretion rate. *British Medical Journal*, ii, 1581
236   Ramcharan, S. (1974). *The Walnut Creek Contraceptive Drug Study Vol I.* Department of Health, Education and Welfare (DHEW) publication No. (NIH) 74-562. Bethesda, Maryland National Institute of Child Health and Human Development, Center for Population Research.
237   Ramcharan, S (1976) *The Walnut Creek Contraceptive Drug Study Vol II.* DHEW publication No (NIH) 76-563 Bethesda, Maryland National Institute of Child Health and Human Development, Center for Population Research.
238   Ramcharan, S , Pellegrin, F A , Ray, R & Hsu, J P. (1981) *The Walnut Creek Contraceptive Drug Study Vol III.* Bethesda, Maryland National Institute of Child Health and Human Development, Center for Population Research
239   Ravenholt, R. T , Kessel, E , Speidel, J J , Talwar, P P. & Levinski, M. J. (1978) A comparison of symptoms associated with the use of three oral contraceptives a double-blind crossover study of Ovral, Norinyl and Norlestrin. *Advances in Planned Parenthood*, 12, 222.
240   Report of the Joint Working Group on Oral Contraceptives. (1976) London HMSO
241   Robinson, R W (1970) Oestrogen, progestogen and combination oestrogen–progesterone effects on clotting factors. *Circulation*, 50, 22 (Supplement 3)
242   Rock, J., Pincus, G. & Garcia, C. R (1956). Effects of certain 19-norsteriods on the normal human menstrual cycle *Science*, 124, 891.
243   Rooks, R B , Ory, H W , Ishak, K G , Strauss, L T., Greenspan, J R , Hill, A P , Tyler, C. W. (1979). Epidemiology of hepatocellular adenoma the role of oral contraceptive use. *Journal of the American Medical Association*, 242, 644.
244   Rosenberg, L , Hennekens, C H , Rosner, B , Belanger, C., Rothman, K J. & Speizer, F E. (1979) Oral contraceptive use in relation to nonfatal myocardial infarction *American Journal of Epidemiology*, 111, 59
245   Rosenberg, L , Shapiro, S., Slone, D., Kaufman, D. W., Helmrich, S. P., Mieetten, O. S , Stolley, P. D , Rosenhein, N. B , Schottenfeld, D. & Engle, L (1982) Epithelial ovarian cancer and oral contraceptives. *Journal of the American Medical Association*, 247, 3210
246   Rothman, K. J & Louik, C (1978). Oral contraceptives and birth defects. *New England Journal of Medicine*, 299, 522.

247 Rowe, P. J. (1975). The design and evaluation of field trials of injectable contraceptives *Journal of Steroidal Biochemistry*, **6**, 921

248 Royal College of General Practitioners (1981) *Family Planning· An Exercise in Preventive Medicine* Report from *General Practice*, **21**

249 Royal College of General Practitioners (1974). *Oral Contraception and Health. an Interim Report from the Oral Contraceptives Study of the Royal College of General Practitioners.* London· Pitman

250 Royal College of General Practitioners (1977). Oral contraceptive study: Effect on hypertension and benign breast disease of progestogen component in combined oral contraceptives. *Lancet*, i, 624

251 Royal College of General Practitioners (1978). Oral Contraceptive Study. Oral contraceptives, venous thrombosis, and varicose veins *Journal of the Royal College of General Practitioners*, **28**, 393.

252 Royal College of General Practitioners (1981). Breast cancer and oral contraceptives: Findings in Royal College of General Practitioner's study *British Medical Journal*, **282**, 2089.

253 Royal College of General Practitioners (1981). Oral Contraceptive Study. Further analysis of morbidity in oral contraceptive users. *Lancet*, i, 541.

254 Royal College of General Practitioners Oral Contraceptive Study (1977). Mortality among oral contraceptive users *Lancet*, ii, 727

255 Royal College of General Practitioners' Oral Contraceptive Study. (1976). The outcome of pregnancy in former oral contraceptive users. *British Journal of Obstetrics and Gynaecology*, **83**, 608.

256 Royal College of General Practitioners' Oral Contraceptive Study (1978) Reduction in incidence of rheumatoid arthritis associated with oral contraceptives. *Lancet*, i, 569.

257 Rozier, J. C. Jr & Underwood, P. B. Jr (1974). Use of progestational agents in endometrial adenocarcinoma *Obstetrics and Gynecology*, **44**, 60.

258 Sagar, S., Stamatakis, J. B., Thomas, D. P & Kakkar, V. V. (1976). Oral contraceptives, Anti-thrombin III activities and post-operative deep vein thrombosis *Lancet*, i, 509

259 Shapiro, Slone, D. & Neff, E. R (1981). Age-specific secular changes in oral contraceptive use. *American Journal of Epidemiology*, **114**, 604

260 Sall, S. Di Saia, P. & Morrow, C. P. (1979). A comparison of medroxyprogesterone serum concentrations by the oral or intramuscular routes in patients with persistent or recurrent endometrial carcinoma. *American Journal of Obstetrics and Gynecology*, **134**, 647

261 Sartwell, P. E. & Anello, C. (1969). Trends in mortality from thromboembolic diseases. In *Second Report on the Oral Contraceptives*, p. 37. Advisory Committee on Obstetrics and Gynecology Food and Drug Administration. Washington, DC· Government Printing Office.

262 Sartwell, P. E., Stolley, P. D , Tanascia, J. A., Pockman, M. F., Rutledge, A. H., & Wertheimer, D. (1976). Oral contraceptive use. *Preventive Medicine*, **5**, 15.

263 Savolainen, E., Saksela, E & Saxen, L. (1981). Teratogenic hazards of oral contraceptives analyzed in a national malformation register *American Journal of Obstetrics and Gynecology*, **140**, 521.

264 Saxena, B. (1977). Levels of contraceptive steroids in breast milk and plasma of lactating women. *Contraception*, **16**, 605.

265 Schwallie, P. C. (1981). The effect of depo-medroxyprogesterone acetate on the fetus and nursing infant· a review. *Contraception*, **23**, 375.

266 Schwallie, P. C & Assenzo, J. R. (1974). The effect of depo medroxyprogesterone acetate on pituitary and ovarian function and the return of fertility following discontinuation *Contraception*, **10**, 81.

267 Schwallie, P. C. & Assenzo, J. R. (1973). Contraceptive use-efficacy study using

Depo Provera administered as an intramuscular injection once every 90 days. *Fertility and Sterility*, **24**, 331.

268 Sennayake, P. & Kramer, D. C (1980) Contraception and the etiology of PID: new prospectives International Symposium on Pelvic Inflammatory Disease. Atlanta, Georgia, April 1980

269 Shapiro, S , Slone, D., Rosenberg, L , Kaufman, D.W., Stolley, P.D. & Miettinen, O (1979) Oral contraceptive use in relation to myocardial infarction. *Lancet*, i, 743.

270 Shapiro, S., Slone, D. & Neff, E R. (1981). Age specific secular changes in oral contraceptive use. *American Journal of Epidemiology*, **114**, 604.

271 Shearman, R P (1981). Oral contraceptives· where are the excess deaths? *The Medical Journal of Australia*, i, 698.

272 Shearman, R. P & Fraser, I. S. (1977). Impact of new diagnostic methods on the differential diagnosis and treatment of secondary amenorrhea. *Lancet*, i, 1195

273 Short, R. V. (1978). Healthy infertility. *Uppsala Journal of Medical Science, Supplement*, **22**, 23

274 Short, R V (1981) The discovery of the ovaries. In *The Ovary*, vol. I New York Academic Press

275 Short, R V. & Drife, J. O (1977) The etiology of mammary cancer in men and animals. *Symposium of the Zoological Society, London*, **41**, 211.

276 Siassi, I. (1972) The psychiatrist's role in family planning. *American Journal of Psychiatry*, **129**, 48

277 Silverberg, S G., Makowski, E L. & Roche, W. D. (1977) Endometrial carcinoma in young women under 40 years of age. comparison of cases in oral contraceptive users and nonusers. *Cancer*, **29**, 592.

278 Sivin, I., Mishell, D. R., Victor, A. & Diaz, S. (1981). A multicenter study of levonorgestrel estradiol contraceptive vaginal rings *Contraception*, **24**, 341

279 Slaunwhite, W R. & Sandberg, A A. (1961). Disposition of radioactive 17-hydroxyprogesterone, 6-methyl-17 acetate-progesterone and 6-methyl prednisolone in the human subjects *Journal of Clinical Endocrinology and Metabolism*, **21**, 753.

280 Slone, D., Shapiro, S., Kaufman, D W , Rosenberg, L., Miettinen, O S. & Stolley, P. P. (1981). Risk of myocardial infarction in relation to current and discontinued use of oral contraceptives. *New England Journal of Medicine*, **305**, 420.

281 Smith, M , Vessey, M. P., Bounds, W & Warren, J. (1976). Progestogen-only contraception and ectopic pregnancy *British Medical Journal*, iv, 104.

282 Sondheimer, S (1981). Metabolic effects of the birth control pill. *Clinical Obstetrics and Gynecology*, **24**, 927

283 Spellacy, W. M & Birk, S A (1974). The effects of mechanical and steroidal contraceptive methods on blood pressure in hypertensive women. *Fertility and Sterility*, **25**, 467

284 Spellacy, W. N., McLeod, A. G W. & Buhi, W C (1970). Medroxyprogesterone acetate and carbohydrate metabolism Measure of glucose, insulin and growth hormone during six months time *Fertility and Sterility*, **21**, 457

285 Spencer, J D., Millis, R R & Hayward, J. L (1978) Contraceptive steroids and breast cancer *British Medical Journal*, i, 1024.

286 Speroff, L. & Vande Wiele, R. L (1971) Regulation of the human menstrual cycle. *American Journal of Obstetrics and Gynecology*, **109**, 234.

287 Stadel, B V C (1981). Oral contraceptives and cardiovascular disease *New England Journal of Medicine*, **305**, 612 and 672.

288 Stamatakis, J. D, Lawrence, D. & Kakkar, V. V. (1977) Surgery, venous thrombosis and anti-Xa *British Journal of Surgery*, **64**, 709.

289 Starup, J. & Visfeldt, J. (1974). Ovarian morphology and pituitary gonadotropins in serum during and after long-term treatment with oral contraceptives. *Acta Obstetrica and Gynecologica Scandinavica*, **53**, 161.

290 Steel, J M. & Duncan, L. J. P (1981) The progestogen only pill in insulin dependent diabetes *The British Journal of Family Planning*, **6**, 108

291 Stem, E., Rorsythe, A. B. & Coffelt, C. F. (1977). Steroid contraceptive use and cervical dysplasia. increased risk of progression. *Science*, **196**, 1460.

292 Stolley, P. D., Tanascia, J. A., Pockman, M. F., Sartwell, P. E., Rutledge, A. H. & Jacobs, M B (1975) Thrombosis with low oestrogen oral contraceptives *American Journal of Epidemiology*, **102**, 197.

293 Sturgis, S H. & Albright, F (1940). The mechanism of estrin therapy in the relief of dysmenorrhoea *Endocrinology*, **26**, 68.

294 Stut, J. C (1973). Extrauterine pregnancy during conception with Depo-Provera *Nederlands Tijdschriff voor Geneeskunde* (Amsterdam), **117**, 343

295 Swenson, I., Khan, A. R & Jahan, F A (1980). A randomized, single blind comparative trial of norethindrone enanthate and depo-medroxyprogesterone acetate in Bangladesh *Contraception*, **21**, 207.

296 Szontagh, F. E. (1970). *Mechanism of Action of Oral Progestogens.* Budapest. Akademiai Kiado.

297 Takahashi, M. & Loveland, D. B. (1974) Bacteria and oral contraceptives· routine examination of 12 076 middle class women *Journal of the American Medical Association*, **277**, 762.

298 Talwar, P. P., Dingfelder, J R & Ravenholt, R. T. (1976). Endometrial control· a comparative study of three oral contraceptives. *International Journal of Gynaecology and Obstetrics*, **14**, 385.

299 Terenius, L. (1974). Affinities of progestogen and oestrogen receptors in rabbit uterus for synthetic progestogens. *Steroids*, **23**, 909.

300 Thomas, D. B. (1972) Relationship of oral contraceptives to cervical carcinogenesis. *Obstetrics and Gynecology*, **40**, 508.

301 Tietze, C (1979). The pill and mortality from cardiovascular disease another look *International Family Planning Perspectives*, **5**, 8.

302 Tieng Pardthaisong, Gray, R. H. & McDaniel, E. B. (1980). Return of fertility after discontinuation of depomedroxyprogesterone acetate and intrauterine devices in northern Thailand *Lancet*, ii, 229

303 Toppozada, M. (1977) The clinical use of monthly injectable contraceptive preparations. *Obstetrics and Gynecology Survey*, **32**, 335.

304 Treloar, A. E , Boynton, R E., Behn, B G. & Brown, B W. (1967) Variation of the human menstrual cycle through reproductive life. *International Journal of Fertility*, **12**, 77

305 Udry, R J. & Morris, N. M (1973). Effect of contraceptive pills on sexual activity in the luteal phase of the human menstrual cycle *Archives of Sexual Behaviour*, **2**, 205

306 Vessey, M. P. (1980). Female hormones and vascular disease – an epidemiological overview *British Journal of Family Planning*, **6**, Supplement 1.

307 Vessey, M. P. & Doll, Sir Richard (1969) Investigation of relationship between the use of oral contraceptives and thromboembolic disease, a further report. *British Medical Journal*, ii, 651.

308 Vessey, M. P , Doll, Sir Richard, Fairbairn, A. S & Glaber, G. (1970). Post-operative thromboembolism and the use of oral contraceptives. *British Medical Journal*, iii, 123.

309 Vessey, M P., Doll, Sir Richard & Sutton, P (1972) Oral contraceptives and

breast neoplasia. a retrospective study. *British Medical Journal*, II, 719.

310   Vessey, M P , Doll, Sir Richard, Johnson, B. & Wiggins, P (1976) A long-term follow-up study of women using different methods of contraception – an interim report. *Journal of Biosocial Science*, **8**, 375.

311   Vessey, M P , Doll, Sir Richard, Jones, K., McPherson, K & Yeates, D. (1982) Oral contraceptive use and abortion before first term pregnancy in relation to breast cancer risk *British Journal of Cancer*, **45**, 327

312   Vessey, M. P , Kay, C R., Baldwin, J. A., Clarke, J. A. & Macleod, I. B (1977). Oral contraceptives and benign liver tumour *British Medical Journal*, I, 1064

313   Vessey, M. P., McPherson, K & Doll, Sir Richard (1981). Breast cancer and oral contraceptives. findings in Oxford Family Planning Association Contraceptive study *British Medical Journal*, **282**, 2093

314   Vessey, M. P , McPherson, K. & Johnson, B (1977). Mortality among women participating in the Oxford Family Planning Association contraceptive study *Lancet*, II, 731

315   Vessey, M P , McPherson, K. C. & Yeates, D. (1981). Mortality in oral contraceptive users. *Lancet*, I, 549.

316   Vessey, M P , Meisler, L., Flavel, R & Yeates, D (1979). Outcome of pregnancy in women using different methods of contraception. *British Journal of Obstetrics and Gynaecology*, **86**, 548.

317   Vessey, M. P., Wright, N. M., McPherson, K & Wiggins, P (1978) Fertility after stopping different methods of contraception *British Medical Journal*, I, 265.

318   Vinikka, L , Hirvonen, E , Ylikorkala, O , Nummi, S. & Virkkunen, J. (1977). Ovulation inhibition by a new low-dose progestogen. *Contraception*, **16**, 51

319   Wallace, R , Hoover, T , Barrett-Conor, E., Rifkind, B M., Hunningloke, D. B., Mackenthun, A. & Heiss, G. (1979). Altered plasma lipid and lipoprotein levels associated with oral contraceptive use. *Lancet*, II, 111.

320   Webber, L S., Hunter, S. M., Baugh, J G., Srinivasan, S. R., Sklov, M. C. & Berenson, G. S. (1982) The interaction of cigarette smoking, oral contraceptive use and cardiovascular risk factor variables in children: the Bogalusa heart study. *American Journal of Public Health*, **72**, 26.

321   Weijers, M J (1982). Clinical trial of an oral contraceptive containing desogestrel and ethinyl estradiol. *Clinical Therapeutics*, **4**, 359.

322   Weiner, J M , Shirley, S., Gilman., N J , Stone, S. M. & Wolf, R M. (1981). Access to data and the information explosion. oral contraception and risk of cancer. *Contraception*, **24**, 301.

323   Weiss, N S. & Sayuetz, T A (1980). Incidence of endometrial cancer in relation to the use of oral contraceptives. *New England Journal of Medicine*, **302**, 551.

324   Wentz, W. B (1974). Progestion therapy in endometrial hyperplasia. *Gynecological Oncology*, **2**, 362.

325   Wessler, S , Gitel, S. N., Wan, L. S. & Pasternick, B S (1976). Estrogen-containing oral contraceptive agents *Journal of the American Medical Association*, **236**, 2179.

326   Whigham, K A. & Howie, P. W. (1979) The effect of an injectable progestogen contraceptive on blood coagulation and fibrinolysis. *British Journal of Gynaecology*, **86**, 806.

327   Wilkins, L., Jones, H. W , Homan, G. H. & Stempsel, R. S. (1958). Masculinization in the female foetus associated with the administration of oral and intramuscular injections of progestins during gestation. Non-adrenal pseudo hermaphroditism. *Journal of Clinical Endocrinology and Metabolism*, **18**, 559.

328 Wingrave, S , Kay, C R. & Vessey, M. P (1980) Oral contraceptives and pituitary adenoma. *British Medical Journal,* **280,** 685

329 Wiseman, A. (1963) Oral contraception. *British Medical Journal,* ii, 55

330 World Health Organization (1977). Expanded Programme of Research, Development and Research Training in Human Reproduction. Task force on Long-acting Systematic Agents for the Regulation of Fertility, Multinational comparative clinical evaluation of two long-acting injectable contraceptive steroids Norethisterone enanthate and medroxyprogesterone acetate I Use effectiveness. *Contraception,* **15,** 153.

331 World Health Organization (1978) Expanded Programme of Research, Development and Research Training in Human Reproduction Task Force on Long-acting Systemic Agents for the Regulation of Fertility, Multinational comparative clinical evaluation of two long-acting injectable contraceptive steroids Norethisterone enanthate and medroxyprogesterone acetate II. Bleeding patterns and side effects. *Contraception,* **17,** 395.

332 World Health Organization (1980) Facts about injectable contraceptives. Memorandum from a WHO meeting. *Bulletin of the World Health Organization,* **60,** 199

333 World Health Organization (1978). *Steroid Contraception and the Risk of Neoplasia* Technical Report Series 619 Geneva· WHO.

334 World Health Organization (1981) *The Effect of Female Sex Hormones on Fetal Development and Infant Health.* Technical Reports Series 657. Geneva WHO.

335 Worth, A. J & Boyes, D A (1971). A case-control study into the possible effects of birth control pill on preclinical carcinoma of the cervix *Journal of Obstetrics and Gynaecology of the British Commonwealth,* **79,** 673.

336 Wynn, V. (1975). Vitamins and oral contraceptive use. *Lancet,* i, 561

337 Wynn, V., Adams, P W. & Godsland, I. (1979). Comparison of effects of different combined oral contraceptive formulations on carbohydrate and lipid metabolism *Lancet,* i, 1045.

338 Zadeh, J A., Karabus, C D. & Fielding, J (1967) Haemoglobin concentration and other values in women using an intrauterine device or taking corticosteroid contraceptive pills *British Medical Journal,* iv, 708

339 Zanartu, J. & Onetto, E (1972) Long-acting injectable progestogens in human fertility control In *Clinical Proceedings of First International Planned Parenthood Federation South-East Asia and Oceania Regional Medical and Scientific Congress,* held in Sydney, Australia, 14–18 Aug. p. 65. Australian and New Zealand Journal of Obstetrics and Gynaecology

340 Zanartu, J , Onetto, E , Medina, E & Dabancens, F. (1973). Mammary gland nodules in women under continuous exposure to progestogens. *Contraception,* **7,** 203.

11 The intrauterine device

1 Aker, D., Boehn, F H , Askew, D. E. & Rothman, H. (1973) Electrocardiogram changes with intrauterine contraceptive device insertion *American Journal of Obstetrics and Gynecology,* **115,** 458.

2 Andolsek, L. (1980). Postabortion IUD insertion In *Medicated Intrauterine Devices Physiological and Clinical Aspects,* ed. E. S. E. Hafez & W. A. A. Van Os, p. 137. The Hague, The Netherlands Martinus Nijhoff

3 Aubert, J. M , Gobeaux-Castadot, M J & Boria, M. C. (1980). Actinomyces in the endometrium of IUD users. *Contraception,* **21,** 577.

4   Batar, I. (1980) Fertility after IUD removal. In *Proceedings of the Medicated IUDs and Polymeric Delivery Systems International Symposium*, ed E. S E Hafez & W A. A. Van Os, p 159 Amsterdam, The Netherlands. Excerpta Medica.

5   Berger, F. S., Keith, L. G. & Edelman, D A. (1980). IUDs and ectopic pregnancy. In *Proceedings of the Medicated IUDs and Polymeric Delivery Systems International Symposium*, ed. E. S. E. Hafez & W. A. A. Van Os, p. 169. Amsterdam, the Netherlands: Excerpta Medica.

6   Black, T. R. L., Goldstuck, N. D. & Spence, A. (1980) Post-Coital intrauterine device insertion – a further evaluation. *Contraception*, **22**, 653

7   Bond, A M. (1980) Malonaldehyde in cervical mucus associated with copper IUD. *Lancet*, i, 1087

8   Bonnar, J , Kasonde, J. M., Haddon, M., Hassanein, M. K. & Allington, M. J (1976). Fibrinolytic activity in utero and bleeding complications with intrauterine contraceptive devices *British Journal of Obstetrics and Gynaecology*, **83**, 160.

9   Bonney, W. A , Glasser, S. R., Clewe, T. M., Noyes, R. W. & Copper, C. L. (1966) Endometrial response to the intrauterine device. *American Journal of Obstetrics and Gynecology*, **96**, 601.

10 Booth, M., Beral, V. A & Guillebaud, J. (1980). Effect of age on pelvic inflammatory disease in nulliparous women using a copper 7 intrauterine contraceptive device. *British Medical Journal*, **281**, 114.

11 Buchman, M. I. (1970). A study of the intrauterine contraceptive device with and without an extracervical appendage or tail. *Fertility and Sterility*, **21**, 348.

12 Burnhill, M. S. (1973) Syndrome of progressive endometritis associated with intrauterine contraceptive devices. *Advances in Planned Parenthood*, **8**, 144.

13 Casanova, J. (1922). *The Memoirs of Jacques Casanova de Seingalt*. London· Navarre Edition

14 Cates, W., Ory, H. W., Rochat, R. W. & Tyler, C W (1976). The Intrauterine device and deaths from spontaneous abortion. *New England Journal of Medicine*, **295**, 115.

15 Cates, W., Ory, H., Rochat, R. W. & Tyler, C W. (1977). Publicity and the public health· the elimination of IUD related abortion deaths. *Family Planning Perspectives*, **9**, 138.

16 Christian, C D. (1974). Maternal deaths associated with an intrauterine device. *American Journal of Obstetrics and Gynecology*, **119**, 441

17 Chowdhury, N. N. R., Mandal, G S & Das, M. (1979). Comparative study of Lippes Loop and CuT inserted in immediate postabortal period *Journal of Obstetrics and Gynaecology of India*, **29**(2), 239.

18 Cole, L. P. & Edelman, D A (1980). A comparison of the Lippes Loop and two copper-bearing intrauterine devices. *International Journal of Gynaecology and Obstetrics*, **18**, 35

19 Davis, H. (1971). *Intrauterine Devices for Contraception*. Baltimore, Maryland Williams and Wilkins.

20 El-Badrawi, H. H , Hafez, E. S E , Barnhart, M. I., Fayad, M. & Shafeek, A. (1981). Ultrastructural changes in human endometrium with copper and nonmedicated IUDs in utero. *Fertility and Sterility*, **36**, 41.

21 Edelman, D A , Berger, G S & Keith, L. E. (1979) *Intrauterine Devices and their Complications* Boston, Massachusetts G. K. Hall and Co

22 Edelman, D. A., Zipper, J., Rivera, M & Medel, M (1979). Timing of the IUD insertion *Contraception*, **19**, 449

23 Erkkola, R. & Liukko, P. (1977) Intrauterine device and ectopic pregnancy *Contraception*, **16**, 569

24 Eschenbach, D A & Holmes, K K (1975) Acute pelvic inflammatory disease current concepts of pathogenesis, etiology, and management. *Clinical Obstetrics and Gynecology*, **18**, 35.

25 Freedman, J. R. (1953) Intrauterine foreign body and pregnancy. *American Journal of Obstetrics and Gynecology*, **66**, 678

26 Goldsmith, A , Goldberg, R., Eyzaguirre, M , Lucero S. & Lizara, L (1972). IUD insertion in the immediate post-abortal period. In *Family Planning Research Conference a Multidisciplinary Approach*, ed. A. Goldsmith & R. Snowden, p. 59. Amsterdam, The Netherlands· Excerpta Medica.

27 Grafenberg, E (1930) In *World League for Sexual Reform*, 3rd Congress, 1929 London. Kegan Paul.

28 Grafenberg, E (1931). Quoted in Davis, H.J. (1971). *Intrauterine Devices for Contraception The IUD*. Baltimore, Maryland. Williams and Wilkins

29 Gray, R. (1976). Pelvic inflammatory disease and intrauterine contraceptive devices. *Lancet*, ii, 521.

30 Guillebaud, J. (1980). Intrauterine devices present and future *International Journal of Gynaecology and Obstetrics*, **18**, 325.

31 Guillebaud, J. & Bonnar, J (1976). Menstrual blood-loss with intrauterine devices *Lancet*, i, 387

32 Guillebaud, J. & Kasonde, J. (1974). 'Lost Threads' with intrauterine devices *British Medical Journal*, iii, 167.

33 Guttmacher, A. (1965) Intrauterine contraceptive devices. *Family Planning*, **13**, 91.

34 Hagenfeldt, K (1980). Mechanism of action of medicated intrauterine devices. In *Blastocyst-endometrium Relationships*, ed F. Leroy, C. A. Finn, A Psychoyos & P. O. Hubinot. New York S Karger.

35 Hata, Y., Ishihama, A., Kudo, N , Nakamura, J , Miyai, T., Makino, T. & Kagabu, T. (1969) The effect of long-term use of intrauterine devices. *International Journal of Fertility*, **14**, 241

36 Hefnawi, F., Hamza, Z , Sheikha, El, Serour, G. & Yacout, M. (1982) Menstrual pattern and blood loss with U-coil inert progesterone-releasing IUDs *Contraceptive Delivery Systems*, **3**, 91.

37 Horowitz, A J. (1973) A study of contraceptive effectiveness and incidence of side effects with the use of the Dalkon Shield. *Contraception*, **7**, 1.

38 Huber, S C , Piotrow, P. T & Orlans, F B (1975). IUDs reassessed· a decade of experience. *Population Reports*, Series **B**, 19.

39 Hue K., Kwon, H Y., Michael, P. M & Watson, W B. (1974) A comparative study of the safety and efficacy of postabortal intrauterine contraceptive device insertion. *American Journal of Obstetrics and Gynecology*, **118**, 975.

40 Hurst, P R , Jefferies, K , Dawson, J K. & Eckstein, P. (1980) *In Vitro* development of preimplantation embryos removed from IUD-bearing mice. *Journal of Reproduction and Fertility*, **54**, 413.

41 Hurst, P. R., Jefferies, K., Eckstein, P & Wheeler, A G (1977) Intrauterine degeneration of embryos in IUD-bearing mice. *Journal of Reproduction and Fertility*, **50**, 187

42 Hurst, P R , Jefferies, K., Eckstein, P., Dawson, K. & Wheeler, A. G. (1977) Leucocytes are consistently associated with degenerating embryos in IUD-bearing Rhesus monkeys *Nature*, **269**, 331.

43 Ishihama, A. & Kagabu, T. (1964) On the cytological and histological studies after long insertion of intrauterine contraceptive device (IUD) *Yokohama Medical Bulletin*, **15**, 201

44 Jafarey, S A , Hardie, J G. & Satterthwaite, A. P (1968). Use of medical-paramedical personnel and traditional midwives in the Pakistan family planning program *Demography*, **5**, 666.

45   Ji, G , Li-yuan, M , Su, Z., Hui-min, F. & Li-hui, H (1981) Menstrual blood
     loss in healthy Chinese women *Contraception*, **23**, 591
46   Jones, R W , Gregons, N M & Elstein, M. (1973). Effect of copper containing
     intrauterine contraceptive devices in human cells in culture *British Medical
     Journal*, ii, 520
47   Kahn, N S. & Tyler, C W (1975). Mortality associated with use of IUDs
     Journal of the American Medical Association, **234**, 57
48   Kamal, I (1979). *Atlas of Hysterographic Studies of the IUD-holding Uterus.*
     Ottawa, Ontario IRDC.
49   Kelly, W. A & Marston, J. H (1967). Contraceptive action of intrauterine
     devices in the Rhesus Monkey. *Nature*, **214**, 735
50   Kessel, E , Bernard, R. & Thomas M. (1976). *IUD Performance and
     Hypothesis Testing in International Clinical Trials.* Research Triangle Park,
     North Carolina: International Fertility Research Program (IFRP).
51   Kondo, H. (1958). Intrauterine contraceptive method report of fertility rate
     and intrauterine ring. *Japan Planned Parenthood Quarterly*, **4**, 3.
52   Laufe, L. E. & Friel, P. G. (1980). Improving IUD performance with
     biodegradable materials In *Biodegradables and Delivery Systems for
     Contraception*, ed. E. S. E. Hafez & W. A. A. Van Os, p.197 Lancaster,
     England· MTP Press
53   Layde, P M., Goldber, M F., Safra, M J & Oakley, G P. (1979). Failed
     intrauterine device contraception and limb reduction deformities a case-
     control study. *Fertility and Sterility*, **31**, 18
54   Lehfeldt, H. (1975) Ernst Grafenberg and his ring *The Mount Sinai Journal of
     Medicine*, **41**, 345.
55   Lehfeldt, H., Tietze, C & Gorstein, F. (1970) Ovarian pregnancy and the
     intrauterine device *American Journal of Obstetrics and Gynecology*, **108**, 1005.
56   Lippes, J (1978) Management of the loss of IUD A conservative approach.
     In *Risks, Benefits and Controversies in Fertility Control*, ed. J.J Sciarra, G. I.
     Zatuchni & J.J. Speidel, p. 404. Hagerstown, Maryland Harper and Row.
57   Lippes, J (1962). A study of intrauterine contraception: development of a
     plastic loop. In *Intrauterine Contraceptive Devices*, ed. C Tietze & S. Lewit, p.
     69 Amsterdam, The Netherlands· Excerpta Medica Foundation.
58   Lippes, J & Zielezny, J. (1975). The Loop after ten years. In *Analysis of
     Intrauterine Contraception*, ed. F Hefnawi & S J Segal, p. 225 New York:
     Elsevier
59   Lu Zilan (1980). Flower intrauterine contraceptive device. *Chinese Medical
     Journal*, **93**, 528
60   Margulies, L. C (1962). Permanent reversible contraception with an
     intrauterine plastic spiral. In *Intrauterine Contraceptive Devices*, ed C. Tietze
     & S. Lewit, p. 61. Amsterdam, The Netherlands Excerpta Medica
     Foundation
61   Mishell, D R., Bell, J. M , Good R G. & Moyer D. L. (1966). The intrauterine
     device· a bacteriologic study of the intrauterine cavity. *American Journal of
     Obstetrics and Gynecology*, **96**, 119.
62   Muramatsu, M (1973). *Statistical Analysis of Long-term Wearers of Ota Ring.*
     Tokyo· The Institute of Public Health.
63   Ory, H, W. & The Women's Health Study (1981). Ectopic pregnancy and
     intrauterine contraceptive devices. new perspectives. *Obstetrics and Gynecology*,
     57, 137.
64   Ota, T. (1980). Personal communication.
65   Pearce, D. J. (1976). Laparascopic removal of IUDs from the abdomen. *British
     Medical Journal*, i, 106.

66 Phaosavasdı, W , Vıcanıchakul, B., Rıenprayura, D , Chutıuvangse, S.,
    Virutanasen, P & Sorıdvongs, W (1975) Pelvıc ınflammatory dısease ın
    contraceptıve acceptors dısclosed at tubal sterılızatıon In *Analysıs of
    Intrauterıne Devıces,* ed F Hefnawı & S J Segal New York Elsevıer
67 Pıotrow, P T , Rınehart, W & Schmıdt, C (1979) IUDs – update on safety,
    effectıveness and research *Populatıon Reports,* Serıes **B,** 80
68 Potts, M & Pearson, R. M (1967) A lıght and electron mıcroscope study of
    cells ın contact wıth ıntrauterıne contraceptıve devıces *Journal of Obstetrıcs
    and Gynaecology of the Brıtısh Commonwealth,* **74,** 129
69 Purnıer, B G A., Sparks, R A , Watt, P J & Elsteın, M (1979). *In Vıtro* study
    of possıble role of the ıntrauterıne contraceptıve devıce taıl ın ascendıng
    ınfectıon of the genıtal tract. *Brıtısh Journal of Obstetrıcs and Gynaecology,* **86,**
    374
70 Rashbaum, W K & Wallach, R C (1971) Immedıate postpartum ınsertıon of
    a new ıntrauterıne devıce *Amerıcan Journal of Obstetrıcs and Gynecology,* **109,**
    1003.
71 Ratnam, S S. & Tow, S. H. (1970) Translocatıon of the loop. In *Post-partum
    Famıly Plannıng A Report on the Internatıonal Program,* ed. G. I. Zatuchnı
    New York McGraw-Hıll Book Co.
72 Reame, N E. (1980) The role of nonphysıcıans ın famıly plannıng In *IUDs
    and Famıly Plannıng,* ed E. S. E. Hafez & W A. A. Van Os Lancaster,
    England MTP Press
73 Rıchter, R (1909). Eın mıttel zur verhutung der Konzeptıon. *Deutsche
    Medızınısche Wochenschrıft,* **35,** 1525
74 Rıvera, R , Gaıtan, J R., Navarro, C L , Valles, J , Almonte, H., Ruız, R. &
    Hernandez, A B. (1978) Effect of the Lıppes IUD on the cırculatıng levels of
    hemoglobın, hematocrıt, serum ıron and ıron bındıng capacıty ın normal
    women. *Contraceptıon,* **17,** 3.
75 Sagıroglu, N. & Sagıroglu, E (1970) Bıologıc mode of actıon of the Lıppes
    Loop ın ıntrauterıne contraceptıon *Amerıcan Journal of Obstetrıcs and
    Gynecology,* **106,** 506.
76 Scott, R B (1968). Crıtıcal ıllnesses and deaths assocıated wıth ıntrauterıne
    devıces *Obstetrıcs and Gynecology,* **31,** 322
77 Smıth, R. P., Goresky, D M. & Etchell, D M (1980) Fıve years prıvate
    practıce experıence of nullıparous women usıng copper IUDs. *Contraceptıon,*
    21, 335.
78 Snowden, R (1977) The Progestasert and ectopıc pregnancy *Brıtısh Medıcal
    Journal,* ıv, 1601
79 Snowden, R., Wıllıams, M. & Hawkıns D. (1977) *The IUD – A practıcal
    guıde.* London Croom Helm.
80 Soonawala, R.P (1974) Intrauterıne contraceptıve devıce *Lancet,* ı, 245.
81 Sparks, R. A , Purnıer, B G , Watt, P J & Elsteın, M. (1981) Bacterıologıcal
    colonısatıon of uterıne cavıty role of taıled ıntrauterıne contraceptıve devıce
    Brıtısh Medıcal Journal, **282,** 1189.
82 Stone, A. & Hımes, N E (1960) *Practıcal Bırth Control Method* New York
    Vıkıng Press
83 Sykes, G S & Shelly, G (1981) Actınomyces-lıke structures and theır
    assocıatıon wıth ıntrauterıne contraceptıve devıces, pelvıc ınfectıon and
    abnormal cervıcal cytology. *Brıtısh Journal of Obstetrıcs and Gynaecology,* **88,**
    934
84 Tacla Fernandez, X , Young, B., Lavın, P A., Baeza, R. & Seaman, V. (1980)
    The IUD and anemıa a study of hematocrıt *Contraceptıve Delıvery Systems,*
    1, 49

85   Tatum, H J (1977). Clinical aspect of intrauterine contraception *Fertility and Sterility*, **28**, 3

86   Tatum, H J., Schmidt, F. H , Phillips, D , McCarty, M. & OLeary, W. M (1975) The Dalkon Shield controversy. structural and bacteriological studies of IUD tails *Journal of the American Medical Association*, **231**, 711.

87   Tietze, C (1968). Use of intrauterine devices by never-pregnant women *American Association of Planned Parenthood Physicians Excerpta Medical International Congress Series No 177*, 84

88   Tietze, C & Lewit, S. (1970). Evaluation of intrauterine devices 9th Progress Report on the cooperative statistical programme *Studies in Family Planning*, **55**, 1

89   Timonen, H & Luukkainen, T (1976) Immediate postabortion insertion of the copper T (TCu 200) with eighteen months follow-up. *Contraception*, **9**, 153.

90   Tuttle, M E , Baker, R W & Laufe, L. E (1980). Slow release apraltinin delivery for control of intrauterine device induced hemorrhage *Journal of Membrane Science*, **7**, 351.

91   Verma, V (1981) Ultrastructural alteration in human endometrium caused by intrauterine contraceptive devices *International Journal of Gynaecology and Obstetrics*, **19**, 211

92   Vessey, M P , Meisher, L , Flavel, R & Yeates, O (1979) Outcome of pregnancy in women using different methods of contraception. *British Journal of Obstetrics and Gynaecology*, **86**, 548

93   Westrom, L , Bengstsson, L P. & Mardh, P A (1976) The risk of pelvic inflammatory disease in women using intrauterine contraceptive devices as compared to nonusers *Lancet*, ii, 221

94   White, M K , Ory, H W , Rooks, J.B & Rochat, R W (1980) Intrauterine device termination rates and the menstrual cycle day of insertion. *Obstetrics and Gynecology*, **55**, 220

95   Wright, N. H , Sujplueum, C., Rosenfield, A G & Varakanain, S (1977) Nurse-midwife insertion of the copper T in Thailand performance, acceptance and programmatic effects *Studies in Family Planning*, **8**, 237

96   World Health Organization (1980) Special Programme of Research, Development and Research Training in Human Reproduction Task Force on Intrauterine Devices for Fertility Regulation Comparative multicentre trial of three IUDs inserted immediately following delivery of the placenta. *Contraception*, **22**, 9

97   Zerner, J , Doil, K L , Drewry, J. & Leeber, D. A (1981). Intrauterine contraceptive device failures in renal transplant patients *International Journal of Reproductive Medicine*, **26**, 99

98   Zipper, J , Tatum, H J , Pasktene, L , Medel, M & Rivera, M (1969) Metallic copper as an intrauterine contraceptive adjunct to the T device *American Journal of Obstetrics and Gynecology*, **105**, 1274

12   Voluntary sterilization

1   Ansbacher, R , Kowk, K Y & Behrman, J.J. (1974) Clinical significance of sperm antibodies in infertile couples. *Fertility and Sterility*, **24**, 305

2   Adams, T W (1964) Female sterilization *American Journal of Obstetrics and Gynecology*, **89**, 395

3   Alexander, N & Anderson, D J (1979). Vasectomy consequences of autoimmunity to sperm antigens *Fertility and Sterility*, **32**, 253

4   Alexander, N. J & Clarkson, T B (1978) Vasectomy increases the severity of diet-induced atherosclerosis in *Maccaca fasciolaris Science*, **201**, 553.

5   Alderman, B (1977) Women who regret sterilization. *British Medical Journal*, ii, 766

6   Ansbacher, R , Keung-Yeung, F , Wurster, J C. (1972) Sperm antibodies in vasectomized men. *Fertility and Sterility*, **23**, 640

7   Astiey Cooper (1830) *Observations on the Structure and Diseases of the Testes* Longman

8   Baird, Sir Dugald (1966) *Conception Control* Amsterdam, The Netherlands. Excerpta Medica Foundation

9   Barglow, P & Lisner, M (1966) An evaluation of tubal ligation *American Journal of Obstetrics and Gynecology*, **95**, 1083.

10   Brosens, I & Winston, R (Eds) (1978). *Reversibility of Female Sterilization*. London. Academic Press.

11   Chaset, N (1962). Male Sterilization *Journal of Urology*, **87**, 512

12   Chen, P -c (1981) *Rural Health and Birth Planning in China*. Research Triangle Park, North Carolina International Fertility Research Program (IFRP)

13   Cheng, M C E & Rochat, R W (1977) The safety of combined abortion-sterilization procedure. *American Journal of Obstetrics and Gynecology*, **129**, 548.

14   Chi, I -c & Cole, L P. (1979) Incidence of pain among women undergoing laparoscopic sterilization by electrocoagulation, the spring-loaded clip and the tubal ring *American Journal of Obstetrics and Gynecology*, **135**, 397

15   Chi, I-c & Feldblum, P J. (1981) Luteal phase pregnancies in female sterilization patients. *Contraception*, **23**, 579

16   Chi, I-c. & Feldblum, P J (1982) Laparoscopic sterilizations requiring laparotomy. *American Journal of Obstetrics and Gynecology*, **142**, 712.

17   Chi, I-c , Laufe, L E & Atwood, R J. (1981) Ectopic pregnancy following female sterilization procedures *Advances in Planned Parenthood*, **26**, 52

18   Chi, I-c , Laufe, L E , Gardner, S D & Tolbert, M A (1980) An epidemiological study of risk factors associated with pregnancy following female sterilization *American Journal of Obstetrics and Gynecology*, **136**, 768.

19   Chi, I-c , Mumford, S D. & Gardner, S. D (1981) Pregnancy risk following laparoscopic sterilization in nongravid and gravid women *Journal of Reproductive Medicine*, **26**, 289.

20   Chi, I-c , Mumford, S D. & Laufe, L E (1980) Technical failures in tubal ring sterilization incidence, perceived reasons, outcome and risk factors *American Journal of Obstetrics and Gynecology*, **138**, 307.

21   Clarkson, M J & Anderson, D J (1979). Vasectomy consequences of autoimmunity to sperm antigens *Fertility and Sterility*, **32**, 253

22   Clarkson, T B & Alexander, M J (1980) Long-term vasectomy. effects on the occurrence and extent of atherosclerosis in rhesus monkeys *Journal of Clinical Investigation*, **65**, 15

23   Craft, I (1976) Hysteroscopy and laparoscopy *British Journal of Hospital Medicine*, **2**, 25

24   Dassenaike, A G S , Saha, A & McCann, M (1976) Female sterilization via minilaparotomy *The Journal of Reproductive Medicine*, **17**, 119

25   Davis, J E (1978) Male sterilization *Clinics in Obstetrics and Gynecology*, **6**, 97

26   Deys, C M & Potts, D M (1972) Condoms and things *Advances in Biosciences*, **10**, 287

27 Diaz, M. O., Atwood, R. J. & Laufe, L. E. (1980). Laparoscopic sterilization with room air insufflation: preliminary report. *International Journal of Gynaecology and Obstetrics*, **18**, 119.

28 Diggory, P. & McEwan, J. (1976). *Planning or Prevention*. London: Marion Boyars.

29 Ferber, A. S., Tietze, C. & Lewit, S. (1967). Men with vasectomies: a study of medical, sexual and psychological changes. *Psychosomatic Medicine*, **27**, 354.

30 Filshie, G. M., Casey, D., Pogmore, J. R., Dutton, A. G. B., Symonds, E. M. & Peake, A. B. C. (1981). The titanium/silicone rubber clip for female sterilization. *British Journal of Obstetrics and Gynaecology*, **88**, 665.

31 Goldacre, M. J., Clarke, J. A., Heasman, M. A. & Vessey, M. P. (1978). Follow-up of vasectomy using medical record linkage. *American Journal of Epidemiology*, **108**, 176.

32 Goldacre, M. J., Vessey, M., Clarke, J.A. & Heasman, M. (1979). Record linkage study of morbidity following vasectomy. In *Vasectomy: Immunologic and Pathophysiologic Effects in Animals and Man*, ed. I. H. Lipers & R. Crozier, p. 567. New York: Academic Press.

33 Goyal, R. M. & Mangal, H. M. (1972). Effects of vasectomy on spermatogensis. *International Conference on Family Planning*, New Delhi, India.

34 Hagedoorn, J. P. & Davis, J. E. (1976). Fine structure of the seminiferous tubules after vasectomy in man. *Physiologist*, **17**, 236.

35 Hampton, P. T. & Tarnasky, W. G. (1974). Hysterectomy and tubal ligation: a comparison of the psychological aftermath. *American Journal of Obstetrics and Gynecology*, **119**, 949.

36 Harrison, R. (1899). *Selected Papers on Stone, Prostate and Other Urinary Disorders*. London: Churchill.

37 Hulka, J. F. (1980). Complications of laparoscopy. *Current Problems in Obstetrics and Gynecology*, **4**, 1.

38 Hulka, J. F., Omran, K., Leiberman, B. A. & Gordon, A. G. (1979). Laparoscopic sterilization with the spring clip. *American Journal of Obstetrics and Gynecology*, **135**, 1016.

39 Janowitz, B., Nakamura, M. S., Lins, F. E., Brown, M. L. & Clopton, D. (1982). Cesarean section in Brazil. *Social Science and Medicine*, **16**, 19.

40 Johnson, M. H. (1964). Social and psychological effects of vasectomy. *American Journal of Psychiatry*, **121**, 482.

41 Kleinman, R. L. (Ed.) (1982). *Female Sterilization*. London: International Planned Parenthood Federation (IPPF).

42 Kwak, H. M., Moon, T. K., Song, C. H., Ahn, D. W. & Chi, I-c. (1980). Timing of laparoscopic sterilization in abortion patients. *Obstetrics and Gynecology*, **56**, 85.

43 Laufe, L. E. (1981). Chemical sterilization with an IUD. *Contraceptive Delivery Systems*, **2**, 343.

44 Laufe, L. E. & Cole, L. P. (1980). Nonsurgical female sterilization. *International Journal of Gynaecology and Obstetrics*, **18**, 333.

45 Laufe, L., Eddy, C., Brosens, J. & Boeckx, W. (1980). Reversible methods of fimbrial enclosure. In *Research Frontiers in Fertility Regulation*, ed. G. I. Zatuchni, M. H. Labbok & J. J. Sciarra, p. 287. Hagerstown, Maryland: Harper and Row.

46 Leavesley, J. M. (1980). A study of vasectomized men and their wives. *Australian Family Physician*, **9**, 8.

47 Lee, H. (1980). Reanastomosis of the vas. *Journal of Andrology*, **1**, 11.

48 Lungren, S. S. (1881). A case of caesarian section twice successfully performed on the same patient. *American Journal of Obstetrics and Gynecology*, **14**, 78.

49   Lu, T & Chun, D (1967) Long-term follow-up study of 1055 cases of female sterilization *Journal of Obstetrics and Gynaecology of the British Commonwealth*, **74**, 875

50   Malaviya, B , Chandra, H & Kar, A B (1975) Chemical occlusion of the monkey oviducts with quinacrine *Contraception*, **12**, 31

51   McCann, M F & Bhiwandiwala, P (1979) Is minilaparotomy appropriate in the United States? *Advances in Planned Parenthood*, **24**, 1

52   McCann, M F & Cole, L P (1980) Laparoscopy and minilaparotomy two major advances in female sterilization *Studies in Family Planning*, **11**, 119

53   Mumford, S D , Bhiwandiwala, P P & Chi, I-c (1980) Laparoscopic and minilaparotomy female sterilization compared in 15,167 cases *Lancet*, ii, 1066

54   Mumford, S D & Bhiwandiwala, P P (1981) Tubal ring sterilization experience with 10,086 cases *Obstetrics and Gynecology*, **57**, 150

55   Mumford, S D & Davis, J E (1979) Flushing of the distal vas during vasectomy *Urology*, **14**, 433

56   Nijs, P & Brosens, I (Eds) (1981) *Reversibility of Sterilization Psycho(patho)logical Aspects* Leuven, Belgium Acco

57   Nikorn Dusitsin, Sumana Chompootaweep, Manthira Tankeyoon & Banpot Boonsiri (1979) The effect of post partum tubal ligation on breast feeding *Journal of Thai Association for Voluntary Sterilization*, **1**, 53

58   Nikorn Dusitsin, Somsak Varakamin, Sopon Chalapate & Gray, R H (1980) Post-partum tubal ligation by nurse-midwives and doctors in Thailand *Lancet*, i, 638

59   Pai, M G , Kumar, B T S , Kaudinga, C & Bhat, H S (1973) Vasovasostomy a clinical study with 10 years follow up *Fertility and Sterility*, **26**, 798

60   Palaniappan, B. (1979) A new technique for minilaparotomy *International Journal of Gynaecology and Obstetrics*, **17**, 260

61   Palmer, R , Dourlen-Rollier, A M , Audebert, A & Geraud, R (1981) *La Sterilisation Volontaire en France et dans le Monde* Paris Massin

62   Peterson, H B , Greenspan, J R , Ory, H W. & DeStafano, F (1981) Tubal sterilization mortality surveillance, United States, 1978–1979 *Advances in Planned Parenthood*, **16**, 71

63   Petitti, D , Klein, R , Kipp, H , Kahn, W , Siegelaub, A & Friedman, G D (1982) Physiologic measures in men with and without vasectomies *Fertility and Sterility*, **37**, 438

64   Phadke, A M & Padukone, K (1964) Presence and significance of autoantibodies against spermatozoa in the blood of men with obstructed vas deferens *Journal of Reproduction and Fertility*, **7**, 163

65   Phadke, A M (1975) Spermiophage cells in man *Fertility and Sterility*, **26**, 760

66   Phillips, J , Hulka, J F , Keith, D , Keith, L & Hulka, B (1976) Laparoscopic procedures AAGL Membership Survey for 1978 *Journal of Reproductive Medicine*, **16**, 105

67   Pichai Bunyaratavej, Bhankasame Kichanantha, Wiset Tangchoi, Somsak Watanapat & Nikorn Dusitsin (1981) Comparison of vasectomy performed by medical students and surgeons in Thailand *Studies in Family Planning*, **12**, 316

68   Ravenholt, R T (1979) Future prospects for voluntary sterilization *Voluntary Sterilization A Decade of Achievement*, ed M. E Schima & I Lubell Amsterdam, The Netherlands Excerpta Medica

69   Royal College of Obstetricians and Gynaecologists. Gynaecological Laparoscopy, The Report of the Working Party of the Confidential Inquiry into Gynaecological Laparoscopy (1978) *British Journal of Obstetrics and Gynaecology*, **85**, 401.

70 Rhodes, D B., Mumford, S. D & Tree, M. J. (1979) Vasectomy efficacy of placing the cut vas in different fascial planes. *Fertility and Sterility*, **33**, 433

71 Rogers, D A , Ziegler, F. L & Levy, M (1972) Psychological reactions to surgical contraception In *Psychological Perspectives in Population*, Ed J T Fawcett, p 306 New York Basic Books.

72 Sackler, A M , Weltman, A S , Pandke, V & Schwartz, R (1973) Gonadal effects of vasectomy and vasoligation. *Science*, **179**, 293.

73 Schmidt, S S (1966) Techniques and complications of elective vasectomy the role of sperm granuloma in spontaneous recanalization *Fertility and Sterility*, **17**, 467.

74 Sciarra, J J , Butler, J C & Speidel, J J (1976). *Hysteroscopic Sterilization.* New York Intercontinental Medical Books

75 Sciarra, J J , Droegemueller, W & Speidel, J.J. (Eds) (1976) *Advances in Female Sterilization* Hagerstown, Maryland Harper and Row.

76 Shrikhande, V M (1981) Vasectomy In *Abortion and Sterilization*, ed J E Hodgson London Academic Press

77 Silber, S J (1977) Microscopic vasectomy reversal *Fertility and Sterility*, **28**, 1191.

78 Smith, K. D , Tcholakian, R K Chowdhury, M. & Steinberger, E (1976) An investigation of plasma hormone levels before and after vasectomy *Fertility and Sterility*, **27**, 145.

79 Soonawala, R P. (1981) Vaginal sterilization In *Abortion and Sterilization*, ed. J.E Hodgson London Academic Press

80 Steinberger, E & Perloff, W H (1965) Preliminary experience with a human sperm bank. *American Journal of Obstetrics and Gynecology*, **92**, 577

81 Steptoe, P (1981) Endoscopic techniques of female sterilization In *Abortion and Sterilization*, ed J E Hodgson London Academic Press

82 Stevenson, T C & Taylor D S (1972) The effect of methyl cyanoacrylate tissue adhesive on human Fallopian tube and endometrium *Journal of Obstetrics and Gynaecology of the British Commonwealth*, **79**, 1028

83 Thompson, B & Baird D (1972) Follow-up of 186 sterilized women In *Foolproof Birth Control, Male and Female Sterilization*, ed L Lader, p 162 Boston, Massachusetts Beacon Press

84 Tingey, R W (1976) A study of laparoscopic sterilization using Yoon's silicone Falope rings *Proceedings of the Royal Society of Medicine*, **69**, 8.

85 Uchida, H (1975) Uchida tubal sterilization *American Journal of Obstetrics and Gynecology*, **121**, 153.

86 Walker, A M , Jick, H , Hunter, J. R , Danford, A & Rothman, K J (1981) Hospitalization rates in vasectomized men *Journal of the American Medical Association*, **248**, 2315

87 Walker, A M , Jick, H , Hunter, J R , Danford, A , Watkins, R. M , Alhadiff, L & Rothman, K J (1981) Vasectomy and non-fatal myocardial infarction *Lancet*, i, 13

88 Wallace, R B , Lea, J , Gerber, W L , Clarke, W R & Lauer, R M (1981) Vasectomy and coronary disease in men under 50, absence of an association *Journal of Urology*, **126** (2), 182.

89 Westoff, C F (1977) Contraception and sterilization in the United States *Family Planning Perspectives*, **9**, 153

90 Westoff, C F & McCarthy, J. (1979) Sterilization in the United States *Family Planning Perspectives*, **11**, 147

91 Yoon, I B , Wheeless, C R & King, T M (1974) A preliminary report on a new laparoscopic sterilization approach the silicone rubber band technique *American Journal of Obstetrics and Gynecology*, **120**, 132

92 Ziegler, F J , Rodgers, D A & Kriegsman, S A (1966) Effects of vasectomy on psychological functioning. *Psychosomatic Medicine*, **28**, 50.
93 Zipper, J. A , Stachetti, E. & Medel, M (1970) Human fertility control by transvaginal application of quinacrine on the Fallopian tubes. *Fertility and Sterility*, **21**, 581
94 Zipper, J A., Prager, R & Medel, M (1973) Biological changes induced by unilateral intrauterine instillation of quinacrine in the rat and their reversal by either use of estradiol or progesterone *Fertility and Sterility*, **24**, 68
95 Zipper, J , Cole, L P., Goldsmith, A., Wheeler, R & Rivera, M (1980) Quinacrine hydrochloride pellets preliminary data in a nonsurgical method of female sterilization *International Journal of Gynaecology and Obstetrics*, **18**, 275.

13 Abortion

1 Asanov, S S (1972) Comparative features of the reproductive biology of hamadryas baboons (*Papio hamadryas*), grivet monkey (*Ceropithecus aethiops*) and the rhesus monkey (*Macaca mulatta*) In *The Use of Non-Human Primates in Research on Human Reproduction*, ed E Diczfalusy & C C Stanley Stockholm, Sweden WHO and Karolinska Institute
2 Ashton, J R (1980). Components of delay among women obtaining termination of pregnancy *Journal of Biosocial Science*, **12**, 261
3 Awan, A K. (1969) *Provoked Abortion Among 1447 Married Women* Lahore, Pakistan Maternal and Child Health Association
4 Baluk, V & O'Niel, P. (1980) Health professional's perceptions of the psychological consequences of abortion *American Journal of Community Psychiatry*, **8**, 67
5 Barnes, H. H. F (1947) Therapeutic abortion by means of soft soap pastes *Lancet*, ii, 825
6 Bongaarts, J. & Tietze, C (1977) The efficiency of menstrual regulation as a method of fertility control *Studies in Family Planning*, **8**, 268
7 Brock, D J H & Sutcliffe, R G (1972). Alpha-fetoprotein in the antenatal diagnosis of anencephaly and spina bifida *Lancet*, ii, 197
8 Bygdeman, M , Christensen, N J , Grien, K & Zheng, S (1981) Self administration of prostaglandin for termination of early pregnancy *Contraception*, **24**, 45
9 Bykov, S G (1927) A method of preventing pregnancy *Vrachebnoe Delo*, **9**, 21
10 Cates, W & Grimes, D A (1981) Deaths from second trimester abortion by dilatation and evacuation causes, prevention, facilities *Obstetrics and Gynecology*, **58**, 401
11 Cates, W., Grimes, D A & Smith, J C (1978) Abortion as a treatment for unwanted pregnancy the number two sexually transmitted condition *Advances in Planned Parenthood*, **12**, 115
12 Confidential Enquiries into Maternal Deaths in England and Wales 1976–1978 (1979) London Her Majesty's Stationery Office (HMSO)
13 Cole, M (1966) Abortifacients for sale In *Abortion in Britain* London Pitman Medical Press
14 Craft, I (1978) Intra-amniotic urea and low-dose prostaglandin E_2 for midtrimester termination *Lancet*, i, 1115.
15 Csapo, A I Pulkkinen, M O (1979). The mechanism of prostaglandin action on the pregnant human uterus *Prostaglandins*, **17**, 282

16   Csapo, A I , Herczeg, J , Pulkkınen, M , Kaıhola, H I , Zoltan, I , Csıllag, M
     & Mocsary, P (1976) Termınatıon of pregnancy wıth double prostaglandın
     ımpact *Amerıcan Journal of Obstetrıcs and Gynecology*, **124**, 1
17   Davıd, H P (1974) *Abortıon Research Internatıonal Experıence* Lexıngton,
     Massachusetts Lexıngton Books
18   Davıd, H P & McIntyre, R (1981) *Reproductıve Behavıour Central and
     Eastern European Experıence* New York Sprınger Publıshıng Company
19   Davıd, H P & Matejček, Z (1981) Chıldren born to women denıed abortıon
     an update *Famıly Plannıng Perspectıves*, **13**, 32
20   Davıd, H , Nıels, K R. & Holst, E. (1981) Postpartum and postabortıon
     experıence *Studıes ın Famıly Plannıng*, **2**, 205
21   Davıd, M . Nıels, K R & Holst, E (1981). Postpartum and postabortıon
     psychotıc reactıons *Famıly Plannıng Perspectıves*, **13**, 88
22   Davıs, G (1974) *Interceptıon of Pregnancy Postconceptıve Fertılıty Control*
     Sydney, Australıa Angus and Robertson
23   Devereux, D (1955) *A Study of Abortıon ın Prımıtıve Socıetıes*. New York
     Julıan Press
24   Dıggory, P (1966) A gynaecologıst's experıence In *Abortıon ın Brıtaın*
     London Pıtman Medıcal
25   Dıggory, P (1981) Revıew of abortıon practıces and theır safety. In *Second
     Trımester Abortıon*, ed M J N C Keırse Boerhaave Serıes for Postgraduate
     Medıcal Educatıon, vol 12 Leıden, The Netherlands Leıden Unıversıty Press
26   Dryden, J (1693) *Juvenal*, **6**, 775.
27   Dytrych, Z Matejček, Z , Schuller, V , Davıd, H P & Frıedman, H. L (1975).
     Chıldren born to women denıed abortıon *Famıly Plannıng Perspectıves*, **7**, 165
28   Edıtorıal (1971) Suıcıde and teenage pregnancy *Brıtısh Medıcal Journal*, ıı,
     602
29   Edıtorıal (1981) Late consequences of abortıon *Brıtısh Medıcal Journal*, **282**,
     1564
30   Edstrom, K (1979) Technıques of ınduced abortıon, theır health ımplıcatıon
     and servıce aspects a revıew of the lıterature *Bulletın of the World Health
     Organızatıon*, **57**, 481
31   Elger, W (1979) Pharmacology of parturıtıon and abortıon *Anımal
     Reproductıve Scıence*, **2**, 133
32   Exodus 21 22–5
33   Fınks, A A (1973) Mıdtrımester abortıon *Lancet*, ı, 263.
34   Fontana, V J , Donovan, D & Wong, R J (1963). The 'maltreatment'
     syndrome ın chıldren *New England Journal of Medıcıne*, **269**, 1389
35   Forssman, H & Thuwe, I (1966) One hundred and twenty chıldren born after
     applıcatıon for therapeutıc abortıon was refused *Acta Psychıatrıca et
     Neurologıca Scandınavıca*, **42**, 71
36   Fortney, J A & Laufe, L E (1978) Menstrual regulatıon–rısks and benefits
     In *Rısks, Benefits and Controversıes ın Fertılıty Control*, ed J. J Scıarra, G I
     Zatuchnı & J J Spıedel, p 274 Hagerstown, Maryland Harper and Row.
37   Fortney, J A & Vengadasalaam, D. (1980) Dısposable menstrual regulatıon
     kıts ın a non-throw-away economy *Contraceptıon*, **21**, 235
38   Freeman, E W (1978) Abortıon subjectıve attıtudes and feelıngs. *Famıly
     Plannıng Perspectıves*, **10**, 150
39   Freeman, E W , Rıckles, K , Hıggıns, G R , Garcıa, Celso-Ramon & Polen, J.
     (1980) Emotıonal dıstress patterns among women havıng first or repeat
     abortıon. *Obstetrıcs and Gynecology*, **55**, 630
40   French, F & Bıerman, J M (1962) Probabılıtıes of fetal mortalıty. *Publıc
     Health Reports*, **77**, 835

41 Goldberg, M F, Edmonds, L D & Oakley, G P (1979) Reducing birth defect risk in advanced maternal age *Journal of the American Medical Association*, **262**, 2292

42 Greer, H S, Lal, S, Lewis, S C., Belsey, E M & Beard, R W (1976). Psychosocial consequences of therapeutic abortion *British Journal of Psychiatry*, **128**, 74

43 Greenhalf, J.O & Diggory, P L C (1971) Induction of therapeutic abortion by intra-amniotic injection of urea *British Medical Journal*, 1, 28

44 Grimes, D V & Cates, W (1976) Deaths from paracervical anesthesia used for first-trimester abortion *New England Journal of Medicine*, **295**, 1397

45 Grimes, D A, Hulka, J F & McCutchen, M.E (1980) Midtrimester abortion by dilatation and evacuation vs intra-amniotic instillation of prostaglandin F_2: a randomized clinical trial *American Journal of Obstetrics and Gynecology*, **137**, 785.

46 Grimes, D A, Schultz, K F, Cates, W F & Tyler, C W (1977) Methods of midtrimester abortion which is safest? *International Journal of Obstetrics and Gynaecology*, **15**, 184

47 Haddow, J. & Macri, T M (1979). Prenatal screening for neural tube defects *Journal of the American Medical Association*, **242**, 515

48 Han Su Shin (1967) IUD programme in Korea *IPPF Medical Bulletin*, **1**(3), 1

49 Hayashi, M & Momase, K (1966). Statistical observation on artificial abortion and secondary sterility In *Harmful Effects of Induced Abortion*, ed. Y. Koya Tokyo Family Planning Federation of Japan

50 Hertig, A (1967) The overall problem in man In *Comparative Aspects of Reproductive Failure*, ed K Benirschke New York Springer-Verlag

51 Hogue, C J R (1978) Review of postulated fertility complications subsequent to pregnancy termination *Risks, Benefits and Controversies in Fertility Control*, ed J J. Sciarra, G I Zatuchni & J J Speidel, p 356 New York Harper and Row

52 Hogue, C J R (1979) Long term sequelae in dilatation and curettage vs vacuum aspiration Report of an epidemiological study in Singapore In *Pregnancy Termination Procedures, Safety and New Developments*, ed. G I Zatuchni & J J Sciarra Hagerstown, Maryland Harper and Row

53 Holtrop, H R & Waife, R S (1976) *Uterine Aspiration Techniques in Family Planning* Boston, Massachusetts Pathfinder Fund

54 Hook, E B (1981) Prevalence of chromosome abnormalities during human gestation and implications for environmental mutagens *Lancet*, II, 169

55 Hulka, J (1969) A mathematical model study of contraceptive efficiency and unplanned pregnancies *American Journal of Obstetrics and Gynecology*, **104**, 443

56 Institute of Medicine (1978) *Legalized Abortion and the Public Health* Washington, DC National Academy of Sciences

57 International Fertility Research Program (1981) *Traditional Abortion Practices* Research Triangle Park, North Carolina, IFRP

58 James, W H (1978) Birth ranks of spontaneous abortion in siblings of children affected by anencephaly. *British Medical Journal*, 1, 72

59 Jaramillo-Gomez, M & Londono, J M (1968) Rhythm a hazardous contraceptive method *Demography*, **5**, 433

60 Johnstone, F D, Beard, R J., Boyd, I E & McCarthy, T G (1976) Cervical diameter after suction termination of pregnancy *British Medical Journal*, 1, 68

61 Karim, S M M (1971). Once-a-month administration of prostaglandin E^2 and F^2 for fertility control. *Contraception*, **3**, 173

62 Karim, S M M & Amy, J.J (1975) Interruption of pregnancy with

prostaglandıns In *Prostaglandıns and Reproduction*, ed S. M. M. Karım, p. 77 Lancaster, England MTP Press

63   Karman, H & Potts, M (1972). Very early abortıon usıng a syrınge as a vacuum source *Lancet*, ı, 1051

64   Kerenyı, T V (1981) Intra-amnıotıc technıques In *Abortıon and Sterılızatıon*, ed J E Hodgson, p 359 London Academıc Press.

65   Kerslake, D & Casey, D (1967) Abortıon ınduced by means of uterıne aspıratıon. *Obstetrıcs and Gynecology*, **30**, 35

66   Kessel, E. (1979) Menstrual regulatıon In *Bırth Control An International Assessment*, ed M Potts & P. Bhıwandıwala, p 187 Lancaster, England· MTP Press

67   Kleınman, R L (1971). *Abortıon Classıfıcatıon and Technıques* London International Planned Parenthood Federatıon (IPPF)

68   Kleınman, R L. (Ed) (1972) *Induced Abortıon* London IPPF

69   Kleınman, R L (Ed) (1980) *Famıly Plannıng Handbook for Doctors* London IPPF

70   Kleınman, R L (Ed) (1976) *Menstrual Regulatıon.* London IPPF

71   Klıne, J , Stem, Z , Strobıno, B , Susser, M & Warburten, D. (1977) Surveıllance of spontaneous abortıons. *American Journal of Epıdemıology*, **106**, 345

72   Klınger, A & Szabady, E (1969) The Hungarıan fertılıty and famıly plannıng study In *Famıly Plannıng and Natıonal Development*, p. 68 London IPPF

73   Laufe, L E (1979) Menstrual regulatıon – ınternatıonal perspectıves In *Pregnancy Termınatıon Procedures, Safety and New Developments*, ed. G. I Zatuchnı, J J Scıarra & J J Speıdel, p 78 Hagerstown, Maryland Harper and Row

74   Lındahl, J. (1959) *Somatıc Complıcatıons followıng Legal Abortıon* Stockholm, Sweden Scandınavıan Unıversıty Books.

75   McLaren, A (1981) 'Barrenness agaınst-nature' recourse to abortıon ın preındustrıal England. *The Journal of Sex Research*, **17**, 224

76   Mackenzıe, I Z , Davıs, A J , Embrey, M P & Guıllebaud, J (1978) Very early abortıon by prostaglandıns *Lancet*, ı, 1223

77   Maıne, D (1979) Does abortıon affect later pregnancıes? *International Family Plannıng Perspectıves*, **5**, 22

78   Maresh, M , Adshead, D , Barber, M & Rowlands, S (1974). Why admıt abortıon patıents? *Lancet*, ıı, 888

79   Mıller, J F , Wıllıamson, E , Glue, J., Gordon, Y B , Grudzınskas, J G. & Skyes, A (1980). Fetal loss after ımplantatıon. *Lancet*, ıı, 554.

80   Muramatsu, M (1970) An analysıs of factors ın fertılıty control ın Japan *Bulletın of the Instıtute of Publıc Health Tokyo*, **19**, 97

81   Nathanson, B M (1972) Ambulatory abortıon, experıence of 26,000 cases *New England Journal of Medıcıne*, **286**, 403

82   Nazer, I (1979) The Tunısıan experıence ın legal abortıon *Internatıonal Journal of Obstetrıcs and Gynaecology*, **17**, 493

83   Obel, E (1979) Pregnancy complıcatıons followıng legally ınduced abortıon wıth specıal reference to abortıon technıque *Acta Obstetrıca et Gynecologıca Scandınavıca*, **58**, 539

84   Omran, A K (1976) *Lıberalızatıon of Abortıon Laws Implıcatıons* Chapel Hıll, North Carolına Carolına Populatıon Center

85   Ovıd (43 BC–AD18) *Nux Elegıa*, lınes 23–4.

86   Panayotou, P P & Kaskarelıs, D M (1972) Induced abortıon and ectopıc pregnancy *American Journal of Obstetrıcs and Gynecology*, **114**, 507

87   Pare, C M B & Raven, H (1970) Follow-up of patıents referred for termınatıon of pregnancy *Lancet*, ı, 635

88 Perry, J (1951) Fecundity and embryonic mortality in pigs *Journal of Embryology and Experimental Morphology*, **2**, 308

89 Peterson, H. B , Grimes, D. A., Cates, W. & Rubin G. (1981) Comparative risk of death from induced abortion at < 12 weeks' gestation performed with local vs general anesthesia *American Journal of Obstetrics and Gynecology*, **141**, 763.

90 Pettersson, F (1968) *Epidemiology of Early Pregnancy Wastage* Stockholm, Sweden Svenska Bokforlaget

91 Pickles, V R. (1957) A plain muscle stimulant in the menstrual fluid *Nature*, 1198

92 Potter, R G. (1971). Inadequacy of a one-method family planning program. *Studies in Family Planning*, **2**, 1

93 Potts, M (1967). Legal abortion in Eastern Europe *Eugenics Review*, **59**, 232

94 Potts, M (1981) Abortion and contraception in relation to family planning services. In *Abortion and Sterilization Medical and Social Aspects*, ed. J. E Hodgson, p 481 London Academic Press

95 Potts, M (1981) Abortion and contraception in relation to family planning services. In *Abortion and Sterilization Medical and Social Aspects*, ed J. E Hodgson, p. 483. London Academic Press

96 Potts, M. & Branch, B (1971) Legal abortion in the USA a preliminary assessment. *Lancet*, II, 651.

97 Potts, M & Diggory, P (1973) Termination of pregnancy. In *Human Reproduction*, ed. E. S. E Hafez & T. N Evans, p 405 Hagerstown, Maryland. Harper and Row

98 Potts, M , Diggory, P & Peel, J (1977) *Abortion*. Cambridge Cambridge University Press.

99 Pritchard, E W (1864). Abortion procured by tents of common sea tangle (*Laminaria digitata*) *Obstetrical Transactions*, **5**, 198

100 Requena, M (1968). The problem of induced abortion in Latin America. *Demography*, **5**, 785

101 Rochat, R W , Jabeen, S , Rosenberg, M T , Measham, A R., Khan, A R., Obaidullah, M & Gould, P (1981). Maternal and abortion related deaths in Bangladesh 1978–79 *International Journal of Gynaecology and Obstetrics*, **19**, 155

102 Rovinsky, J (1972) Abortion recidivism *Obstetrics and Gynecology*, **39**, 649

103 Sawazaki, C & Tanaku, S. (1966) The relationship between artificial abortion and extrauterine pregnancy In *Harmful Effects of Induced Abortion*, ed Y Koya Tokyo Family Planning Federation of Japan

104 Shapiro, S , Levine, H S & Abramowicz, M (1971) Factors associated with early and late fetal loss *Advances in Planned Parenthood*, **6**, 45

105 Simms, M (1980). *Abortion in Britain before the Abortion Act* London Birth Control Trust

106 Simpson, J Y (1863) *Clinical Lectures on Diseases of Women* Philadelphia, Pennsylvania Blanchard and Lea

107 Simon, N & Senturia, A (1966) Psychiatric sequelae of abortion *Archives of General Psychiatry*, **15**, 378

108 Sood, S V (1971) Termination of pregnancy by the intrauterine injection of utus paste *British Medical Journal*, II, 215

109 Sook Bang (1968) Comparative study of the effectiveness of a family planning program in rural Korea Doctoral Thesis, University of Michigan

110 Stamm, H (1967) Statistiche Unterlageen zum Problem der Geb urtenkontrolle unite der Familien planung *Ars Medici*, **11**, 748

111 Stein, Z , Susser, M & Guterman, A U (1973) Screening programme for prevention of Down's syndrome *Lancet*, I, 305

112 Stringer, T., Anderson, M , Beard, R. W Fairweather, D. U. I & Steele, S J.
     (1975) Very early termination of pregnancy (menstrual extraction). *British
     Medical Journal*, iii, 7
113 Stubblefield, P. G. (1981). Midtrimester abortion by curettage procedures· an
     overview. In *Abortion and Sterilization Medical and Surgical Aspects*, ed. J. E.
     Hodgson, p. 277. London Academic Press
114 Tietze, C. (1973) Two years experience with a liberal abortion law. its impact
     on fertility trends in New York City. *Family Planning Perspectives*, **5**, 36.
115 Tietze, C (1977). Legal abortions in the United States: rates by race and age
     1972–74. *Family Planning Perspectives*, **9**, 12.
116 Tietze, C. (1981). *Induced Abortion a World Review, 1981*, 4th ed. New York
     Population Council.
117 Tietze, C., Guttmacher, A. F. & Rubin, S. (1959) Unintentional abortion in
     1494 planned pregnancies. *Journal of the American Medical Association*, **142**,
     1348
118 Tietze, C. & Lewit, S (1972). Joint program for the study of abortion (JPSA):
     early medical complications of legal abortion. *Studies in Family Planning*, **3**,
     97.
119 Tohan, N., Tejani, N., Varansai, M. & Robins, J. (1979). Ripening the term
     cervix with laminaria. *Obstetrics and Gynecology*, **54**, 588.
120 Tongplaew Narkavonkit (1979) Abortion in rural Thailand. *Studies in Family
     Planning*, **10**, 223.
121 Trichopoulos, D., Handanos, N. & Danezis, J. (1976). Induced abortion and
     secondary infertility. *British Journal of Obstetrics and Gynaecology*, **83**, 645.
122 Tyack, A. J , Parson, R J , Millar, D. R., Pennington, G & Hall, R. (1973).
     Plasma progesterone changes in abortion induced by hypertonic saline in the
     second trimester of pregnancy. *Journal of Obstetrics and Gynaecology of the
     British Commonwealth*, **80**, 548
123 Tyler, C W (1981). Epidemiology of abortion *Journal of Reproductive
     Medicine*, **26**, 459.
124 UK Collaborative study on alpha-fetoprotein in relation to neural tube defects
     (1977). *New England Journal of Medicine*, **294**, 365.
125 Van der Slikke, J. W & Treffers, P. E. (1978). Influence of induced abortion on
     gestational duration in subsequent pregnancies. *British Medical Journal*, i, 270.
126 Van der Tak, J. (1974). *Abortion, Fertility and Changing Legislation An
     International Review*. Lexington, Massachusetts Lexington Books.
127 Van der Vlugt, T. & Piotrow, P. T. (1973). Menstrual regulation – what is it?
     Population Reports, Series F.
128 Van de Warkle (1870). The detection of criminal abortion. *Journal of the
     Boston Obstetrical Society*, **4**, 292, **5**, 229, **5**, 350.
129 Viel, B. (1976) *The Demographic Explosion*. New York John Wiley & Sons.
130 WHO Task Force on Sequelae of Abortion (1979). Gestation, birth weight and
     spontaneous abortion in pregnancy after induced abortion *Lancet*, i, 142.
131 Wagatsuma, T. (1965). Intraamniotic injection of saline for therapeutic
     abortion. *American Journal of Obstetrics and Gynecology*, **93**, 743
132 Walter, G. S (1970). Psychologic and emotional consequences of elective
     abortion. *Obstetrics and Gynecology*, **36**, 483.
133 Ward, J W., Cuckle, H. S., Catz, C., Dayton, D & Reimer, C. B. (1981).
     Alpha-fetoprotein screening and diagnosis of fetal open neural tube defects·
     the need for quality control. *American Journal of Obstetrics and Gynecology*,
     141, 1.
134 Wilcox, A. J., Treloar, A. E. & Sandler, D. P. (1981). Spontaneous abortion
     over time comparing occurrence in two cohorts of women a generation apart
     American Journal of Epidemiology, **114**, 548.

135 Wu, T & Wu, H C (1958) Suction curettage for artificial abortion
preliminary report of 300 cases *Chinese Journal of Obstetrics*, **6**, 26
136 *Report of the Committee on the Working of the Abortion Act* (1974) Vols I, II
and III London Her Majesty's Stationery Office (HMSO)

14 Medical aspects

1 Alan Guttmacher Institute (1976) *11 Million Teenagers* New York AGI
2 Barnes, C G (1974) *Medical Disorders in Obstetric Practice*, 4th Ed Oxford
Blackwell Scientific Publications
3 *British Medical Journal* (Editorial) (1982) Will breast self-examination save
lives? **284**, 142
4 Cartwright, A (1970) *Parents and Family Planning Services*, p 64 London
Routledge and Kegan Paul
5 Diggory, P (1982) Modern serological tests for syphilis *Update*, **24**, 1546
6 Diggory, P L C (1982) Breast cancer and the Pill *Lancet*, i, 995
7 Diggory, P L C (1981) The long term effects upon the child of perinatal
events In *Changing Patterns of Child Bearing*, ed R Chester, P L C Diggory
& M Sutherland London Academic Press
8 Fraser, I S (1979). Ovarian function and its control In *Human Reproductive
Physiology*, ed P Shearman Oxford and Melbourne Blackwell Scientific
Publications
9 Hale, R W & Char, D. F B (1982) Sexual and contraceptive behaviour on a
college campus a five year follow-up *Contraception*, **25**, 126
10 Kelsey, J L (1978) Oral contraceptives and breast disease, an epidemiologic
study *American Journal of Epidemiology*, **10**, 236
11 Lenton, E A , Weston, G A & Cooke, I D (1977) Long term follow-up of
apparently normal couples with a complaint of infertility *Fertility and
Sterility*, **28**, 913
12 Macgregor, J E & Teper, S (1978) Uterine cervical cytology and young
women *Lancet*, i, 1029
13 Macgregor, J E (1982) Screening for pre-clinical cervical cancer In *Pre-
clinical Neoplasia of the Cervix* Proceedings of the Ninth Study Group of the
Royal College of Obstetricians and Gynaecologists, ed J. A Jordan, F Sharp
& A Singer London Royal College of Obstetricians and Gynaecologists
(RCOG)
14 Matthews, P N , Mills, R. R & Hayward, J L (1981) Breast cancer in women
who have taken oral contraceptives *British Medical Journal*, **282**, 774
15 Monif, G R G & Chez, R A (1980) How to culture for gonorrhoea
Contemporary Obstetrics and Gynaecology, **16**, 165
16 Mumford, J P (1974) Drugs affecting oral contraceptives *British Medical
Journal*, ii, 333
17 Noyes, R W & Chapnic, E M (1964) Literature on psychology and
infertility *Fertility and Sterility*, **15**, 543
18 Poffenberger, R.S , Fasal, S , Simmons, M E & Lamber, J B (1977) Cancer
risk related to use of oral contraceptives during fertile years *Cancer*, **39**, 1887
19 Population Reference Bureau (1976) Adolescent Pregnancy and Childbearing
– Growing Concerns for Americans Washington, DC.
20 Royal College of General Practitioners (1981) Family planning An exercise in
preventive medicine Reports from *General Practice*, 21.
21 Schofield, M (1968) Pap smear screening at what intervals? *Contraceptive
Technology Update*, **3**, 3

22   Schofield, M (1968) *The Sexual Behaviour of Young People* Penguin Books Harmondsworth, Middlesex, England
23   Skinner, G (1982) Sero-epidemiological evidence of association between type 2 herpes simplex virus and carcinoma of the cervix, in *Pre-Clinical Neoplasia of the Cervix* Proceedings of the Ninth Study Group of the Royal College of Obstetricians and Gynaecologists, ed. J A. Jordan, F Sharp & A Singer London RCOG
24   Tumson, I S , Dudley, D K L & Walters, J H (1981) Genital herpes simplex *Canadian Medical Journal*, **125**, 231
25   Vessey, M P , Doll, R & Sutton, P. M (1971). Investigation of possible relationship between oral contraceptives and benign and malignant breast disease *Cancer*, **28**, 1395.
26   Vessey, M.P , Doll, R , Jones, K , McPherson, R. & Yeats, P (1979) An epidemiological study of oral contraceptives and breast cancer *British Medical Journal*, I, 57
27   Udry, R , Bauman, K E & Morris, N M (1975) Changes in premarital coital experience of recent decade-of-birth cohorts of urban American women *Journal of Marriage and the Family*, II, 783
28   WHO (1975) Pregnancy and Abortion in Adolescence World Health Organization Technical Report Series No 583 Geneva WHO.

15   Legal and administrative aspects of family planning

1   Ang Eng Suan , Yusof, K & Sinnathuray, T A (1979) Time and motion study of family planning clinic attached to a university hospital *Singapore Journal of Obstetrics and Gynaecology*, **10**, 23
2   American Law Institute (1962) *Model Penal Code*, art 230
3   Anonymous (1981) China's new marriage law *Population and Development Review*, 7, 369.
4   Anonymous (1979). Menstrual aspiration *British Journal of Family Planning*, **5**, 48
5   Baird, D (1965) The Fifth Freedom *British Medical Journal*, XII, 1141
6   Bayliss, P. (1982) Personal communication
7   Bhiwandiwala, P P , Cook, R J , Dickens, B M & Potts, M (1982) Menstrual therapies in Commonwealth Asian Law *International Journal of Obstetrics and Gynaecology*, **20**, 273
8   Bourne, A (1962) *A Doctor's Creed* London Gollancz
9   Chile *International Digest for Health Legislation* (1977) **28**, 2
10   Cook, R J & Dickens, B M (1978). A decade of change in abortion laws 1967–77 *American Journal of Public Health*, **68**, 637 and (1977), *Three Studies of Abortion Laws in the Commonwealth* London Commonwealth Secretariat
11   Cook, R J (1976) Distribution of oral contraceptives legal changes and new concepts of preventive care *American Journal of Public Health*, **66**, 590
12   Cooper, T (1980) Compensation for human research subjects reform ahead of its time *Journal of Legal Medicine*, **3**, 1
13   David, H P (1970) *Family Planning and Abortion in the Socialist Countries of Central and Eastern Europe* New York Population Council
14   David, H P & McIntyre, R J (1981) *Reproductive Behaviour Central and Eastern European Experience* New York Springer Books
15   Fletcher School of Law Diplomacy (1975) *Law and Population* (Lectures and Reading Materials) Medford, Massachusetts Tufts University
16   Goldthorpe, J (1977). *British Medical Journal*, I, 562, and Director of Public Prosecutions, letter to Medical Defence Union Solicitors, 5 April 1979

17 India L A Bill No XXV of 1976
18 Johsson, V (1937) The Icelandic Birth Control and Feticide Act *Journal of Contraception*, **2**, 219
19 Lee, L T (1976) Compulsory sterilization and human rights *Populi*, p. 32
20 Lee, L. T (1977). Legal aspects of menstrual regulation *Studies in Family Planning*, **8**, 273
21 Lucas, R (1970). Laws of the United States In *Abortion in a Changing World*, vol 1, ed R. E Hall, p 127 New York Columbia University Press
22 Mabrouk, M (1975) Development of the right to abortion in Tunisia In The Symposium on Law and Population, Tunis New York United Nations Fund for Population Activities (UNFPA)
23 Meisel, A — Roth, L H (1981) What we do and do not know about informed consent *Journal of the American Association*, **246**, 2473
24 Meyer, H S (1981) Science and the 'Human Life Bill' *Journal of the American Medical Association*, **246**, 837
25 Mohr, J. (1978) *Abortion in America* Oxford Oxford University Press
26 Moore-Cavar, E C (1974) *International Inventory of Information on Induced Abortion* New York Columbia University
27 Muir, B (1980). Contraception for the young legal restrictions *New Zealand Journal of Family Planning*, **1**, 32
28 Nazar, I R (Ed) (1971) *Induced Abortion a Hazard to Public Health* Beirut International Planned Parenthood Federation (IPPF).
29 New Zealand Report of the Royal Commission of Inquiry (1977) *Contraception, Sterilization and Abortion in New Zealand* Wellington Government Printer
30 Ottensen-Jensen, O. (1971) Legal abortion in Sweden thirty years experience. *Journal of Biosocial Science*, **3**, 173
31 Paul, E W , Pilpel, H F & Weschsler, N F (1976) Pregnancy, teenagers and the law 1976 *Family Planning Perspectives*, **6**, 142
32 Paul, E W & Schaap, P (1980) Abortion and the law *New York Law School Law Review*, **25**, 497
33 Paxman, J M (1980) Roles of non-physicians in fertility regulation an international overview of legal obstacles and solutions *American Journal of Public Health*, **70**, 31
34 Paxman, J M (1980) *Law and Planned Parenthood* London IPPF
35 Pi-chao Chen (1981) *Rural Health and Birth Planning in China* Research Triangle Park, North Carolina International Fertility Research Program (IFRP)
36 Pilpel, H (1974) Voluntary sterilization a human right In *The Symposium on Law and Population, Tunis*, p 105 New York UNFPA
37 Potts, M (1967) Legal abortion in Eastern Europe *Eugenics Review*, **59**, 232
38 Potts, M (1974) Laws regulating the manufacture and distribution of contraceptives In *The Symposium on Law and Population, Tunis*, p 82 New York UNFPA
39 Potts, M , Diggory, P & Peel, J (1977) *Abortion* Cambridge Cambridge University Press
40 Rosenfield, A G (1974) Laws related to professional paramedical role in contraception In *The Symposium on Law and Population, Tunis* p 93 New York UNFPA
41 Saudi Arabia Royal Decree, 28 April 1975
42 Schesinger, R (1969) *The Family in the USSR* London Routledge and Kegan Paul
43 Schima, M E & Lubell, I (1976) *New Advances in Sterilization The Third World Conference on Voluntary Sterilization, Tunis* New York Association for Voluntary Sterilization

44 Sharma, M L (1976) *Abortion Law in India* Bombay Family Planning Association India
45 Simms, M & Hindel, K (1971) *Abortion Law Reformed* London Peter Oliver
46 Stephan, J & Kellogg, E H (1973) The world's laws concerning voluntary sterilization for family planning purposes *Californian Western International Law Review*, **5**, 72
47 Stephan, J & Kellogg, E H (1974) *The World's Laws on Contraceptives*, Law and Population Monograph No 17 Medford, Massachusetts Tufts University
48 Sturgis, S H (1970) Contraception since Comstockery *New England Journal of Medicine*, **283**, 595
49 Sweden Ordinance No 109, 3 April 1975 and No 1, 12 January 1978.
50 Tomsic, V (1976) Status for women, family planning and population dynamics In *The Symposium on Law and Population, Tunis*, p 27 New York UNFPA
51 Udry, J. R. (1974). *The Media and Family Planning*. New York. Ballinger.
52 United Kingdom Sexual Offences Act 1965, sec 5
53 United Kingdom Television Act 1954, sec 4(5) and Independent Television Authority (1960) *Principles of Television Advertising* London
54 United Kingdom (1978). Hansard **916**, no 160, col, 1161
55 United Nations Fund for Population Activities (1976) *Survey of Contraceptive Laws Country Profiles, Checklist and Summaries* Declaration on Social Progress and Development New York UNFPA
56 United States Virginia Code An. tit 32 ch 27 423 1972.
57 United States *Griswald* v *Connecticut* 381 US, 475 (1965) *Eisenstadt* v *Baird* 405 US, 438 (1972)
58 United States *Roe* v *Wade* Supreme Court of the United States (22 Jan 1973) NO 70-18
59 United States S J Res 110 (1981) Human Life Federalism Amendment
60 United States S J Res 17 Human Life Amendment
61 United States S 1741 and S188 (1981) 'Human Life' Statute
62 United States *Federal Register* (1982) **47** (35), col 7699
63 Williams, G (1958) *The Sanctity of Life and Criminal Law* London Faber and Faber
64 World Health Organization (WHO) (1981) International code on marketing breast milk substitutes *WHO Chronicle*, **35**, 112
65 Yugoslavia (1974) Constitution of the Socialist Federal Republic of Yugoslavia Art 191

16 Conspectus

1 Atkinson, L , Schearer, B , Harkavy, O & Luncal, R (1980). Prospects for improved contraception *Family Planning Perspectives*, **12**, 173.
2 Bernard, R P , Kendall, E M. & Manton, K. G (1980). International maternity care monitoring a beginning In *Clinical Perinatology*, ed S. Aladjem, A K Brown & C Sureau St Louis, Missouri C V Mosby.
3 Bracken, M B & Kasl, S. V (1973) Factors associated with dropping out of family planning clinics in Jamaica *American Journal of Public Health*, **63**, 262
4 Callahan, D (1970) *Abortion Law, Choice and Morality* London Macmillan
5 Chandrasckhar, S (1981) '*A Dirty Filthy Book*' Berkeley, California University of California Press

6 Csapo, A I (1974) Prostaglandin impact for menstrual induction *Population Reports*, Series G, 33
7 Darwin, C (1871) *The Descent of Man and Selection in Relation to Sex* London
8 de Kretser, D M (1978) Fertility regulation in the male *Bulletin of the World Health Organization*, 56, 353
9 de Raddo, J & Wardell, W M (1981) Research activity on systemic contraceptive drugs by US pharmaceutical industry 1963–76 *Contraception*, 23, 345
10 Deys, C M & Potts, D M (1972) Condoms and things *Advances in the Biosciences*, 10, 287
11 Djerassi, C. (1970) Birth control after 1984 *Science*, 169, 941
12 Djerassi, C (1979) The Politics of Contraception, p. 76 New York W W Norton Company
13 Doll, Sir Richard, Gray, R., Hafner, B & Peto, R (1980) Mortality in relation to smoking 22 years observation in female British doctors. *British Medical Journal*, 280, 967
14 Doll, Sir Richard & Peto, R (1981). *The Causes of Cancer* Oxford Oxford University Press
15 Dunbar, B S & Raynor, B D (1980) Characterization of porcine zona pellucida antigens *Biology of Reproduction*, 22, 941
16 Elgar, W (1979). Pharamacology of parturition and abortion *Animal Reproduction Science*, 2, 133
17 Elstein, M, Gordon, A D G & Buckingham, M S (1977) Sexual knowledge and attitudes of general practitioners in Wessex *British Medical Journal*, i, 369
18 Gray, M (1979) *Margaret Sanger* New York Richard Marek
19 Greep, R O, Koblinsky, M A. & Jaffe, Y (1976) *Reproduction and Human Welfare A Challenge to Research* Cambridge, Massachusetts MIT Press
20 Grunberg, R (1979) *The 12-Year Reich A social history of Nazi Germany 1933–45* New York Holt, Rinehart & Winston
21 Hahn, D W, Ericson, E W. & Lai, M T (1981) Antifertility activity of *Montanoa tomentosa Contraception*, 23, 133
22 Hearn, J P (1976) Immunization against pregnancy *Proceedings of the Royal Society*, London, B, 195, 149
23 Heller, C G, Moore, D J & Paulsen, C A. (1961). Suppression of spermatogenesis and chronic toxicity in men by a new series of bis (dichloroacetyl) diamines *Toxicology and Applied Pharmacology*, 3, 1
24 Hollerbach, P E (1980) Power in families, communication and fertility decision-making. *Population and Environmental Behavioural and Social Issues*, 3, 146.
25 Howard, R A, Matherson, J E & Owen, D L (1978) The value of life and nuclear design In *Probabilistic Analysis of Nuclear Reactor Safety*, ed D Okrent & E. Cramer Illinois American Nuclear Society
26 International Fertility Research Program (1981) *Traditional Abortion Practices*. Research Triangle Park, North Carolina IFRP.
27 International Fertility Research Program (1981) *Surgical Family Planning Methods the Role of the Private Practitioner* Research Triangle Park, North Carolina IFRP
28 Jochle, W (1974) Menses inducing drugs Their role in antique, medieval and renaissance gynecology and birth control *Contraception*, 10, 425.
29 Koch, U J, lorenz, F, Danehl, K, Ericsson, R & Hasan, S M (1976) Continuous oral low-dosage cyproterone acetate for fertility regulation in the male *Contraception*, 14, 117.

30   Langer, W L (1974) Infanticide a historical survey. History Childhood Quarterly, **1**, 353

31   Laufe, L E , McCann, M F (1978) Training an integral adjunct to the introduction of newer methods of fertility regulation *International Journal of Gynaecology and Obstetrics*, **15**, 302

32   Lichtenstein, S , Slovic, P , Fischhoff, B , Layman, M & Combs, B (1978) Judged frequency of lethal events *Journal of Experimental Psychology Human Learning and Memory*, **4**, 551.

33   Luker, K (1975) *Taking Chances* Berekely, California University of California Press

34   Maine, D (1981) *Family Planning its Impact on the Health of Women and Children* New York Center for Population and Family Health, Columbia University

35   Metropolitan Life Insurance Company (1974) Homicide in the United States *Statistical Bulletin*, **55**, 1

36   Metropolitan Life Insurance Company (1979). Sports Hazards *Statistical Bulletin*, **60**, (3), 1

37   Metropolitan Life Insurance Company (1980) Accidental poisoning *Statistical Bulletin*, **61**, (2), 8

38   Metropolitan Life Insurance Company (1981) Fatalities in the US railroads. *Statistical Bulletin*, **52**, (4), 1

39   Moorehead, W & Oei, T O (1978) Talc in drugs. *New England Journal of Medicine*, **298**, 1365

40   Murphy, F X (1981). Catholic perspectives on population issues II *Population Bulletin*, **35**, 1

41   National Coordinating Group on Male Antifertility Agents (1978) Gossypol a new antifertility agent for males. *Chinese Medical Journal*, **4**, 417

42   Nazer, I. R , Karmi, H S & Zayid, M Y. (Eds) (1974). *Islam and Family Planning Proceedings of the International Islamic Conference, Rabat, Morocco, Dec. 1971.* Beirut, Lebanon International Planned Parenthood Federation, Middle East and North Region

43   Nillius, S J , Bergquist, C & Wide, L (1980). Chronic treatment with the gonadotrophin-releasing hormone agonist D-Ser (TBU)-EA-LRH for contraception in women and men *International Journal of Fertility*, **25**, 239

44   Noonan, J T (1967) *Contraception A History of its Treatment by Catholic Theologians and Canonists* Cambridge, Massachusetts Harvard University Press

45   Pearson, R M , Hong, C Y , Penhall, R K , Turner, P , Zahman, S & Zipper, J (1983) Studies on the effects of drugs on sperm motility In *Proceedings of the First Inter-American Congress on Clinical Pharmacology and Therapeutics 1982*, ed M Velasco Caracas, Venezuela

46   Pi-chao, Chen (1981) *Rural Health and Birth Planning in China* Research Triangle Park, North Carolina IFRP

47   Potts, M , Speidel, J J & Kessel, E (1978) Relative risk of various means of fertility control when used in less developed countries In *Risks, Benefits and Controversies in Fertility Control*, ed J J Sciarra, G I Zatuchni & J J Speidel, p 229 Hagerstown, Maryland Harper and Row

48   Potts, M & Wheeler, R (1981) The quest for a magic bullet *Family Planning Perspectives*, **13**, 269

49   Roberts, Archbishop I E (Ed.) (1964) *Contraception and Holiness* New York Herder and Herder

50   Robinson, W , Shah, M & Shah, N M (1981) The family planning program in Pakistan what went wrong? *International Family Planning Perspectives*, **7**, 85

51   Rochat, R W (1976) Abortion, the Bible and the Christian physician *Christian Medical Journal,* **7,** 19

52   Rowland, B (1981) *Medieval Woman's Guide to Health.* London· Croom Helm

53   Rubin, G , McCarthy, B., Shelton, T., Rochat, R W & Terry, T (1981). The risk of childbearing re-evaluated *American Journal of Public Health,* **71,** 712

54   Schally, A V (1978). Aspects of hypothalamic regulation of the pituitary gland· its implications in the control of the reproductive process Science, **202,** 18

55   Shedlin, M. (1979). Assessment of body concepts and beliefs regarding reproductive physiology *Studies in Family Planning,* **10,** 393

56   Shandilya, L N & Clarkson, T B (1982) Hypolipedemic effects of gossypol in cynomolgus monkeys (*Maccaca fascicularis*) *Lipids,* **17,** 285

57   Sheehan, K. L , Casper, R. F & Yen, S S C (1982). Luteal phase defects induced by an agonist of luteinizing hormone-releasing factor· a model for fertility control. *Science,* **215,** 170

58   Short, R V (1980) Sexual selection in the great apes In *Reproductive Biology of the Great Apes,* ed. C E. Graham, p 319 New York Academic Press.

59   Simpson, J Y (1871) *Anaesthesia, Hospitalism, Hemaphrodeltism and a Proposal to Stamp out Small Pox and other Contagious Diseases.* Edinburgh.

60   Smout, T C (1980) Aspects of sexual behaviour in nineteenth century Scotland In *Bastardy and its Comparative History,* ed. P Laslett London Edward Arnold

61   Stevas, N St John (1971). *The Agonizing Choice Birth Control, Religion and the Law* London Eyre and Spottiswoode

62   Stevens, V C., Powell, J E , Lee, A C. & Griffin, D (1981). Antifertility effects of immunization of female baboons with C-terminal peptides of the β-subunit of human chorionic gonadotrophin. *Fertility and Sterility,* **36,** 98.

63   Stopes, M (1957) *Wise Parenthood.* 25th edn. London: Putnam and Co

64   Sutherland, H G (1936) *Birth Control Exposed* London Cecil Palmer

65   Taha, A & Ball, K (1980) Smoking and Africa the coming epidemic. *British Medical Journal,* i, 991

66   Talwar, G P. (1978). Anti-HGG immunization. *Contraception,* **18,** 19

67   Taylor, M. C & Berelson, B. (1968) Maternity care and family planning as a world program *American Journal of Obstetrics and Gynecology,* **100,** 885

68   Tietze, C (1977) New estimates of mortality associated with fertility control. *Family Planning Perspectives,* **9,** 74

69   *Times,* London. 8 Dec. 1981

70   Tomkinson, J S (1976) The cost of motherhood *British Medical Journal,* p 383

71   Tsai, S P , Lee, E S & Hardy, R J (1978). The effect of a reduction in leading causes of death, potential gains in life expectancy *American Journal of Public Health,* **68,** 966

72   Wan, L S., Stiber, A J & Turkel, J (1981) Termination of very early pregnancy by vaginal suppositories (15S)-15-methyl prostaglandin F_2 methyl ester. *Contraception,* **24,** 603

73   Williamson, N (1976) *Sons or Daughters? A Cross-Cultural Survey of Parental Preferences* Beverly Hills, California Saga Publication.

Index

abortifacients, 280–1, 383, *see also*
    prostaglandins
abortion and age of woman, 286–7,
    complications, 297, 301, 303, 307–13,
    day-care, 301–3, definition, 275; ectopic
    pregnancy after, 311, by educational
    level, 388–90; emotional benefits,
    312–13, ethical considerations, 319, 400,
    and fetal abnormalities, 290–1, illegal,
    and morbidity and mortality, 308,
    incidence of, 2, 3, 4, 28, 30, 33, 283,
    286–90, and intrauterine device
    insertion, 229–30; legal, and mortality,
    308–10, legal status in world, 7, 8, and
    legislation, 262, 286–90, 302, 308, 319,
    355–60, 400, maternal mortality, 286,
    302, 303, 306–10, 319, 320, 378; of
    minors and informed consent, 362;
    objection to, by doctor, 362, 363, and
    the Pill, 170, psychological
    consequences, 311–12; rates, 315–16,
    reasons for, 290; refused, and the child,
    313–14; and reproductive patterns, 19,
    20, 21, 23; therapeutic, 308, 356, of
    unplanned pregnancy, 317
abortion methods and anaesthesia, 293,
    294, crochet hook, 283, curettage and
    fluid injection, 281; dilatation and
    curettage, 292, 293–5, 300;
    hysterectomy, 306, 311, illegal, 281, 282,
    by massage, 283–5, mechanical, 281–3,
    medicinal, 280–1, 383, menstrual
    regulation, 295–9, mid-trimester, 303–7;
    prostaglandins, 291–2, by urinary
    catheters, 281, vacuum aspiration, 14,
    292–3, 299–300
abortion, spontaneous· and chromosome
    abnormalities, 171, 275, and congenital
    abnormalities, 276; epidemiology, 277–9;
    and intrauterine devices, 237, 244;

maternal factors, 276–7, and periodic
    abstinence, 103; and teratogens, 275–6
abstinence, 74, and lactation, 75
actinomycosis and intrauterine devices,
    237
Acts of Parliament, *see under* legislation,
    individual countries
advertising, 28, 107, 114, 352, legislation,
    113, 352; and preventive medicine,
    371–2, *see also* marketing
Africa abortions, 8, 279; abstinence and
    lactation, 75; birth intervals and
    lactation, 85, 90; periodic abstinence, 97;
    population growth, 38, 39
alimentary disorders· and contraceptive
    usage, 328–9
Allbutt, Arthur, 7, on cervical cap, 121;
    The Wife's Handbook (1886), 4
amenorrhoea· and contraceptive use,
    324–5, and Depo-Provera (DMPA) use,
    206; and the Pill, 146, 168–70, 324
amenorrhoea, postpartum, 85; and child
    spacing, 90, and lactation, 87
amniocentesis fetal abnormality detection,
    290–1; mid-trimester abortion, 304–5
anal intercourse, 81, 82
anovulation: anorexia nervosa, 18, and
    breast-feeding, 17, 19, 85–6, and
    nutritional status, 17–18, 85
antibodies in human milk, 87–8, and
    immunological contraception, 384–5,
    and sperm after vasectomy, 264, 384
Asia. age of marriage and legislation, 349,
    legal status of abortion, 8, Lippes loop
    performance, 224; population growth,
    39
Augustine, St and coitus interruptus, 76;
    periodic abstinence, 97
Australia Pill and cardiovascular disease,
    181–2; popularity of the Pill, 212

Baird, *Sir* Dugald, 267, 367
Bangladesh abortion, 8, 310, 359,
    contraceptives, 92, 113, 211, 385;
    maternal mortality, 262, 310, 387;
    menstrual regulation and legislation,
    360, minilaparotomy and female
    sterilization, 254, population growth, 38;
    spermicide effectiveness, 130, voluntary
    sterilization and mortality, 261–2
Behcet's syndrome, 325
Bernardine, St: on coitus interruptus, 76
Besant, Annie, 26, 399
birth control clinics· cervical caps versus
    diaphragms, 61, 121–2; first, 9–11;
    hostility towards, 35, 399; social class of
    clientele, 35, *see also* family planning
    services
birth-rates: and abortion legislation,
    285–6, 287, and Bradlaugh–Besant trial,
    26–7; and contraceptive use, 397,
    differentials among ethnic and social
    groups, 33–4; during the Depression, 30,
    and induced abortion, 315–16;
    legislation on rewards and penalties,
    366–7, reasons for decline of, 24–5, *see
    also* population explosion; population
    size
blood dyscrasias: and contraceptive use,
    165, 179, 328
Bradlaugh, Charles, 3, 26
Bradlaugh–Besant trial, 26–7
Brazil: abortion, 8; family size, 20;
    popularity of Pill, 213; population
    growth, 38; voluntary sterilization 247,
    355
breakthrough bleeding and drug
    interaction, 165, and the Pill, 146, 150,
    161, 165
breast-feeding advantages of, 86–9, and
    anovulation, 17, 19, 85–6, antibodies in
    human milk, 87–8; and child spacing,
    85, 90–1, contraceptive protection
    during, 92–3, epidemiology of, 89–91,
    patterns through the ages, 23, versus
    bottle-feeding, 86–9, 96
breasts benign disease and the Pill, 186,
    187, 199, 209, control of hormone
    secretion, 85; development and lactation,
    84–6, discomfort of, and the Pill, 146,
    160, 161, diseases of, and contraceptive
    use, 329–30; and progesterone, 142; self-
    examination of, 332–3, *see also* cancer,
    breast

Canada abortion, 8, 288, 311, 359,
    periodic abstinence, 101·
cancer, breast. and age of childbearing,
    184, 185, 388, and contraceptive use,
    330, in men, 184; and the Pill, 183–90,
    330, and progestogens, 209; self-
    examination, 332–3
cancer, cervical and contraceptive use,
    133, 134; cytological screening, 333–4;
    and diethylstilboestrol, 195, 276; and
    herpes genitalis, 133, 337; mortality,
    333; and the Pill, 190–2
cancer, endometrial. and Depo-Provera
    (DMPA), 204, 208–9, and the Pill, 192,
    199
cancer, ovarian: and Depo-Provera, 208,
    and late childbearing, 388; and the Pill,
    193, 199
Candida albicans. and spermicides, 123,
    vaginal infection, 326
carcinogenicity: of drugs and devices, tests
    for, 65–7
cardiovascular disease· and bottle-feeding,
    88, and contraceptive use, 327–8, and
    the Pill, 69, 172–83, 213, 328; and
    smoking, 173–4, 178, 179, 213, 391
Catholics: and abortion, 282–3, 290, 315,
    363, 400; coitus reservatus, 80;
    contraceptive use, 395–6; family size,
    397; love in marriage, 2, 395; and
    periodic abstinence, 97–8, 397
celibacy. and religion, 74–5, of young
    unmarried, 75
cervical caps, 123–4; care and use of,
    128–30; extent of use, 122, 123; fitting
    of, 125–6, 128, history of, 121–2, quality
    control, 56; reliability, 61; sizes, 124
cervical erosion· and contraceptive use,
    327
cervical mucus method, 100–1
cervicitis· and contraceptive use, 327
children· battered, 313, born after abortion
    refusal, 313–14; and divorce laws, 350
Chile lactation and the Pill, 94,
    sterilization legislation, 355
China abortion, 8; age of marriage and
    fertility control, 74, 349, birth-rate, 375,
    coitus reservatus, 80; family planning,
    48–9, 366, intrauterine device use, 218;
    Pill use, 165, 210, 212; population
    growth, 38, 43, 48–9, sexual behaviour
    and contraceptive availability, 398–9,
    vacuum aspiration, 292–3, voluntary
    sterilization, 245, 247
Chlamydia and pelvic inflammatory
    disease, 237
Chylamydia prachomatis non-specific
    urethritis, 336
chloasma and the Pill, 161
chlormadinone, 66, 204
chromosome abnormalities and
    spontaneous abortion, 171, 275
Coca Cola, 80, 283
coitus interruptus alleged side-effects, 79;

extent of use, 32, 75–7; reliability, 58,
60, 61, 77–8, 92, safety, 78–9
coitus reservatus, 79–80
coitus saxonicus, 80–1
Colombia family size, 45, periodic
abstinence, 98, 102, popularity of Pill,
213
colpotomy female sterilization, 254
Comstock, Anthony, 3–4, 28
Comstock Act (1873), 4, 53, 121, 352–3
conception· during menstrual cycle, 18–19,
and frequency of intercourse, 18
condoms· caecal, 107, 110; choice of,
115–17, coloured, 108, 112,
complementary to other methods, 377;
costs of, 109; electronic testing, 109,
extent of use, 32, 33, 110–11, history,
28, 106–7, lubricated, 108–9,
manufacture methods, 107–10,
marketing, 107, 111–14; other uses for,
113, pelvic inflammatory disease, 133,
plain and teat ended, 112; plastic, 110,
quality control, 55–6, 109, reliability, 58,
60, 64, 92–3, 114–15, side-effects,
116–17; sizes, 55, 109, use and care of,
117–18, and venereal infections, 115–16
congenital abnormality and intrauterine
devices, 238, and periodic abstinence,
102–3, and the Pill, 170, 171, 172; and
spontaneous abortion, 276
Cooper, Astley· vasectomy in dogs, 15,
245
cotton seed oil. and infertility, 381
counselling, 83, 322–4, 337–43; attitude of
advisors and method acceptance, 31–2,
323, 361–2, 373–4, communication
barriers, 339; effectiveness of different
methods, 60, 64, 323; on intrauterine
device use, 226–7, on Pill use, 149–51,
166–7, and psychological disorders,
338–9, sexual problems, 338, 339, for
the unmarried, 340–3, and voluntary
sterilization, 247–8
culdoscopy: female sterilization, 254–5
cystitis, 339–40

Darwin, Charles R human fertility
control, 2–3
Deladroxone, 94
Depo-Provera (depomedroxyprogesterone
acetate or DMPA), 94, 95, 203–4, choice
of, 211, effectivenss, 205, male Pill, 381,
masculinizing effect, 208, and neoplasia,
67, 208–9; and physiology, 205, side-
effects, 205–6, subsequent fertility, 207,
teratology and effect on infant, 207–8,
usage and medical disorders, 328, 329
desogestrel, 152
diabetes and contraceptive use, 328; and

endometrial cancer, 192; and the Pill,
156, 164, and vaginal moniliasis, 326
Diamond method, 81
diaphragms, 123–4, 125, care and use of,
128–30; evaluation, 134–5, extent of use,
32, 122–3; fitting of, 125–8; history of,
121–2, Mensinga Pessarie, 28, 121, pelvic
inflammatory disease, 133, quality
control, 56, toxic shock syndrome, 133
diethylstilboestrol· and cervical and
vaginal cancer, 195, 276, post-coital
contraception, 202
dilatation and curettage (D and C), 292,
293–5, 300
dilatation and evacuation (D and E), 304
diosgenin· and steroid synthesis, 136–7
disease studies prospective and
retrospective, 67–9
divorce adolescent marriages, 340, and
children, 350
DMPA, *see* Depo-Provera
doctors· on abortion, 274, 301, 312, 362,
363; on contraceptive information, 349,
398; education of medical students, 14,
family planning and preventive
medicine, 331–2, informed consent,
361–2, role as family planning advisers,
371, view of the Pill, 159, 168; on
voluntary sterilization, 246, 247; *see also*
counselling
Doderlein's bacillus, 325, 326
Draper, *General* William, 13
Dutch cap, *see* diaphragms
dysmenorrhoea and contraceptive use,
329; and the Pill, 156–7

ectopic pregnancy and Depo-Provera
(DMPA), 207; Fallopian tube
reanastomosis, 260, induced abortion,
311, and intrauterine devices, 223, 226,
238–9, pelvic inflammatory disease, 243,
and periodic abstinence, 103, and the
Pill, 198, 199; steroid implants, 207
education of medical students, 14
effectiveness, *see* use-effectiveness
Egypt: family size, 20; lactation and the
Pill, 94, population growth, 38, 40–1, 43
emmenagogues, 280, prostaglandins as, 383
Enavid failure rate, 153, and libido, 159,
production of, 137
endometriosis and contraceptive use, 329;
late childbearing, 388; and the Pill, 198
epilepsy· and contraceptive use, 165, 329
ethics. biological issues and fertility
control, 393–4, of doctor and advice to
patient, 363, immorality and
contraceptives, 398–9, induced abortion,
319–21, religious issues and fertility
control, 394–6, of self-referral, 11–12,

technological issues and fertility control,
  396–8
ethinyloestradiol, 152, 165, 180, post-coital
  Pill, 202, structure, 139, 140

Fallopian tubes, 251, 252, blockage and
  infertility, 345, electrocoagulation, 255,
  258, 266, methods of approach, 253–7,
  occlusion techniques, 257–9, 268–9,
  271–2, reanastomosis, 259–60, Yoon
  ring, 258, 266, 272
Family Health International (FHI,
  formerly The International Fertility
  Research Program, IFRP), 223, 269,
  271, 379
family limitation, 29–30, abortion and
  contraception integrated, 22–3, 314–18,
  376–7, 384, acceptability of method,
  58–9, accessibility of services, 44–5, 46,
  47–8, advice on, and medical practice,
  371, beliefs and myths, 369, and
  Bradlaugh–Besant trial, 26–7; and
  breast-feeding, 83, 85–6, 90–1; a human
  right, 12, 364–5, 367, 400–1, impetus
  for, 25–6, 36, as a learning process,
  368–71, and legislation, 347, 367, in
  nineteenth century, 2–4, optimum use of
  methods, 375–9, and patterns of
  contraceptive choice, 30–3, risks and
  benefits of contraceptives, 71–3, sexual
  risk-taking, 369–70, spread through
  social classes, 5, 26, 33, 35; twentieth-
  century transition 4–6
family planning services abortion and
  contraception integrated, 22–3, 314–18,
  376–7, 384, and the Catholic Church,
  396, condom distribution, 112–13; in
  developing world, 44–50, 51–2, *see also*
  individual countries, financial aid to,
  51–2, 401, legislation, 354, 363–4, and
  National Health Service, 35; 1926
  debate on, 12; and preventive medicine,
  330–7, quality of, 373, restraints on, 9,
  12, 53–4, 122–3, 362, 373–4, risks and
  benefits of contraceptives, 71–3;
  twentieth-century transition, 6–13, and
  under-privileged, 34–5, *see also* birth
  control clinics, marketing
family size in absence of birth control, 20,
  64, Catholic and non-Catholic and
  contraceptive use, 397, control by
  rewards and penalties, 49, 366–7,
  desired, 12, 24, 30, 31, 44, 45; in
  nineteenth century, 3, and replacement,
  22, 24, in Victorian era, 22
fellatio, 81
fertility after steroidal contraception,
  168–70, 207; assessment of, 19–20, and
  fecundity, 17–22, patterns through the

ages, 23
fertility control by abortion and
  contraception combined, 22–3, 314–18,
  376–7, 384, age of marriage, 19, 48, 74,
  availability of method versus education,
  24, and breast-feeding, 85–6, 90–1; and
  free condom distribution, 112–13, a
  human right, 12, 364–5, 367, 400–1, and
  intrauterine device use, 241–2, optimum
  use of methods, 375–9; research and
  development, 379–85; and sexual
  behaviour patterns, 398–9
fertility decline and Bradlaugh–Besant
  trial, 26–7, and access to fertility
  regulation, 24, 48, 49, in the developing
  world, 51, legislation and family size,
  366–7, underlying causes, 24, 25–6, 36
fertility differentials, 33–5, 37
fibroids and contraceptive use, 329, and
  intrauterine devices, 226; late
  childbearing, 388, and the Pill, 194; and
  spontaneous abortion, 276
Florey, Howard W., 10, 65
follicle-stimulating hormone. and
  oestrogens, 140, 141
Food and Drug Administration (US
  FDA), 55, 64, 72, 137, 176, 180, 203,
  351, 393

galactorrhoea: and amenorrhoea, 169
gall bladder disease and the Pill, 196
gingivitis, hypertrophic· and the Pill, 160–1
glucose tolerance tests and the Pill, 156
gonorrhoea, 335–6; and condom use,
  115–16, and Pill use, 334, 335, and
  spermicides, 132–3
gossypol and infertility, 381
Guttmacher, Alan, 13, 216

haematosis. and vasectomy, 250, 262
haematuria and coitus saxonicus, 81
handguns, 390
Hegar's sign, 299
hepatitis, infectious. and the Pill, 164, 197
hepatocellular adenoma: and the Pill, 69,
  194; *see also* liver
herpes genitalis, 337; and spermicides, 132,
  133
high-density lipoprotein (HDL): and the
  Pill, 155–6, 173, 178
holding back, 80
homosexuality disease transmission, 133;
  syphilis, 336
hormonal pregnancy tests, 170, 171
Hutterites· fertility rate, 20, 21
17-hydroxyprogesterone acetate, 204
hypertension· and the Pill, 163–4, 179, 328,
  smoking, Pill use and myocardial
  infarction, 174

hysterectomy, 257, 306, and abortion, 306, 311, extent of, 246
hysteroscopy female sterilization, 256-7
hysterotomy, 305-6

immune responses: and contraceptive methods, 384-5; and sperm after vasectomy, 264
implantation and intrauterine devices, 220, and spontaneous abortion, 275, *see also* ectopic pregnancy
India: abortion, 8, 283, 288, 359, age of marriage and legislation, 349; coitus interruptus, 77, colpotomy, 254; compulsory sterilization, 366-7, condom marketing, 113; family planning, 49-50, periodic abstinence, 101; population growth, 38, 43, 49, 50
Indonesia abortion, 8, family size, 45, fertility decline, 375
infanticide, 3, 25, 369
infertile period, 98, 99, 397
infertility causes, 343; and cotton seed oil, 381, female, 343-4, incidence of, 343, investigations, 344-5, male, 344, psychological factors, 345, and scrotal hyperthermia, 82, treatment, 345
injectable steroids, 202-9; effectiveness, 205, and neoplasia, 208-9, and physiology, 205, quality control, 57, reliability, 60, side-effects, 205-7, and subsequent fertility, 169, teratology and effect on infant, 207-8
International Planned Parenthood Federation (IPPF), 13, 162
intrauterine devices (IUDs) age and performance, 223, 225, complementary to other methods, 377, copper in, 222, 241, costs of, 222, 351; counselling on use of, 226-7, design, 221-3; effectiveness, 58, 60, 220, 223, 316, expulsion of, 93, 223, 224, 225, 229, 241, 242, 243; extent of use, 32, 48, 218; and fertilization, 218, 219, history, 14-15, 28, 216-18, and implantation, 220; and leucocyte migration, 218-20, 222; mode of action, 218-21, and mortality, 234-5, 244, 378; progestogens in, 222, 223, 224, quality control, 56-7, reasons for removal, 220, 243, side-effects, 228, 234-41; storage and sterilization, 225-6; and subsequent fertility, 241-2, tails of, 223, 237; for the unmarried, 341
—*insertion* follow-up, 233-4, and infection, 235-7; introducers, 222-3, 225, 231, and menorrhagia, 240-1; and pain, 232, 240, and perforations, 93, 229, 233, 239-40, techniques, 230-1, time of, 93, 228-30
—*medical conditions*. actinomycosis, 237,

ectopic pregnancy, 223, 226, 238-9, endocervicitis, 226; fibroids, 226, menorrhagia, 227, 233, 240-1, 332, menstruation, 225, 233; pain, 220, 232, 240, pelvic inflammatory disease, 69, 197, 235-6, 237, 242-4, pregnancy, 237-8; spontaneous abortion, 244
—*types* Copper omega, 221, Copper 7, 221, (performance) 224, 225, (time of insertion) 228, 229, Copper T, 221, (time of insertion) 228, 229, Dalkon shield, 222, 234, 235, Delta loops, 229; Flower, 221, 224, Grafenberg ring, 217, 221, Lippes loop, 218, 221, 222, (insertion) 229, 231, (performance) 224, 225, Margulies coil, 218, Multiload copper, 221, 229, 250; Novogard, 221, Ota ring, 221, 243, Petal, 229; Progestasert, 221, 224; Saftı coil, 221; Wishbone, 216, 221; Zipper ring, 218, 222
Ireland. divorce in, 350, legislation and contraceptive distribution, 353, voluntary sterilization, 33; Irish Censorship Act (1929, 1946), 353; Criminal Law Amendment Act (1935), 353
IUDs, *see* intrauterine devices

Japan abortion, 8, 288, 316, 359, condom use, 110-11, extent of contraceptive use, 32, 213, 316, intrauterine device use, 225, 243, marketing 385; periodic abstinence, 98, spermicide use, 121; vacuum aspiration, 293; Pharmacy Law, Section 12, 351

Kaposi's syndrome, 133
Karman curette, 295-6
Knowlton, Charles. birth control movement, 3, *Fruits of Philosophy* (1832), 3, 26, 27
Korea birth-rate, 315; family size, 45, induced abortion, 283, periodic abstinence, 98
'Kung women breast-feeding and birth intervals, 85

lactation and abstinence, 75, antibodies in milk, 87-8; and contraception, 84-6, 91-5, fertility control, 90-1; milk content changes, 88; and ovulation, 86-7, and the Pill, 94, and tubal ligation, 262; *see also* breast-feeding
laminaria tents: cervical dilatation, 294-5, 304
laparoscopic sterilization, 255-6, 271; complications and failure rates, 272; and menstrual loss, 266; surgical hazards, 263

laparoscopy infertility investigation, 344–5
laparotomy female sterilization, 253–4
Latin America abortion and educational
    level, 288–90; Lippes loop performance,
    224, menstrual regulation and
    legislation, 360, non-vaginal intercourse,
    81, population growth, 39, voluntary
    sterilization, 245
legal cases *Bradlaugh–Besant*, 26–7; *Carey
    v. Population Services*, 352, *Harris v.
    McRae*, 358; *de Marchi*, 353; *Mary
    McGee*, 353, *Morgentaler*, 365; *Planned
    Parenthood v. Danforth*, 358; *Roe v.
    Wade*, 365; *The United States v. One
    Package*, 353; *Vuitch*, 365, *Williams v.
    Zbaraz*, 358, *Woolnough*, 365
legislation advertising, 113, 352; age of
    marriage, 349, and child adoption, 350;
    consent to sexual intercourse, 349;
    contraceptive provision by non-
    physicians, 363–4; and contraceptives,
    350–4; contraceptive use by minors, 362;
    control of medical practice, 347–8; and
    family planning, 347, 364–5, 366–7,
    392–3, family planning services, 354;
    informed consent, 361–2; malpractice
    suits, 348–9, menstrual regulation, 360,
    patents, 351, pre-marketing testing,
    64–5, voluntary sterilization, 354–5; *see
    also under individual countries*
    –*Acts of Parliament* Abortion Act (1967),
    6, 302, 363; Children's and Young
    Persons' Acts (1963, 1969), 349, Family
    Planning Act (1967), 7, 14, 354, Family
    Planning Amendment Act (1972), 354,
    Obscene Publications Act (1857), 26,
    352, Offences against the Person Act
    (1861), 356, (amendment to, 1967),
    356–7, 360; Sex Discrimination Act, 362;
    Sexual Offences Act (1965), 349,
    Television Act (1954), 352
legislation, abortion, 262, 286–90, 355–60;
    400; and birth-rate, 285–6, 287, and
    contraceptive use, 287–8; liberal
    abortion, 307, 308, 312, 319
Lippes, Jack on loop development, 218,
    on loop expulsion, 341; on pelvic
    infection, 236, on perforation, 239, 240
Lippes loop, 218, 221, 222, performance,
    224, 225
liver and the Pill, 142, 155
liver diseases and the Pill, 69, 164, 194,
    197
luteinizing hormone (LH), 85, and
    oestrogens, 140, 141
lynesternol phenyl-propionate, 204

male Pill, 379–82
Malthus, Thomas *Essay on the Principle*

of Population (1798), 2
marketing, 385; condoms, 111–14;
    legislation, 351–3, and post-marketing
    surveillance, 67–71; *see also* advertising
marriage of adolescents and divorce, 340;
    age of, and fertility regulation 19, 48,
    74, legislation on age of, 349; legislation
    and consummation of, 360–1, sociology
    of, and contraceptive choice, 111
Marvelon (Pill), 152
medroxyprogesterone acetate, 145,
    structure, 139; in vaginal rings, 209
melanoma, malignant: and the Pill, 194
menarche, age of, 17, 388; and breast
    cancer, 185; and sexual exploration, 340
menopause age of, 18
menorrhagia and intrauterine devices, 227,
    233, 240–1, 332
Mensinga pessarie, 28, 121
menstrual cycles: breast size changes, 84;
    and conception, 18–19, and hormone
    levels in blood, 140, 141; number of,
    and breast cancer, 185; serum
    lipoprotein variation, 156
menstrual regulation (MR): complications,
    297; contraindications, 296, extent of
    use, 298–9; Karman curette, 295–6,
    legislation, 360; procedure, 296–7
menstruation, 141–2, amount of loss, 240,
    disturbances and Depo-Provera, 205–6;
    and intrauterine devices, 225, 233,
    irregularities in, 99, long intervals of,
    and risks, 388; myths and taboos, 151,
    158, 227; pattern changes after
    laparoscopic sterilization, 265, 266
mestranol (synthetic oestrogen), 140, 165
methylcyanoacrylate. occlusion of
    Fallopian tubes, 269
Mexico· abortion, 8, 283; advertising, 352;
    coitus interruptus, 92–3; population
    growth, 42, 43; steroid manufacture,
    137, 138
Mexico City: population growth, 42
migraine· and the Pill, 160, 177, 329
Mohammed· and coitus interruptus, 76,
    394
moniliasis, vaginal, 326, and Depo-Provera
    (DMPA), 206, and the Pill, 160
mortality, 340; and cancer, 332, 333, 391;
    causes and risks, 390–3
mortality, infant, 386; and birth-rate, 24–5;
    teenage mothers, 341, through the ages,
    23
mortality, maternal and abortion, 266,
    302, 303, 306–10, 319, 320, 378, and
    abortion legislation, 286, 319; at
    childbirth, 386, 389; and contraceptive
    use, 378, 389, lack of family planning
    services, 387, risks of, 386–7; teenage, 341

MR, *see* menstrual regulation
mucorrhoea, cervical· and the Pill, 160
myocardial infarction and the Pill,
174–5, 179, 180

Neisseria gonorrhoea· and pelvic
inflammatory disease, 236; and
spermicides, 132
neoplasia and steroidal contraceptives,
183–96, 208–9, *see also* cancer, breast,
cancer, endometrial, cancer, ovarian
Neo Sampoon (spermicide), 130
NET-EN, *see* norethisterone enanthate
Netherlands· abortion, 302, 356, out-
patient abortion, 302, popularity of the
Pill, 213
New Zealand Contraception, Sterilization
and Abortion Act, 362
nonoxynol-9 spermicide, 125, and venereal
disease, 132, 133
norethisterone enanthate (NET-EN), 204,
and breast disease, 165, effectiveness,
205; fertility return, 207; synthesis, 137,
weight gain, 206, 207
norgestrel, 137, 165
D-norgestrel, 222, post-coital
contraception, 202
L-norgestrel. effectiveness, 205; in silastic
capsules, 204; in vaginal rings, 210, and
weight gain, 206
19-norsteroids, 94
nutrition age of menarche, 17–18, age of
menopause, 18; and anovulation, 17–18

17β-oestradiol· extraction of, 136;
structure, 139
oestrogens· and breast cancer, 186, in Pills,
143–4, structure and activity, 139, 140,
141, synthetic, 139, 140; and
thromboembolism, 94, 172
Ogino–Knaus theory, 98
Onan· and coitus interruptus, 75, 78
once-a-month Pill, 210, 383
Oneida Community: and coitus
interruptus, 79–80
oral contraceptives, *see* Pills, steroidal
contraceptives
Ovacon and coagulation, 180
ovaries cysts and the Pill, 193, oocyte
production and natural wastage, 275.
394, and the Pill, 154, role in sexual
cycle, 136, *see also* cancer, ovarian
ovulation, 98–9, and cervical mucus
changes, 100, in menstrual cycle, 19,
141, and the Pill, 144, 157; and
temperature rise, 100, 142
Owen, Robert D and birth control
movement, 3, on sexual instinct, 15;

Moral Physiology (1831), 3, 15
oxytoxic drugs dilatation and curettage,
300

PA, *see* periodic abstinence
Pakistan: abortion, 8, 277–8, 359; family
planning, 375–6; menstrual regulation
and legislation, 360
Pearl pregnancy rate: calculation of, 61
pelvic inflammatory disease (PID). and
contraceptive use, 133, 197–8, 199; and
ectopic pregnancy, 243; and intrauterine
devices, 69, 197, 235–6, 237, 242–4; and
the Pill, 197–8, 199; risk factors, 244
periodic abstinence (PA), 93, 104–5,
cervical mucus method, 100–1; extent of
use, 32, 101–2; history, 97–8; ovulation
method, 98–9; reliability, 58, 60; side-
effects, 102–3; symptothermic method,
101, temperature method, 100; use-
effectiveness, 103–4
Peru anal intercourse, 81, 82; family size,
45
PGs, *see* prostaglandins
Philippines· abortion, 8, 281–4; bottle-
feeding and neonatal infection, 87;
contraceptive reliability, 58, family size,
20; periodic abstinence, 98; population
growth, 40; sterilization legislation, 355
PID, *see* pelvic inflammatory disease
Pill, male, 379–82
Pills: accidental ingestion, 167; and adrenal
glands, 154–5; assessment of, 145–9;
benefits and risks, 148–9, 198–201,
388–9; and coital frequency, 390;
complementary to other methods, 377;
compositions of, 142–4; and contact
lenses, 161, continuous taking of, 151;
and control of uterine bleeding, 151;
counselling on use of, 149–51, 166–7;
decline in use of, 149; development of,
137–8; duration of use, 168;
epidemiology, 148–9; failure rates and
dose, 153; and high-density lipoproteins,
173; and hospital admissions, 199,
interaction with other drugs, 165, and
libido, 159; and the liver, 142, 155;
matching user with, 165–8; and
menstruation, 158; mode of action,
144–5, mortality and age of woman,
378; other 'uses' for, 167, packaging,
149, and perinatal mortality, 171,
popularity, 32, 146, 149–50, 211, 212,
213, prescription of, 162–3, 363, and
prolactin levels, 94; quality control, 57,
152–3, reliability, 58, 60, 64; and
religion, 153, and serum composition,
155–6, side-effects, 145–7, 156–61,
smoking and cardiovascular disease,

173-4, 178, 179, 213; and subsequent
fertility, 168-70; and teenagers, 200, for
the unmarried, 341-2, use of, and
distribution method, 151, 152; and
vitamin levels, 150, and weight gain,
146, 160, *see also* steroidal
contraceptives
–dosage, 153, 167; and breakthrough
bleeding, 165; and failure rate, 153, low,
144, 151, 153, 165, 175, 200, and
myocardial infarction, 175, 200
–medical conditions acne, 158; alopecia,
158, 161; amenorrhoea, 146, 168-70,
benign breast disease, 186, 187, 199,
209; blood clotting, 173, 180; blood
pressure, 163-4; breakthrough bleeding,
146, 150, 161, 165; breast cancer,
183-90, 330, breast discomfort, 160, 161;
breast size changes, 84; cardiovascular
disease, 69, 172-83, 213, 328;
cerebrovascular disease, 172, 182,
cervical cancer, 190-2; chloasma, 161,
congenital abnormality, 170, 171, 172;
contraindications, 163, 164, 179;
diabetes, 164; duration of lactation, 94,
dysmenorrhoea, 156-7; ectopic
pregnancy, 198, effect of offspring,
170-7; endometrial cancer, 192, 199,
endometriosis, 198; fibroids, 194,
galactorrhoea, 94, gall bladder disease,
196; headaches, 160, 161, hepatocellular
adenoma, 69; 194, hirsutism, 158;
hypertension, 163-4, 179, 328;
hypertrophic gingivitis, 160-1, infectious
hepatitis, 164, 197, liver disease, 69, 164,
194, 197, malignant melanoma, 194;
migraine, 160, 177, Mittelschmerz, 157;
moniliasis, 160; mucorrhoea, 160;
myocardial infarction, 174-5, 179, 180,
200; neoplasia, 183-96, 208-9, ovarian
cancer, 193, 199, ovarian cysts, 193,
pelvic inflammatory disease, 197-8, 199,
pre-existing disease, 163-5; premenstrual
tension, 157; respiratory distress
syndrome, 171, rheumatoid arthritis,
196, subarachnoid haemorrhage, 177,
thromboembolic disease, 94, 175-8;
tuberculosis, 165, 328
–types, 142-4, biphasic, 142, 151, once-a-
month, 210, 383, post-coital, 202;
progestogen-only, 201-2, tricycle, 151,
triphasic, 142, 143, 151-2, 154
pituitary adenomas of, and the Pill, 169,
194, function of, and the Pill, 154, 381
polyps, 327
Population Council, 204, 223, 379
population explosion, 15, 37-52; economic
implications, 39-44, and financial aid to
family planning, 51-2, 401; urbanization
and slum development, 41-2
population size. access to fertility
regulation, 24; and breast-feeding, 91;
and coitus interruptus, 76, 77, in
developed and less developed regions,
39-40; fertility and mortality rates, 22-3;
legislation and family size, 366-7;
Malthus on, 2-3; and optimum use of
control methods, 375, world, by age and
sex, 39, 40
porphyria: and the Pill, 164
pre-ejaculatory secretion, 78
pregnancy: after sterilization, 263, age of
first, and breast cancer, 184, 185, and
conception, 18-19; contraindications
and contraceptive use, 327-30; and
diabetes, 164, and drug avoidance, 171,
duration assessment, 296, during oral
contraception, 170; and intrauterine
devices, 237-8; sexual risk-taking,
369-70; and smoking, 171, 172, 391-2
pregnancy, unplanned· and the child,
313-14, method failure, 62, 317
premenstrual tension. and the Pill, 157,
329
prescription· by non-physicians, 363, of the
Pill, 162–3
Proclamation of Teheran (1968), 364
progesterone: and abortion, 276; activity
of, 140-1, 142
progestogens· in intrauterine devices, 222,
223, 224; and lactation, 94; manufacture
of, 137, 138; in Pills, 143-4, steroids
related to, 142, structure and action of,
139, 140-2
prolactin: levels of, and breast-feeding, 85,
milk secretion in men, 84; and the Pill,
94
prostaglandins (PGs)· induced abortion,
305, 383; late period induction, 291-2,
383, side-effects, 291-2, 383
Protestants: and abortion, 315; on
contraception, 1; on fertility control, 395
psychiatric factors· and contraceptive use,
329, 338-9; and induced abortion,
311-12; and infertility, 345; and
voluntary sterilization, 265-8

quinacrine: occlusion of Fallopian tubes,
269
quinestrol once-a-month Pills, 210
quinine pessaries, 28, 119

Ravenholt, Reimart, 13, 212
religion and abstinence, 74-5; and fertility
control, 394-6, and Pill taking, 153;
prejudice, and delay in progress, 5, 374;
see also Catholics, Protestants
research and development: female

reproduction, 382–3; immunological contraception, 384–5, male Pill, 384–5
respiratory distress syndrome: and the Pill, 171
rheumatoid arthritis· and the Pill, 196
rhythm method, 98, 99, 397
Russia· abortion, 8, 33, 288, 356; contraception, 33, population growth rate, 39, vacuum aspiration, 292–3

safe period, 98, 99, 397
safety: carcinogenicity tests, 65–7; pre-marketing testing, 64–5
Salvarsan, 5
Sander–Cramer test· for spermicides, 54
Sanger, Margaret, 6, 12, 35, 217, 371, and the Comstock Act, 353; and the Dutch cap, 121, life and work of, 10–11, 13, oral contraception development, 137
scrotal hyperthermia and infertility, 82
semen· freeze storage, 261, and health in women, 6, 374
sickle-cell anaemia. and Depo-Provera (DMPA), 328, and the Pill, 165
side-effects, 67–71; fear of, 343; female sterilization, 261–2, injectable steroids, 205–7; intrauterine devices, 228, 234–41; periodic abstinence, 102–3; of the Pill, 145–7, 156–61; prospective studies of, 68–9, prostaglandins, 291–2, 383; relative risk and attributable risk, 69; retrospective studies of, 67–8; spermicides, 131, vasectomy, 261
smoking cancer, 391, and cardiovascular disease, 173–4, 178, 179, 213, 391; counselling against, 332; and haemorrhagic stroke, 177; mortality and morbidity, 393; Pill use and diseases, 173–4, 389; and pregnancy, 171, 172, 391–2, and spontaneous abortion, 276
sperm capacitation of, 120, 144, 382; destruction in situ by ultrasound, 82–3; freeze storage, 261; phagocytosis, and intrauterine devices, 219; production and natural wastage, 275, 394, toxic chemicals and male Pill, 380–2; and vasectomy, 264
sperm granuloma, 264
spermicides. in condom lubricants, 108–9; development of, 10, 53; and disease organisms, 132, effectiveness of, 130; evaluation, 133–4; extent of use, 121; foaming, 55, 130, history, 119; mode of action, 120, nonoxynol-9, 125, pelvic inflammatory disease, 133; quality control, 54–5; side-effects, 131; and sponges, 125, types, 121; use with condom, 117, and vaginal contraceptives, 129

Sri Lanka· abortion legislation, 359; age of marriage and legislation, 349, menstrual regulation and legislation, 360; periodic abstinence, 98
Stein-Leventhal syndrome and endometrial cancer, 192
sterilization, female, 15, 251–9, and abortion, 252, choice of technique, 271–2, colpotomy, 254; complications, 262–3, 265; conventional laparotomy, 253; culdoscopy, 254–5; Fallopian tube blockage, 268–9; fimbrial enclosure, 268, hysterectomy, 257; hysteroscopy, 256–7, and lactation, 95; laparoscopy, 255–6, 263, 266, 271, 272; minilaparotomy, 253–4, mortality, 261–2; postpartum, 251–2, 253–4, and quinacrine, 269; reversal, 259–60; side-effects, 261–2
sterilization, male, *see* vasectomy
sterilization, voluntary· and coital frequency, 267; complementary to other methods, 21–2, 49, 377–8; counselling, 247–8, cultural acceptability, 269–70; extent of, 32, 33, 211, 245–7, 272–3; female versus male, 270–1; and health, 266; legislation, 354–5; psychological factors, 265–8; regrets about, 265–6, 267, 268; reliability, 60; reversal, 259–61; *see also* sterilization, female; vasectomy
steroidal contraceptives· administration, 142–5; and the baby, 95, during lactation, 93–5; effectiveness, 153–4; history, 136–8; injectables, 202–9, in intrauterine devices, 222, 223, 224, manufacture of, 137, 138, microencapsulation, 204–5, nasal aerosol, 142; and physiology, 154–6; subdermal implants, 203, 204; and 'unnatural' modifications of reproduction, 214–15; and vaginal rings, 209–10; *see also* Pills
steroids: availability, 48, metabolism of, and racial differences, 149; placental, and lactation, 85, structure and metabolic pathways, 138–9; *see also individual steroids*
Stopes, Marie, 35; birth control clinic, 10, 11, 372; cervical cap, 61, 121–2, 374; life and views of, 6; *Birth Control Today* (1934), 6, *Married Love* (1918), 6; *Wise Parenthood* (1918), 6
strokes: and Pill use, 176–7
sympto-thermic method, 101
syphilis, 336; incidence and Pill use, 334, 335

teenagers abortion and legislation, 362; birth weight of babies, 341; consent to sexual intercourse and legislation, 349,

contraceptive advice to, 341, 349;
contraceptive use and legislation, 362;
infant mortality, 341; marriage and
legislation, 349; and the Pill, 200,
premarital sex and pregnancy, 340–1,
342; sex and contraceptive availability,
352
temperature method, 100
testosterone· and male Pill, 381
Thailand. abortion, 284, breast-feeding,
90; condom marketing, 113–14,
contraceptive services, 46;
minilaparotomy and female sterilization,
254
thyroxine. and the Pill, 155
toxic shock syndrome, 71; diaphragm use,
133
Treponema pallidum and syphilis, 336
Trichomonas vaginalis· infection by, 326–7,
and spermicides, 132
trophoblast disease, 195
tubal motility. and intrauterine devices,
218, and the Pill, 144, 154
tuberculosis. and the Pill, 165, 328

United Nations Fund for Population
Activities (UNFPA), 13
United States Agency for International
Development (AID), 13, 52, 212, 379
United States of America: abortion, 8,
28–9, 278, 287, 288, 309, 356, 357–9,
400; age of menarche, 17; age of
menopause, 18; breast-feeding, 90,
cancer and steroidal contraceptives,
186–9, cardiovascular disease and the
Pill, 181, coital frequency and the Pill,
390; coitus interruptus, 76, 78; coitus
saxonicus, 81; condoms, 108, 110,
112–13, 114–15; contraceptives, 29–30,
32, 53–4, 58–9, 351; Depo-Provera
(DMPA), 203–4, 209; diaphragm use,
122–3, dilatation and evacuation, 304,
ectopic pregnancy and intrauterine
devices, 238–9; family planning services,
3–4, 11, 12–13, 354, (restraints on) 9,
53–4, 122–3, 362, fertility decline, 22;
financial aid to international family
planning, 51–2, gall bladder disease and
the Pill, 196, informed consent, 361–2,
intrauterine device development, 218,
malpractice suits, 348–9, out-patient
abortion, 302, periodic abstinence, 98,
103–4, the Pill, 148, 149, 212, 213,
population growth, 39, 42, 43, pre-
marketing testing, 64–5; research and
development, 379, spermicides, 131, 132,
sterilization legislation, 355, teenagers
and contraceptive use, 362,
thromboembolic disease and the Pill,

176, voluntary sterilization, 245, 246
–*legislation* Act of the Suppression of
Trade in and the Circulation of,
Obscene Literature and Articles of
immoral Use (1873) (the Comstock
Act), 4, 53, 121, 352–3; Federal Food,
Drug and Cosmetic Act, 351, Federal
Society Security Act, 362, Public Health
Service Act (1970) Title X, 9, 14
urbanization: population growth and slum
development, 41–2
urethra, male: internal contraceptive for,
81–2
urethritis, 336–7
use-effectiveness: clinical studies, 63;
condoms, 114, 118; criteria of, 60–1;
determination of, 61–4, life-table
analysis method, 62; Pearl pregnancy
rate, 61, 62, periodic abstinence, 103–4,
and theoretical effectiveness, 57–60,
unplanned pregnancies, 62

vacuum aspiration (VA), 299–300, 384,
history, 14, 292–3
vagina· longitudinal division of, 81
vaginal discharges: and contraceptive use,
325–7
vaginal rings and steroidal contraception,
209–10
vasectomy, 15, 95, 245, 248–51; and
cardiovascular disease, 264–5;
complications, 262–5; confusion with
castration, 267–8; diagram, 249; follow-
up, 251; future developments, 268; and
haematosis, 250, 262; immunological
consequences, 264; legislation, 354–5;
and macrophage influx, 264; methods,
248–51, mortality, 261, qualifications of
operators, 251, reversal possibility, 250,
260–1; sexual satisfaction after, 266, 267;
side-effects, 261, sperm granuloma
formation, 264
Vatican Council: marriage and
procreation, 2, 395–6
vault cap, 123, 124, care and use of,
128–30; fitting of, 128; sizes, 124
venereal disease· and condom use, 115–16;
and other contraceptives, 132–3, 334–5;
screening for, 334–7
venous thromboembolic disease and Pill
use, 175–8
Victoria, *Queen* on birth control, 7,
vacuum aspiration abortion, 14, 292
Victorian era· family limitation, 25–6
vimule cap, 123, 124, care and use of,
128–30, criteria for use, 126, fitting of,
128, sizes, 124
Viravaidya, Mechai contraception in
Thailand, 46

visiting Pill, 202
vitamin levels: and oral contraceptives, 150
Volpar· spermicide, 10

weight gain. and the Pill, 146, 160; and
    steroidal contraceptives, 206

withdrawal, *see* coitus interruptus
World Fertility Survey (WFS), 44, 46

Yoon ring, 258, 266, 272

Zipper ring, 218, 222